MW01294202

The Philosophy, Theory and Methods of J. L. Moreno

J. L. Moreno, M.D., is recognized as the originator of sociometry and psychodrama, and was a prodigious creator of methods and theories of creativity, society, and human behavior. The methods and techniques he authored have been widely adopted; the theories and philosophy upon which the methods are founded have not, as they are frequently couched in language which is not easily understood. Moreno's sociometry, his theory of society, is kept alive only by a handful of psychodramatists. Group psychotherapy and psychodrama are both widely practiced but often based on non-Morenean theory, probably because of the inaccessibility of Moreno's work.

This book outlines Moreno's early years (his religious phase), the philosophy on which his methods are founded, and the theories upon which Moreno's three major methods, psychodrama, sociometry, and group psychotherapy are based. The book provides a more systematic presentation of Moreno's work and presents his philosophy and theory in a clearer, more understandable manner.

John Nolte has a doctorate in clinical psychology from Washington University, and was trained in psychodrama by J.L. and Zerka Moreno. He served as Director of Training for the Moreno Institute after Moreno's death. From 1994 to 2008, he was a training consultant and staff member of Trial Lawyers College, Dubois, Wyoming.

Explorations in Mental Health

Books in this series:

The Philosophy, Theory and Methods of J. L. Moreno

The Man Who Tried to Become God

John Nolte

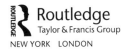
Routledge
Taylor & Francis Group

NEW YORK   LONDON

First published 2014
by Routledge
711 Third Avenue, New York, NY 10017

and by Routledge
2 Park Square, Milton Park, Abingdon, Oxon OX14 4RN

*Routledge is an imprint of the Taylor & Francis Group,
an informa business*

© 2014 Taylor & Francis

The right of John Nolte to be identified as author of this work has been asserted by him in accordance with sections 77 and 78 of the Copyright, Designs and Patents Act 1988.

Library of Congress Cataloging-in-Publication Data
Nolte, John.
    The philosophy, theory and methods of J.L. Moreno : the man who tried to become God / by John Nolte.
        pages cm. — (Explorations in mental health ; 8)
    Includes bibliographical references and index.
    1. Moreno, J. L. (Jacob Levy), 1889–1974.   2. Psychotherapists—United States.   3. Drama—Therapeutic use.   4. Sociometry.   I. Title.
    RC438.6.M67N66 2014
    616.89'1653—dc23
    2013050057

ISBN13: 978-0-415-70287-4 (hbk)
ISBN13: 978-0-203-79517-0 (ebk)

Typeset in Sabon
by IBT Global.

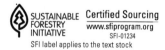
SUSTAINABLE FORESTRY INITIATIVE
Certified Sourcing
www.sfiprogram.org
SFI-01234
SFI label applies to the text stock

Printed and bound in the United States of America
by IBT Global.

To:

Beth,
Cathy,
Mike, and
Jane

who have taught me so much about spontaneity and creativity.

Contents

Figures and Tables

FIGURES

TABLES

Acknowledgments

I felt for a long time a deep obligation to Dr. J. L. and Zerka Moreno for what they had given me, a new way of life and a new way of practicing my profession as a psychologist. I wondered how I could repay them. The money I had spent in training, even though it was a lot for me, seemed insignificant compared with the gifts I had received. What could I give to them? I asked myself over and over. The answer was simple when it struck me: I can best express my appreciation by passing along to others that which I have received. I believe that I have had some success in doing that through the many psychodramas I have directed over 50 years and the many participants I have met in training workshops. This book is acknowledgment of that debt as well as a tribute to both J. L. and Zerka Moreno.

The American Society of Group Psychotherapy and Psychodrama and its president, David Moran, have generously given permission to quote extensively from the following books by J. L. Moreno:

Words of the Father
Psychodrama, First Volume
Who Shall Survive?

And from the journal, Group Psychotherapy, Psychodrama & Sociometry:

The Autobiography of J. L. Moreno, MD

Paul Hare's "Bibliography of Work of J. L. Moreno" (1986) was of substantial assistance in locating Moreno's articles, books, and edited works. The online *Bibliography of Psychodrama* (http://www.pdbib.org/), originally compiled and updated by Jim Sacks with contributions by Valerie Greer, Jeanine Gendron, and Marie-Therese Bilaniuk, and now updated by Michael Wieser, was also a great help, especially in finding articles not by Moreno. I also made generous use of René Marineau's 1989 biography, *Jacob Levy Moreno 1889–1974*, Paul and June Hare's *J. L. Moreno* (1996), and Rosa Cukier's *Words of Jacob Levy Moreno* (2007) during the writing of this book. Thanks also to Marcia Hinkley for her helpful comments and for proofreading the text.

I owe the greatest debt to my wife and life partner, Nancy Drew. Without her substantial encouragement, I would never have completed this book. She contributed to my efforts in many ways. She is a recognized contributor to the field of qualitative research and it is because she shared her knowledge of philosophy, especially phenomenology and existentialism, that I came to understand how important Moreno's existential philosophy was to understanding his work. In addition, Nancy served as an excellent editor, reading draft after draft and repeatedly identifying passages that needed more work. To the extent that this book is readable, much credit goes to her. Nancy also encouraged me, at times prodded me, to keep at it in spite of the fact that writing sometimes interfered with other activities that we both would have preferred to be doing.

Introduction

Jacob Levy Moreno (1889–1974) was a prodigiously creative individual whose self-assigned life mission was amelioration of the problems of human society. From an early age he was sensitive to injustice and inequality and believed that all people should have an opportunity for the fullest expression of their talents. As a teenage tutor of the children of wealthy Viennese bourgeois families, he encouraged his charges to give their toys to poor children who were not as fortunate as they. As a university student, Moreno, along with four chums, established the House of Encounter in Vienna, where they provided both shelter and assistance to poor people from all over the Austro-Hungarian Empire who were trying to emigrate to other countries. As a scientist, he became an inventor of methods through which he hoped to better the plight of marginalized, excluded, and disadvantaged groups of people as well as treat mental illness.

Moreno first founded a spontaneous form of drama that he considered to be a social therapy. He was the originator of the methods of sociometry and psychodrama and is also credited, along with others, as one of the fathers of group psychotherapy. Each of his methods, at one time or another, was widely received and appreciated, but the philosophy and theory upon which they were based, including the *raison d'être* of the methods, generally got left, in Moreno's words, on the back shelves of the library. Moreno was perturbed that his methods and techniques were so readily adopted while the philosophical and theoretical origins from which they came and the aims to which they were dedicated were brushed aside. This book reflects my understanding of Moreno's philosophy, his methods, and the theory upon which they are founded.

My introduction to psychodrama came in the fall of 1959 when I was a relatively new clinical psychologist on the staff of Missouri State Hospital #1, in Fulton. Several staff members from the St. Louis State Hospital were visiting to demonstrate the psychodramatic method. Leon Fine, who had been a fellow graduate student at Washington University, Abel Ossario, and Barbara Seabourne, both of whom I knew well and considered good friends, led this team. I attended the workshop only because of my positive connections with the presenters. I was not interested in psychodrama and, from the little I had read, I considered it a superficial and gimmicky process.

To my surprise, I found the first session quite engrossing. Three hours passed by quickly. I walked across the campus to lunch with my friend and fellow staff psychologist, John Miller. We were talking animatedly about what we had seen and what the director had done and speculating why. Suddenly, realizing how caught up I was in the session we had just come from, I stopped. "John," I said to Miller, "if something gets me this riled up, I think I need to learn more about it."

It took me two years to arrange for a two-week visit to the Moreno Institute, the only official training center at the time. Before that happened, I met the Morenos when they presented a program at the Psychiatric Receiving Center in Kansas City. Dr. Moreno gave a brief talk and then Zerka, his wife, directed a psychodrama. The chief psychologist of the center volunteered to be the protagonist. Afterwards he told the group, "That was worth six months of analysis." The staff had lunch with the Morenos and I was invited. I was seated next to Zerka and was invited by her to cut the meat on her plate, one of the few activities that she had not mastered after the amputation of her right arm. I told her that I had been quite impressed by the session that she had directed, and that was the truth. Inwardly, I reaffirmed my intention to train at the Moreno Institute.

I finally arrived at the Moreno Institute in June 1962. The Institute was an accredited psychiatric hospital at that time, and a woman had been admitted as a patient the day before the training workshop began. She claimed that she had been divorced from her husband of many years and remarried to a doctor by radio waves. Her complaint was that her first husband would not let her go live with the doctor. The initial stages of her treatment were part of the training workshop.

Although by 1962, Zerka was responsible for most of the training sessions, J. L. Moreno came to the theater from time to time, and only he directed the sessions in which Dorothy, the newly admitted patient, was the protagonist. She was unwilling to stay voluntarily and was to be legally committed at the request of her husband. That is usually accomplished by having a patient examined by two psychiatrists, who then attest to the need for psychiatric treatment. A standard psychiatric examination is typically a threatening and uncomfortable process. Moreno had a different plan. He invited two colleagues to make the examination. They came to the theater, as did the training group and Dorothy. Moreno introduced her to the group and invited her to show us, onstage, some activities of her daily life. Among other things, she worked as a clerk in the drugstore owned by her husband (her ex-husband, according to her). Several of us in the group took the roles of customers and she graciously attended to our purchases. After some action, Moreno interviewed her. She told her story and Moreno promised that he would do his best to help her. It was obvious that she had absolute trust in him and believed him implicitly. It was also obvious to the two committing psychiatrists that she was delusional, a fact that justified commitment in 1962.

This was the first evening of training, and I received my first lesson from Moreno. The psychologists from whom I had learned the skills of my profession were all good people. They were not only intelligent, but considerate, thoughtful human beings. They had taught me to be respectful of the patients that I saw, no matter how emotionally disordered they might be and they taught by example. I had, however, never seen the best of these good professionals listen to the delusions of a patient with the respect and concern with which Moreno listened to this woman. He offered no skepticism nor did he challenge her account of what had happened. He did not try to convince her of the absurdity of her story. Instead, he promised to help her in every way that he could. He was sincere, and she realized this. I realized that I had been taught to be polite; Moreno demonstrated what it meant to be caring.

The training group had two sessions a day in the theater and I was amazed by what happened on the psychodrama stage under Zerka's direction. Events in people's lives were explored in astounding detail. Painful experiences were revisited, the hurt drained out and emotional wounds healed. Monsters were slain. Demons were exercised. Shackles were struck off. This was the type of psychotherapy that I could appreciate and one I wanted to master.

We met in the evening in the Moreno living room, where we would discuss the day's activities. Moreno used our discussion as the stimulus to talk about his ideas and often his experiences. On the two weekends of the training workshop, additional people came to the theater. Jim Enneis, director of the psychodrama program of St. Elizabeth Hospital, the federal psychiatric hospital, brought his first training group to the Institute. Don Clarkson was a member of that group, and he and I have been close friends since. In addition to Enneis, Hannah Weiner and Dick Korn, early leaders in the psychodrama movement, appeared for a day or two. I was tremendously impressed by their skills as psychodrama directors. I hoped that I could become as skilled someday.

On Friday evening of each week, the training group went into New York City for the open session of the New York City Moreno Institute. The New York City Theater was in a small building on West 78th Street. Open sessions, conducted by Moreno Institute graduates, were held nightly. Twice a week the Morenos presented a session that was open to anybody who wanted to attend and pay a modest fee. J. L. Moreno would give a short talk about his work and then warm up the group by engaging with individual members, one of whom would be invited to explore a problem situation through psychodrama. He would then call on Zerka to direct, and a full-blown personal psychodrama session would ensue.

Like many conventionally trained psychotherapists, I found this practice unsettling. We are trained that the privacy of the client is sacrosanct. In the public psychodrama session, the protagonist very likely has no previous experience with the method and is unaware of how powerfully the method facilitates self-revelation of very private, personal information. Done before a group of people whom the protagonist does not know seemed like a violation of confidence and ethically questionable. Today, open sessions have virtually ceased, and the Morenos' son, Jonathan Moreno, a bioethicist, has written that it is indeed unethical by today's standards.[1] Since then, I have talked with a number of protagonists of open sessions and have yet to hear anything unfavorable about the experience. Several have acknowledged being taken aback immediately after the drama was over, but feeling quite all right after hearing from group members during the sharing phase of the session. And I have conducted many open sessions myself.

When Zerka Moreno first invited me to be the protagonist of a session, I politely declined. I had come to the Institute to learn how to direct, not to do my own psychodramas. I did not then know how much of psychodrama had to be learned from the role of the protagonist. Eventually I was persuaded to take the stage. After a few minutes, Zerka, who is renowned for her intuition, asked me a question. Without warning a huge ball of pain welled up, entirely filling my body. I had no control over it no matter how hard I tried, and I sobbed for minutes. It was a pain connected to a failed relationship from 10 years previously. I had my first lesson in the immense power of the psychodrama stage.

I spent an intense two weeks in a different world. I had been working as a psychotherapist for several years, but for the first time, I saw emotional healing taking place in minutes right before my eyes. I wished that I could stay in this magical milieu forever. It wasn't possible, of course. I had obligations, a job, a family elsewhere. I did not yet see that the ultimate goal of this training was not to remain in this freedom-enhancing culture of the Moreno Institute, but to spread that culture where I lived.

Upon returning home, I started two psychodrama groups in the hospital, applying the basic psychodrama skills that I had picked up at Beacon. I was a long way from being a competent psychodramatist, yet the groups accomplished a great deal, more than I had been achieving in my other activities as a psychotherapist. In addition, the sessions were interesting to the group members and to me, a quality not always found in conventional talk psychotherapy. My attempts at directing also prepared me to learn when I returned to the Moreno Institute for more training. This was the Moreno model of training: a period of training followed by an interval of practice, then another training experience. I continued to return to the Moreno Institute many times until Moreno's death.

I not only wanted to learn the skills of directing psychodrama; I was intensely curious as to how and why psychodrama accomplished what it did. It was clear to me that in psychodrama sessions I was learning more about human functioning than I had been taught in all my university classes, and more than I had learned through conventional psychotherapy. I read

Moreno's books and articles and I listened to him very closely when he discussed his ideas with a training group. I struggled with *Who Shall Survive?* and the first two *Psychodrama* volumes, finding many of the ideas intriguing but often not completely understandable. I read *Words of the Father* and was deeply moved by some passages. I could relate some to them, but I did not understand their importance to Morenean oeuvre.

Although Moreno was a prolific writer with nearly 300 citations (Hare, 1986), nowhere does he produce a clear, well organized, and straightforward account of his triadic system (sociometry, group psychotherapy, and psychodrama). The second edition of *Who Shall Survive?* (1953c) has the most complete presentation of his ideas and methods, and the autobiographical supplement (1953a) helps understand Moreno. However, I suspect that there are few people who can claim to have carefully read the whole 724 pages; fewer still, including myself, can claim to have thoroughly understood everything in this volume.

I became convinced that Moreno had seen deeply into the workings of the cosmos and I wanted to know what he had perceived. He answered most of the questions that I asked by quoting or pointing out passages that I had already read in his books and articles. He died before I knew how to ask him the questions I really wanted him to answer.

When I was introduced to phenomenological and existential philosophy, much of Moreno's work became more comprehensible. Based on that experience, it is my hypothesis that one reason for poor reception of Moreno's work is that psychotherapists and most methods of psychotherapy are informed and formed by a positivist, objectivist philosophy. The medical model of mental illness prevails and is concretized in the diagnostic and statistical manuals (DSMs). Even humanistic and existential psychotherapists make use of the latest DSM. They also tend to think about their clients in terms of a personality theory or a theory of psychopathology that comes from a positivist, objectivist point of view. Moreno is much more understandable from a phenomenological, existential perspective.

NONCLINICAL PSYCHODRAMA

Moreno had known from the beginning that psychodrama was far more than a method of psychotherapy. He encouraged and engaged in nonclinical applications, beginning with his search for the king of Austria. He encouraged students to engage in the employment of psychodrama in nonpsychotherapy settings even though he largely wrote about psychodrama as a method of psychotherapy.

I looked for opportunities to use psychodrama outside the hospital. Over the years, I have done such things as team building in business organizations and role training with doctors, nurses, and psychotherapy trainees. I once conducted a workshop for nursing school instructors on the use of action techniques in teaching student nurses. This group figured out how to teach the cardiac electrical system in action in a way much more interesting than lecture and diagrams.

In 1994, an opportunity to conduct personal growth psychodrama with a group of lawyers came my way. The situation was this: Gerry Spence, a well-known and very successful lawyer—some of his colleagues consider him the best contemporary lawyer in the country—put into action a longtime dream to establish a postgraduate course in trial law. He called it the Trial Lawyers College. Spence (1998) charged the law schools of this country with neglecting to teach trial skills to their students. He pointed out that doctors go through years of internship and residency before they are allowed to practice on their patients. On the other hand, a young lawyer just out of law school who has passed the bar exam is allowed to represent anybody who will hire him, no matter how important or complex the case. His idea was that he and a group of other famous and successful older lawyers would teach their skills to younger lawyers.

Spence had himself developed a unique style of courtroom practice—as have most highly successful trial lawyers—and wished to pass this along to younger colleagues who were struggling to master the complex skills involved in trial work. Spence's approach to trial practice had been inspired by his participation in activities of the human potential movement in the 1960s, into which he had been guided by his close friend, social worker John Johnson, the head of the mental health program in the Wyoming county where Spence had been the county attorney. Spence had also sampled psychodrama at programs sponsored by John Ackerman, president of the National College for Criminal Defense. He believed that the self-understanding obtained through personal growth work was critically important to the system that he had developed, and the Trial Lawyers College began with three days of psychodramatic personal growth activity. Don Clarkson, with whom Spence had previously worked, and I were engaged to conduct this work. The college was a month long course, situated on Spence's ranch in high desert country of Wyoming.

As time for the college approached, I became concerned about the response we might have to psychodrama, especially as the group members were of a very different profession and were attending the college to learn the skills of trying lawsuits in courtrooms, not to participate in psychodrama. It was wasted concern. After the initial shock of being thrown into something most of them had never heard of, the lawyers dived in with great gusto. They seemed more enthusiastic about psychodrama than many mental health professionals. Having never heard of psychodrama, they were curious why it was not more widely known and applied. They were especially curious why more psychotherapists did not use it. The most common theory they put forward was that it was too effective and psychotherapists were afraid they would cure their clients too quickly and lose out economically. I assured them that this was not the reason.

When I recognized that the purpose of the college was training in professional skills, I suggested to Spence that psychodrama might have more to offer than just personal growth. I had role training in mind, of course. Spence was quite open to the idea and welcoming to me. I spent the next 14 years attending Trial Lawyers College events. The lawyers, both staff and students, were appreciative of the action methods that Clarkson and I introduced and found many creative ways of using them in trial preparation and even in trial. Some of them recognized the value of personal psychodrama to better understand themselves and others. They also recognized how much they learned about group dynamics through the psychodrama sessions. Most saw the usefulness of psychodrama in understanding their clients' experiences. They also learned the importance of looking at the trial situation from the perspective of the other participants, the judge, the jurors, the opposing counsel, and even the clerks and bailiffs. Many attended psychodrama training workshops, sometimes for personal growth and usually to learn enough of the method to conduct reenactment interviewing as a means of learning about their clients' experiences at a deeper level than conventional interview can accomplish.

I was associated with the Trial Lawyers College from 1994 to 2007. Psychodrama became an integral component of the program. Two more psychodramatists, Kathryn Larimer and Kathryn St. Clair, were added to the staff. During that span of time, we introduced psychodrama to more than 2,000 people. Many of the graduates of Trial Lawyers College are making use of the psychodrama method in one way or another.

The Trial Lawyers College was one of the most rewarding undertakings in my life. It also confirmed for me that, because psychodrama is so widely perceived as a method of psychotherapy, there are an infinite number of possible nonclinical applications of psychodrama just waiting to be discovered.[2]

ABOUT THIS BOOK

Hundreds of people have contributed to the sociometric, psychodramatic, and group psychotherapy literature. Many books on psychodrama and several on sociodrama and sociometry have appeared in the last 40 years. Because my purpose in writing has been to explicate J. L. Moreno's ideas, especially his philosophy and theories, I have relied heavily on his articles and books. This is not to be taken as a dismissal of the work of others.

I have gone beyond Moreno's original thinking in only one place. That is the addition of David Bohm's interpretation of quantum theory, which, in my opinion, solves a major issue of Moreno's Canon of Spontaneity-Creativity. In explaining spontaneity, Moreno invokes the notion of non-conservable energy to explain spontaneity. As I explain in a discussion of this entity, conventional physics has no place for such an energy. Bohm's concept of the implicate order provides an explanation, a physical basis for Moreno's theorizing.

Adam Blatner, in his several editions of *Foundations of Psychodrama*, the fourth of which was published in 2000, has made the most ambitious attempt to present a full picture of Moreno's work. However, Blatner's major aim seems to be relating Moreno's thinking to mainstream philosophy, theory, and practice of psychotherapy and group psychotherapy. His motivation seems to be making Moreno more palatable to conventional thought and practice in the hope of enticing more people to get involved in psychodrama. In doing so, he has, in my opinion, overlooked or downplayed some of Moreno's most creative contributions.

The major sources for this book are Moreno's articles in the journals *Sociometry* and in *Group Psychotherapy*, as well as the books Moreno either wrote or edited. Fortunately, all issues of *Sociometry* can be found online through a service called JSTOR (http://www.jstor.org/?), a digital library that makes more than 2,000 journals available through college and university libraries. Unfortunately *Group Psychotherapy* is not among them. In addition to the above resources, there is all that I have learned from both Morenos during the 12 years that I was a student of the Moreno Institute. Finally, there is what I have learned from the practice of psychodrama.

CONVENTIONS

Three Morenos are mentioned in this book: Jacob Levy Moreno, Zerka Toeman Moreno, and Jonathan D. Moreno. Whenever the name Moreno stands alone without initials, it refers to J. L. Moreno. I use J. L. Moreno only when it is needed for clarification or sometimes at the beginning of a chapter or section.

NOTES

1. I have found an approach to demonstrating psychodrama that I believe to be ethical. A description can be found in my book, *The Psychodrama Papers*.

2. I also learned to have great respect for a badly maligned group of people: the trial lawyers who represent people as plaintiff lawyers in civil trials and defense lawyers in criminal trials. These are the only kinds of lawyers trained by the Trial Lawyers College. Instead of sly, conniving, unscrupulous manipulators, I found the large majority of the students to be thoughtful, highly ethical, caring professionals who worked against the odds to see that their clients received justice.

Part I

The Religious Phase

It was in the early part of our century that a young man tried to become God. The place was Vienna; the period of his appearance was between 1908 and 1914. He made a deep impression upon his contemporaries. He had his gospel, his apostles, his apocrypha. The religious books in which his doctrine was expressed had profound reverberations throughout the intellectual world. The cruel wars and revolutions through which mankind has passed since have destroyed or dispersed most of the original witnesses, but some of them are still living and I am one of them.

—J. L. Moreno, *The Autobiography of J. L. Moreno, MD*

1 The Man in the Green Cloak

Vienna, just after the turn of the 19th century, was an exhilarating city in which to live—as long as you were a member of the well-to-do merchant class. Vienna was second only to Paris as a European center of culture and the arts, and an extraordinary profusion of intellectual and scientific productivity emerged in the city in the years just before and after the turn of the century. It was also the city of social movements, including Zionism, Austro-Marxism, German Nationalism, and Existentialism. Anti-Semitism was also rampant. Paris was known as the City of Lights, Vienna as the City of Dreams.[1]

Anyone living in Vienna in the years between 1908 and 1914 might occasionally have come across a young man wearing a dark green cloak. One of the places where he frequently appeared was the *Augarten*, the grounds of the palace of Emperor Franz Joseph that served as a public park for the people of Vienna. This was a place where nannies and nursemaids took their young charges, and where older children often came to play.

A mysterious youth who came to be recognized as the Young Man in the Green Cloak could often be found sitting at the foot of a tree, making up fairy tales to tell the children who came to play in the *Augarten*. They gathered around him, eager to hear what wondrous story he would next invent. He never told the same story twice, and often he engaged the children in creating with him new stories or new versions of old stories. Moreover, he had this air of mystery about him. Nobody knew his name or where he lived. Though he might make known when his youthful audience would expect to see him again, he often showed up unannounced. He was like one of the characters from the fairy tales he told.

The Young Man in the Green Cloak was Jacob Moreno Levy, who would later rearrange his name to become J. L. Moreno, and whose methods, philosophy, and theories are the subject of this book. About 18 years old at the time of his engagement with the children in the *Augarten*, he had been emancipated from his family for several years, supporting himself by tutoring the children of bourgeois families of Vienna. In the *Augarten*, he not only told fairy tales. He engaged the children he met there in creative play. He saw himself as removing these children from their everyday drab surroundings (they were mostly children of the working class for whom Vienna could be and more often was a city of nightmares than the City of Dreams) and taking them bodily into a fairyland of unlimited wonder.

It was here, observing the spontaneity and creativity of children, that his theory linking spontaneity with creativity began to take shape. "In children," Moreno says:

> you see spontaneity in its living form. It is written all over the child, in his act-hunger, as he looks at things, as he listens to things, as he rushes into time, as he moves into space, as he grabs for objects, as he smiles and cries. In the very beginning, he sees no barrier in objects, no limits of distance, no resistance or prohibitions. But as objects hinder his locomotion and people respond to him with "no, no, no," he starts on his reactive phase, still reaching out, but with growing anxiety, fear, tension, and caution. (1989a, p. 37)

Moreno later claimed that he was instigating a revolution among the children, a revolution against social stereotypes and class distinctions, a revolution for spontaneity and creativity. What he observed was that as children grow older, they became less spontaneous, less creative, more anxious and cautious. He wanted to teach them how to retain their spontaneity and remain creative in the face of society's attempt to mold them into its templates.

THE RELIGION OF ENCOUNTER

Even if one did not frequent the *Augarten*, by 1914, the Man in the Green Cloak might have been seen in the company of one or more of his four close friends, all students at the University of Vienna. They were constantly walking the streets and roads of Vienna, always talking, always engaging with everyone they met along the way. Although they affected anonymity in their time, we now know their respective identities. The tall member of the group was Chaim Kellmer, a philosophy student. A man with many questions about life in general and his life in particular, he had come from Romania to the university to seek answers. Like Moreno, he, too, supported himself as a tutor. He was considered by many to be a wise person and many sought his counsel and advice.

When Moreno and Kellmer met, both found a deep kinship of spirit that initiated what Moreno later described as the Religion of Encounter. Three other like-minded students joined them to form a unique group. There was András Pető of Budapest, a medical student who eventually achieved renown for developing new methods of treating handicapped children. Jan Feda from Prague, who became a friend of Thomas Masaryk, founder and first president of Czechoslovakia, also became one of the group.

The third was Hans Brauchbar of Vienna, also a medical student who later moved to Russia and, in Moreno's words, "disappeared." These five comprised the total membership of the Religion of Encounter. They were indefatigable talkers, preoccupied with ideas about the nature of God and the Second Coming of Christ. In spite of their constant conversation, they were absolutely dedicated to the notion that their actions were far more meaningful than their words.

Moreno describes the group in his autobiography:

> We were all committed to the sharing of anonymity, of living and giv-ing, living a direct and concrete life in the community with all we met. We left our homes and families and took to the streets. We were name-less but were easily recognized by our beards and our warm, human, and gay approach to all comers. None of us would accept any money for the services we rendered to others, but we received many gifts from anonymous donors. (1989a, p. 42)

Vienna, in addition to being a hotbed for modernism in the arts, was a hotbed of movements. Nazism, Zionism, Communism, and Existentialism. Moreno and his group belonged to the latter. The first principle, he wrote, was the all-inclusiveness of being and the constant effort of maintaining the natural spontaneous flow of being from one moment to the next with-out interruption. The second principle was that all existing things are by nature good and blessed. Other ideas include the concept of the moment as a category in itself rather than as a function of past and future, and the notion of the situation, which is to say that we always find ourselves in a setting that has meaning for us and that challenges us or demands that we act. A further principle is spontaneity and creativity as the guides of ethical conduct rather than the social rules of cultural conserves.

In the pre–World War I years, the Austro-Hungarian Empire was becom-ing increasingly unstable and, as a result, hordes of people from its many nationalities poured into Vienna on their way to more promising countries. America and Palestine were particularly high among their destinations. These emigrants were most often poor and uneducated. Making their way through governmental bureaucracy was nearly impossible without help. Shelter and sustenance were often even more urgent problems.

The five members of the Religion of Encounter procured a house in central Vienna and opened it to all comers. They refused payment from those who found their way to the house and who seldom had the means to pay anyway. The House of Encounter not only provided food and shel-ter, but also helped the emigrants understand and fill out their emigration papers and deal with the government bureaucratic agencies. Moreover, the emigrants, far from their homes and native countries found much desired comfort in companionship and mutual emotional support. The house was supported entirely by donations received by Moreno and his friends.

In his autobiography, Moreno writes that he was amazed that so many people crowded into that house and shared with one another whatever they had, and did so without fighting or hard feelings. Every evening was a meeting time in which problems were discussed and any grievances were addressed. Later, Moreno would point to these meetings as the model for the encounter group movement that prevailed in America during the 1960s and 1970s.

MORENO AND THE CONCEPT OF GOD

From an early age, Moreno was intrigued with the concept of God. "The most famous person in the universe was God and I liked to be connected with Him" (1989a, pp. 19–20). He sometimes traced the origins of psychodrama, the best known of the several methods that he would originate, to an incident from his childhood. When he was about four years old, his parents were visiting friends on a Sunday afternoon, and he was playing with neighbors' children in the basement of his house. "Let's play God and his angels," little Jacob suggested, and the other children agreed. They piled chairs upon an oak table that was in the basement to represent heaven, and Jacob chose to play God, climbing up to the highest level:

> The children circled around the table, using their arms as wings, singing. One or two of the larger children held up the mountain of chairs we had assembled. Suddenly one of the children asked me, "Why don't you fly?" I stretched my arms, trying it. A second later, I fell and found myself on the floor, my right arm broken. (1946b, p. 2)

> The psychodrama of the fallen God. This was, as far as I can recall, the first "private" psychodramatic session I ever conducted. I was the director and protagonist in one. (1989a, p. 20)

Moreno experienced the first of two powerful mystical events when was 14. Late one night walking the streets of Chemnitz, where his parents had moved, he had what he called an epiphany. He found himself before a statue of Christ. As he thought about how Christ had lived his life, and how chaotic Moreno's own then seemed, he realized that he had to make a decision. "The question was, how would I choose: was my identity the universe or was it with the particular family or clan from which I had sprung? I decided for the universe" (1989a, p. 22). This was what Jesus had done and for which he had paid the ultimate consequence. From that moment on, Moreno wrote, he began to believe that he was an extraordinary person with an extraordinary mission to fulfill through his life.

Moreno also formulated his struggle with the questions of existence this way:

I began to try to find meaning in an existence, which appears meaning-less in itself. If there is nothing else in life except a dreamlike passing into nothing, at least we can protest against an unreasonable fate, an unpardonable sin, a mistake of the cosmos to have thrown us out here, into the desert of this planet, perceiving, feeling, thinking, without any chance or hope to become something which really matters. My quest therefore, was: "Am I, this perishable thing, a hopeless existence or am I at the center of all creation, of the entire cosmos?"

I asked myself: "Who is this me? A name? A bit of nothing, vanish-ing like a rainbow in the sky never to return? Or is this me the most real thing there is, the Creator of the world, the first and final being, the all-inclusive thing? In other words, am I nothing, or am I God?" (1972b, pp. 197–198)

The publishing of thoughts like this, after he had achieved some fame and stature as a psychiatrist and originator of the sociometric and psychodra-matic methods, led to accusations of megalomania and accusations that he was delusional.

As a teenager, Moreno may have struggled more passionately perhaps than most of us with the questions that all of us ask at some time or another, those basic existential questions: "Who am I? Why am I here?" Moreno's search may have been more profound than that of most young people his age. He read extensively:

Extensive and feverish reading of religious, philosophical, and esthetic literature set the internal, psychic scene for the decisive period to come. The reading of religious books centered around the Old and New Tes-taments, Saints Paul, Augustine, Origen, Benedict, Francis, Meister Eckhart, Angelus Silesius, Fredrich Novalis, the Apocrypha, the Sohar and Jezirah, Blaise Pascal. Søren Kierkegaard's writings were having great impact throughout Europe at the beginning of the twentieth cen-tury, and I, too, fell under his spell. (1989a, p. 29)

He was also engrossed in philosophers, Spinoza, Descartes, Leibnitz, Kant, Fichte, Hegel, Marx, Schopenhauer, and Nietzsche, and novelists and poets, Dostoevsky, Tolstoy, Walt Whitman, and Goethe. He found himself growing increasingly distressed by the works of all these "saints, prophets and geniuses." It was not their ideas that were excellent and beautifully voiced, he said, but their behavior as individuals and as representatives of the values they proclaimed:

They predicted disaster unless a prescribed course of action was fol-lowed, but they left it to crafty and opportunistic politicians to run the world. With few exceptions, they did not act themselves. They hid behind profound books and beautiful sermons. They seemed to think that having written their books or having preached their sermons, their jobs were ended. None of them made the jump out of the book into reality. (1989a, p. 30)

INVITATION TO AN ENCOUNTER

The outbreak of World War I disrupted many social institutions, of course, and the House of Encounter was one of its victims. The five friends were scattered. Kellmer, who had volunteered for the medical corps—he was willing to rescue but not to kill others—died from tuberculosis before the war was over. Not long after, in 1914, Moreno published *Ein Ladung zu Einer Begegnung* (*Invitation to an Encounter*), the first of his writings to articulate his ideas and the philosophy of the Religion of the Encounter.

Invitation to an Encounter is a curious work for several reasons. Paradoxically, it is a book that criticizes the practice of writing books. Books, Moreno argues, are substitutes for actual meetings between a creator of ideas, the author, and an audience, the readers. The author sends his thoughts out into the world where readers may be influenced, one way or another, by them. But there is no mutuality, no reciprocity. The reader cannot interact with the author, asking questions, arguing, or expressing his own ideas. The spontaneous encounter between the two that leads both to learn and grow from each other is aborted.

In this piece Moreno addressed for the first time the notion of the "conserve," defined as the end result of a spontaneous-creative act, using the book as a prime example. The result of a spontaneous-creative act, the book, once written can be technologically reproduced endlessly without re-invoking the creativity that gave rise to its original emergence. One of Moreno's concerns about Western society was that it had become so involved and intrigued with its conserves that it had neglected to understand and nourish the spontaneous-creative process from which conserves emerge.

Invitation to an Encounter was offered as something of an antidote. It was intended to be what the title says, an invitation to the reader, to any and every reader, to seek out the author for a true encounter, an exchange of views face-to-face. This idea also reflects a basic principle of the Religion of the Encounter, whose five members often walked the streets of Vienna and the roads of the countryside, seeking interaction with anyone and everyone they met along the way. During the 1960s, when the so-called hippie movement developed in America and other Western nations, Moreno would claim that his chums of the Religion of Encounter were the first hippie movement.

Invitation to an Encounter includes the passage that Moreno quoted a number of times and that was reprinted in a preliminary page of *Psychodrama, First Volume*, under the title, "Motto":

More important than science is its result
One answer provokes a hundred questions.
More important than poetry is its result,
One poem invokes a hundred heroic acts.

More important than recognition is its result,
The result is pain and guilt

More important than procreation is the child.
More important than evolution of creation is the
Evolution of the creator

In the place of the imperative steps the imperator.
In the place of the creative steps the creator
A meeting of two: eye to eye, face to face.
And when you are near I will tear your eyes out
And place them instead of mine,
And you will tear my eyes out,
And will place them instead of yours
Then I will look at you with your eyes
And you will look at me with mine.

Thus even the common thing serves the silence and
our meeting remains the chainless goal:
The undetermined place, at the undetermined time,
the undetermined word to the undetermined man.

As all students of the Morenean methods learn, the seven italicized lines above define the concept of encounter. The German word *Begegnung* is difficult to translate, Moreno wrote, and there is no single English word to convey all its meaning:

It means meeting, contact of bodies, confronting each other, facing each other, countering and battling, seeing and perceiving, touching and entering into each other, sharing and loving, communicating with each other in a primary, intuitive manner by speech or gesture, by kiss and embrace, becoming one—*una cum uno*. The word *Begegnung* contains the root for the word, *gegen*, which means "against." It thus encompasses not only loving, but also hostile and threatening relationships. Encounter which derives from the French *rencontre* is the nearest translation of *Begegnung*. (1960b, p. 15)

The commonly used term *interpersonal relationship* is a pretty sterile and tepid concept compared with "encounter," which denotes two active individuals who live and experience each other:

In a meeting the two persons are there in space, with all their strengths and all their weaknesses, two human actors seething with spontaneity, only partly conscious of their mutual aims. It became clear to me then that only people who meet one another can form a natural group and an actual society of human beings. It is people who meet one another who are the responsible and genuine founders of social living. (Moreno, 1946b, p. 251)

Each party to an encounter has a profound impact upon the other and both will be changed as a result of the meeting. However, victory and defeat are not the purpose of encounter. Quite to the contrary, the ultimate goals are understanding and co-creating between two people. That comes, Moreno contends, when each sees the other as the other sees him/herself. As Marineau (1989, p. 48) points out, the definition of the encounter is also a dramatic and accurate poetical description of the psychodramatic technique of role reversal, unquestionably the most important and most powerful of all psychodramatic techniques. In a psychodrama, the individual is typically asked to take the roles of significant others in his/her life, to put him/herself in their place, to perceive the situation from the perspective and position of the other, to behave as they do and then to justify their behaviors. This procedure seldom fails to reveal new information that increases the protagonist's understanding of the situation and event more completely. A basic concept of psychodrama, the role reversal, is thus anticipated in Moreno's writings some years before he developed either the method or the technique.

"Motto" is additionally interesting in that Moreno acknowledges the positive aspects of the conserve. Although *Invitation to an Encounter* is critical of adulation of the conserve, it recognizes the conserve's usefulness. Both the scientific answer "that provokes a hundred questions" and the poem "that invokes a hundred heroic acts" are conserves, and the conserve often serves to stimulate the warming up process to the level of new creativity. It is easy in a casual reading of Moreno to get the idea that he is only critical of conserves. Such is not the case. His criticism is of the tendency to value the conserve above the creative process that brings it into existence, and it is this faulty perspective on values that, he believes, has resulted in great problems for humankind.

In Western culture delusional paranoid individuals occasionally believe that they are Jesus Christ reincarnated (e.g., see Rokeach, 1964). As a matter of fact, anybody who claims to be Christ is immediately suspected of being delusional. Moreno in his later life was sometimes introduced to professional audiences as "the man who thought that he was God" or "the man who played God." This usually evoked smiles and sometimes nervous laughter from the audience. Few understood the significance of this part of Moreno's life or what he learned by what he sometimes referred to as his role reversal with God. Psychiatric colleagues accused him of megalomania and even of being psychotic.

It was an interesting concept, reversing roles with God, considering that perhaps he was God who had decided to incarnate himself, not as his Son, but as himself. Moreno's son, Jonathan, suggests that he may have been inspired by Alfred Einstein's thought experiments through which Einstein had intuited his great insights about the universe. Moreno himself supports this hypothesis with this passage from the early pages of *Who Shall Survive?*:

> My first scientific dream was that if I were God, the Creator of the universe, I would be able to start an adequate science of the universe. Or, if I would have been at least there and near the source on the first day of creation, his auxiliary ego and participant observer—instead of being born into the twentieth century of an elusive mankind's history—my account of the meaning of the universe would have some semblance of reality. This fanciful dream of getting into the midst of creation, of "ongoing life and production," has never forsaken me and is behind all my actional and written communications and my insistence that all measures and tests of humanity should be constructed after the model of God involved in the creation of the universe.
>
> When I had the courage to put the idea of the Godhead to an empirical test I concluded from it one thing: just like a science of the Godhead also a science of culture cannot be produced at a distance and post mortem by philosophers and historians; it must initiated and inspired by the creators of the cultures themselves. (1953c, pp. 21–22)

The first thing most of us think about when we are contemplating the notion of God is God's omnipotence. So it is easy to imagine that someone playing God, or reversing roles with God, would experience this omnipotence and behave in an imperious or grandiose manner. God-playing instead impressed upon Moreno a tremendous sense of humility and responsibility. He experienced in the God-role a responsibility for the universe and for all things in it. Of greater significance is the fact that Moreno was acting out his ideas and values, not just writing about them as he had criticized others for doing. The Religion of the Encounter was certainly a central part of putting into action with others his ideas and values.

Moreno described this period as follows:

> At that time and for many of the years that followed, I had the sensation that I was the chief actor, the protagonist, in a drama with great scenes and exits, one act climaxing in the other, culminating in a great and final victory. It was drama, but it was not theater. I was my own playwright and producer. The scenes were real, not like those in a theater. But they were not quite as real as in a simple life. They were of a higher reality. They were created by my imagination with the help of actual people and actual objects in the midst of real life. I escaped the

fate of the schizophrenic who operates in a vacuum and has to fill the void with hallucinated figures up to the point of making himself believe that these figures interact with him.

In contrast to this, I was able to arouse the people around me to identify themselves with me and to create, with their aid, a supraworld in which I could test my prophetic role in a comparatively safe environment, made to order for me. (1989a, p. 32)

This psychodrama in life thus preceded psychodrama as a method that he could teach others to use in the creating of themselves and a more satisfying world.

The impact of World War I upon Moreno (as it must have been for all Viennese) could hardly have been greater. At the turn of the century, the Austro-Hungarian Empire was one of the superpowers in today's terms. Austria was the head state of the empire, and Vienna was the capital of both. The empire was one of the longest-lasting and most solid-appearing geopolitical entities in the Western world. It possessed vast territories, had existed for 900 years, and had a history of constitutional stability. Then came the Great War and: "In 1918, the political work of centuries collapsed like a card castle" (Janik & Toulmin, 1973, p. 16). What had been a single supernation was now a handful of separate nationalities. The political bonds holding the empire together vanished overnight. Vienna was in a far from equilibrium state, approaching anarchy for several years. Everybody must have felt the urgency and a sense of potential doom. This was the energy that gave rise to the many, often contradictory, social movements. Moreno thought that if the collective spontaneity of the nation could be mobilized, a workable solution would emerge.

NOTES

1. The major sources for the content of this chapter include Moreno (1946b, 1953a, 1989a); Janik and Toulman (1973); Marineau (1989); and Hare and Hare (1996).

2 Young Man of Many Parts

The years between 1909, when Moreno entered the University of Vienna, and 1925, when he immigrated to America, the years, which comprise what he called the religious phase of his life, were extremely productive ones for Moreno. He threw himself spontaneously into situations in which he perceived groups of people in trouble, often in despair and needing help. He worked to identify the causes of their problems and searched for the means to resolve their problems. Several of these experiences would become the seminal events upon which his later scientific work in America was based. The House of Encounter described in the first chapter is one example of how he took on the social problems of his immediate environment. There are at least seven other events, not counting the completion of his medical degree from the University of Vienna, which characterize Moreno's transition from the religious to the scientific phase of his life. They are:

1. Conducting group therapy with the prostitutes of Vienna.
2. Resolving social turbulence in a refugee community.
3. The first psychodrama, a search for the new king of Austria.
4. Founding of the literary journal *Daimon*.
5. Creating the theater of spontaneity.
6. Discovering the therapeutic application of spontaneity techniques.
7. Invention of a sound and picture recording device.

ORGANIZING THE PROSTITUTES OF VIENNA

Although Vienna was a cultural center second only to Paris in Europe, and a major seat of medical and scientific training and research, Viennese society had its drawbacks and was rife with sham and hypocrisy. The Austro-Hungarian Empire, one of the superpowers of the era and a police state under the rule of Emperor Franz Joseph, was nearing disintegration and dissolution into a dozen independent states. World War I finally brought an end to the empire, and, simultaneously, it brought social and political turbulence to Vienna.

Viennese society may have been more prudish than Victorian England. Certainly Viennese society had similar attitudes toward sexuality as did English society. For all intents, sexuality did not exist as far as polite Viennese society was concerned. One would never, in public, allow any hint that men and women engaged in those activities without which humankind would become extinct after one generation. Even in the privacy of the bedroom, women were considered incapable of obtaining anything but pregnancy from the sexual act, and a bourgeois woman would probably be ashamed to admit it if she found anything exciting or enjoyable about copulation. Of course, a society that represses mention of sex ensures that its members will be obsessed with thoughts of sex.

It was also expected among the bourgeoisie that a man establish himself socially and economically before he considered marriage. By the time he had achieved this, perhaps late 20s or early 30s, he was likely beyond the highest peak of his sexual desires. Before reaching an economically independent state, if a young man had sex it was likely with a prostitute. It would be unthinkable to have sex with a woman of one's own class to whom one was not married, with a woman whom he might consider marrying. Young women, of course, were denied any such outlet for their sexual desires, and the resulting suppression and repression of feminine sexuality gave psychoanalysis much of its flavor. Besides, marriage for the middle class was largely a pragmatic and commercial event, the joining of families of wealth to create families of even greater wealth. Love and affection, if they entered the picture at all, were secondary considerations. The situation was not one that would enhance sexuality for even the married woman. All of these characteristics of Viennese society created and supported a very strong demand for commercial sex.

This demand was met by the availability of young women of a lower class, a result of economic circumstances. For the upper- and middle-class citizens, Vienna may well have lived up to its characterization as the City of Dreams. For the working class, the dreams were more often nightmares. Factory workers, both men and women, might work 10- to 12-hour days, seven days a week, with the women receiving lesser wages than the men. Children were also employed in factories at still lesser wages. By law they had to be given a day a week off. As if the working conditions weren't bad enough, living conditions offered little respite. Housing was in short supply and expensive relative to wages. Apartments were crowded, often with more than one family occupying a few rooms. Many had no running water and indoor toilets were rare. They were poorly heated and drab (Janik & Toulmin, 1973).

A young woman had few possibilities for escaping the deprivations of poverty. Selling her body was one of them. Some turned to the trade for a bed to sleep in. Perhaps the lucky ones became *süssmadchen*, mistresses kept by the well-to-do merchant or professional man. The prostitutes were reviled on all sides. A red-light district had grown in the Am Spittelberg and became a ghetto for prostitutes.

Here was an entire class of people segregated from the rest of society, not because of their religion or ethnic character, but because of their occupation. They were unacceptable to the bourgeois, the Marxists, even the criminals. . . . they had no civil rights. There were no laws . . . protecting their interests. (Moreno, 1989a, p. 48)

Viennese society thus made prostitution both immoral and a social necessity, illegal but protected by the police in return for bribes paid them by the prostitutes. Newspapers called for campaigns to eliminate the practice of prostitution in the front pages—and took discreet ads in the classified sections from its practitioners. Exposed to venereal disease, prostitutes found it difficult to find doctors who would treat them. They were arrested, often arbitrarily and even after they had paid bribes to the police, but they could not find lawyers to advocate for them.

These were the conditions that existed when Moreno one day encountered "a pretty girl who smiled at me. She was wearing a striking red skirt and a white blouse decorated with red ribbons to match her skirt" (1989a, p. 48). As they were just striking up a conversation, a policeman arrested the girl and took her to the police station. Moreno followed and waited for her to reappear. She had been out on the street "in uniform" too early in the day, she informed him. Prostitutes, by the rules laid down by the "little gods at the police station" were not supposed to wear the bright and provocative clothing that identified their profession until after dark. Although Moreno doesn't say so, this woman probably had to pay a bribe in the guise of a fine at the police station. This young woman became Moreno's entrée into the world and the houses of the Am Spittelberg prostitutes.

Moreno persuaded a physician, a specialist in venereal diseases, and a newspaper publisher to accompany him and began making visits to the women who lived there, meeting with groups of 8 to 10 at a time. Initially they found the women suspicious of their motives. Were they coming to reform them like workers of Catholic charities sometimes did? Would these visits lead to prosecution? Eventually Moreno and his colleagues became accepted as they were recognized as wanting to help on the prostitutes' own terms.

Initially the meetings of small groups of prostitutes focused on immediate problems: problems with the police who harassed them, arrested them, and shook them down for money; having venereal disease but being unable to find a doctor who would treat them; pregnancies and the babies that resulted; exploitation by pimps and madams. The new visitors helped them find doctors who would treat them and lawyers who would represent them. The women also began to recognize how they could help each other. They started donating money to a collective emergency fund. "From the outside it looked like we had 'unionized' prostitutes" (Moreno, 1989a, p. 49).

However, Moreno had more in mind than resolving these immediate and concrete problems. He recognized that the ostracism and stigmatization that the prostitutes experienced, the perception by others that they were despicable, sinful, and unworthy of social contact, had a pervasive effect upon their perceptions of themselves. They could not avoid internalizing these altitudes and perceiving themselves as others perceived them. "I had in mind what LaSalle and Marx had done for the working class, ideology aside. They made the workers respectable by giving them a sense of dignity. . . . I had in mind that something similar could be done for the prostitutes" (Moreno, 1989a, p. 48). Near the end of the year 1913, Moreno reports, the prostitutes held a mass meeting in a large hall, the Sofiensaal, in Vienna. They had become a true organization with elected leaders. "It was one of my early efforts at applying group therapy to one of the most difficult of human problems, that of prostitution" (1989a, p. 49).

Mitterndorf

The year 1914, World War I, death knell of the Austro-Hungarian Empire, broke out. Moreno's medical student colleagues all enlisted in the army, but Moreno was turned down. In later years, Moreno accounted for this by promulgating the myth that he had been born on a ship on the Black Sea and so had no birth certificate. We now know that this is not a literal truth, and Marineau (1989) goes to some length to provide a rationale for the myth. The fact is that Moreno was born in Bucharest, and his birth was duly recorded in Rathaus archives (Bratescu, 1975).

But it is also true that Moreno Levy, Moreno's father, was born in Turkey. Turkey was aligned against Austria in the war, and it is likely that his Turkish heritage was the reason why he was turned down for army duty. That fact did not, however, prevent the government from hiring him as a medical officer. His first assignment was to Mitterndorf, a village constructed for refugees from Tyrol, a southern district upon which the Italian army was marching. The Tyroleans were Italian-speaking Austrian subjects and were essentially interned at Mitterndorf, both to protect them from the Italian army and because the Austrian government did not completely trust them to withstand the invading army.

The Austrian government had constructed Mitterndorf expressly for the Tyrolean refugees. It was a village designed and built for that purpose. Housing, of course, was provided (Moreno describes the living quarters as cottages, and Marineau calls them barracks) with several families placed in each dwelling. Other buildings had been constructed, a church, a hospital, a commissary, and so forth. Those in charge of the project probably believed that they had anticipated everything the refugees could need. The planners had considered safety from the enemy, sanitation, and subsistence. They must have anticipated that the Tyroleans would welcome Mitterndorf as a place of safety and security.

Actually, Moreno tells us, it was an internment camp, somewhat like those in which Japanese-Americans on the West Coast were placed during

World War II. Although provided with the basic needs and comforts of life, the villagers were not free to leave. German police who looked down upon their Italian charges and often dealt with them with a heavy hand administered the camp. Moreno was placed in charge of sanitation, initially; later he became superintendent of the children's hospital.

But the village did not function as smoothly as the planners must have imagined it would:

> The structure of the camp gave rise to the most tremendous corruption I have ever witnessed. It was a regular Sodom and Gomorrah. There was an enormous black market, of course. The women were particularly abused—so many abortions and illicit pregnancies. The German police were the worst in this respect. (Moreno, 1989b, p. 65)

Moreno had already developed what would become a lifelong contempt and disdain for absolute arbitrary authorities such as the police and, together with a psychologist, Ferruccio Bannizoni, who was part of the administration and functioned as a mediator between the administration and the villagers, wrote many letters to the Ministry of the Interior, who had ultimate responsibility for the village, complaining about the police and requesting that they be disciplined. They were moderately successful.

With Bannizoni, Moreno began to investigate the psychological currents swirling through the social components of life in Mitterndorf, such elements as nationality, politics, sex, status (such as staff vs. villager), and so forth. It was during this study that the basic idea of sociometry emerged. The Tyroleans had been arbitrarily assigned to living quarters, to their various duties in the village and factory. Moreno's radical idea, which he proposed to the Minister of the Interior, was that the villages should be given a choice in whom they shared living quarters with, that they should choose who would live close to them and to whom they would live in proximity.

> I moved families around on the basis of their mutual affinities for one another. Thus the groundwork by which the community was organized was changed for the better. My theory was borne out by the fact that when people were able to live with those to whom they were positively attracted, the families tended to be helpful to one another and the signs of maladjustment diminished both in number and in intensity. We also rearranged work groups in the factories whenever possible to create greater harmony and productivity among the workers. (Moreno, 1989b, p. 66)

The development of sociometry was gradual. After the war concluded, Moreno returned to the university, completed his degree, and began his practice as the village doctor of Voslau. He maintained important ties in Vienna and when he established the *Stegreiftheater* in Vienna in 1921, he paid very close attention to his players and how they interacted with each other. He constructed inter-action diagrams that depicted various aspects of their interactions. In 1923, he published *Rede über die Begegnung* (*A Speech about the Encounter*) in which he relates the story of a doctor who sets out to treat a man in a certain village. He is delayed in reaching the patient because along the way he meets so many others whose maladies are interlocked with the original patient's illness and whom he feels obligated to stop and treat. He discovers that people cannot be treated singly but all must be treated together. This notion is expressed again, in 1934, in the first sentence of his major opus, *Who Shall Survive?*: "A truly therapeutic procedure cannot have less an objective than the whole of mankind." It was at Mitterndorf that Moreno first got the idea of the preferential nature of the structure of society. This was his first, and perhaps simplistic, use of sociometry in social planning. Moreno's next opportunity for developing sociometry as a science of society as well as a method of social assignment would not come for another 15 years or so, after he had moved to America. Then he would conceive of sociometry as the umbrella for his other major innovations, group psychotherapy and psychodrama.

Throughout his life Moreno championed the cause of the weak and power-less against arbitrary authority. He saw sociometry as a means of ameliorating dissension and redistributing power within a group so that all its members shared sociometric wealth.

SEEKING A NEW KING OF AUSTRIA

During his tenure at Mitterndorf, Moreno went into Vienna whenever he could take a few hours away from his duties. There he became a member of two Viennese café groups. One, Café Herrenhof, was a gathering place for young intellectuals, poets, and writers, the core of literary expressionism in Austria. The other, Café Museum, was composed of mostly actors and actresses, although several writers also were a part.

Austria at this time was still attempting to find social and political stability in the aftermath of the First World War that had resulted in the destruction of the Austro-Hungarian Empire, for which Austria, and especially Vienna, had served as the capital. It was now a head with its body lopped off. With the elimination of its exiled emperor as well as the loss of the empire itself, Vienna was a swirling cauldron of sociopolitical movements as disparate as Zionism and German Nationalism, Austro-Communism and Christian Socialism, all competing for ascendency. The country was in a state of near anarchy, and, indeed, there were those who actively advo-cated anarchy—no government at all. A common topic discussed by the group at Café Museum was how the theater could influence and change society for the better.

It is in this setting that Moreno suggested an audacious idea. The father of one of the actresses in the group at Café Museum, Anna Höllering, owned a theater, the Komoedian Haus. He agreed to loan the theater to Moreno for the night. Moreno and his friends announced a great event, one that the new king himself would attend to be introduced to the country and his subjects. Posters proclaimed the event and the group sent invitations to various dignitaries, political leaders, and elected officials, literary figures, theater people, representatives of religious and cultural organizations, and, of course, the press.

The theater was packed with people, perhaps 1,000 or so. At 7:00 p.m., the curtain rose on a stage, empty except for a red plush armchair with a high back and gilded frame representing a throne. A gilded crown was in the chair. Moreno walked onto the stage and introduced himself as the king's jester. "But where is the king?" he asked. "It was announced that he would be here. Here is his throne. Perhaps he is sitting in the audience. Perhaps he is sitting next to you." He proceeded to invite members of the audience, representatives of all groups, to try out for the role of the king, the leader of the people, the head of Austria, and express their ideas for leading the country. He asked them to sit on the throne and discuss their ideas of what needed to be done for the country to achieve stability again.

> It was an attempt to treat and purge the audience from a disease, a pathological cultural syndrome that the participants shared. Postwar Vienna was seething with revolt. It had no stable government, no emperor, no king, and no leader. Like Germany, Russia, the United States, indeed, the entire populated earth, also Austria was restless, in search of a new soul.
>
> But psychodramatically speaking, I had a cast and I had a play. The audience was my cast, the people in the audience were like a thousand unconscious playwrights. The play was the plot into which they had been thrown by the historical events and in which each played a real part. If I could only turn the spectators into actors, the actors of their own collective drama, that is the dramatic social conflicts in which they were actually involved, then my boldness would be redeemed and the session could start. (Moreno, 1946b, p. 1)

The audience was to be the jury that would select its leader. Not expecting to be personally involved and attending primarily to see who the new king of Austria was, few people responded to the challenge. Many, frustrated and disgusted with what they were witnessing, left the theater. Franz Werfel, the writer and friend of Moreno, was there with his following of university student anarchists, cheering Moreno on and causing quite a fuss in the process. The test, he says afterward, must have been too difficult. Nobody was chosen. According to Moreno, the press was quite disturbed by the event and reported it with much criticism. He lost many friends as a result of the performance and the bad press that followed. His self-evaluation was: "nemo profeta in patria" (1946b, p. 2).

It is this date, April 1, 1921, upon which psychodrama was born, Moreno maintains, and every serious student of psychodrama learns this fact, even though the event itself is what Moreno would later call sociodrama, and even though there were events preceding and subsequent to this one that are considered as germane to the origins of psychodrama. The one that most closely resembles therapeutic psychodrama occurred a couple of years after this official "birth" of psychodrama.

DAIMON

Another piece of the transition period between Moreno's religious and scientific phases is his part in founding *Daimon*, the first journal of Austrian expressionist authors. Moreno, while he was still stationed at Mitterndorf, became a member of the group of intellectuals, and writers who met at Café Herrenhof during the war. After World War I, authors became disgruntled with publishers, mostly in Germany, whom, they felt, made big profits off their works and paid them minimally. This led to the establishment of the *Genossenschaftsverlag*, a writers' cooperative publishing house. At Moreno's instigation, the group established a periodical, *Daimon*, of which Moreno served as the editor.

The first issue was published in 1918. In 1919, the journal was renamed as *Der Neue Daimon* and later became *Gefährten*. The journal published works by some of the best-known authors and poets of the time, including Otokar Brezina, Max Brod, Francis Jammes, Paul Kornfeld, E. A. Rheinhardt, Fredrich Schnack, Jaakob Wasserman, Ernst Weiss, Franz Werfel, Alfred Wolfenstein, A. P. Gutersloh, Martin Buber, Arthur Schnitzler, Robert Musil, Franz Lehar, Franz Blei, and others who were a part of the Café Herrenhof group (Kohl & Robertson, 2006). Marineau adds Fritz Lampl, Albert Ehrenstein, Hugo Sonnenschein, and Alfred Adler to the list. A web page of the Vienna City Library discusses the publication and adds even more names to the list.

Austrian Expressionism emphasized subjectivity and communication via expression of intense emotion, both in art and literature. Expressionist art and literature represent rebellion and struggle against bourgeois values as well as established authority. Especially it was rebellion against the artificiality and sham that pervaded Viennese culture. The official pronouncement was art for art's sake. The expressionists insisted that art reflect the authentic experience of the artist. It is easy to see the influence of expressionism in the psychodramatic method in which the subjective life experiences of a protagonist are given tangible dramatic expression on the psychodramatic stage. The expressionist writers expressed many existential ideas.

The journal under its various names was short-lived. It was last published in 1922. This may have been partly because of Moreno's fading interests in the journal that he was so instrumental in founding. Marineau

(1989) suggests that Moreno was not so comfortable with the tendency of the intellectuals of the times to talk and debate rather than take action. In any case, his interests were turning more toward the theater and the group of actors who met at the Café Museum.

STEGREIFTHEATER: THE THEATER OF SPONTANEITY

The idea was to use the theater as an agent of social change. The first step had been the search for the king. Sometime after this, perhaps in 1922, Moreno rented a hall on Maysedergasse in Vienna and here, with actors from the group that met at the Café Museum, he began the *Stegreiftheater*, the theater of spontaneous drama. Sometimes he devised a theme or plot for the drama. Sometimes the actors or the audience made suggestions for the drama. In any event, the dramas were created in the moment without playwright or script, without rehearsal, and with minimal props and scenery.

The press reviewed the theater, and good reviews resulted in large audiences. However, the theater encountered a dilemma inherent in spontaneous work of this sort. When things go well and the actors really engage with each other, with their roles, and with the themes of the drama, spontaneous drama is magnificent and electrifying. The audience members are deeply moved and appreciative. However, sometimes the spontaneity of the actors fails and the drama falls flat. It is not a satisfying performance and the audience is disappointed. Moreno found that when the spontaneity players were at their best, many people, including some of the critics, were saying, "That was a very powerful performance, but obviously it had to be rehearsed. Why do you insist upon saying that it was not?" And when the players had an off night, when things did not go well, some people would say, "That was terrible, but then what do you expect when the actors have no script and don't prepare?"

In part to prove that the dramas were indeed spontaneously created, the group added "The Living Newspaper" to their repertoire. For this, stories from the latest editions of the Vienna newspapers served as the plots of some dramas. Obviously there would not be time for the drama to be scripted and rehearsed. Good or not so good, these pieces were obviously produced spontaneously since there was not time for script writing, casting, or rehearsal.

Although the *Stegreiftheater* was successful in terms of generating a following and played to a large audience every performance, Moreno was not entirely satisfied. He did not see the theater having the effect upon Viennese society that he had anticipated and hoped for. He ascribed this to the rigidity of Austrian society and decided that he must try out his ideas in a more democratic society, the United States. When he did come to America, it took several years before he was able to establish Impromtu, the name he gave to the American spontaneity theater.

Again, Moreno met with significant interest but not enough to satisfy him. There were also significant difficulties. Audiences suspected that well-played scenes were not spontaneously created and took poorly played scenes as evidence that spontaneity methods would not work. Moreno was disheartened when he saw his best players resorting to conserve even when acting extemporaneously. He also found them abandoning the theater of spontaneity and going to the legitimate stage or becoming movie actors. At this point he writes, "*I turned 'temporarily' to the therapeutic theatre, a strategic decision which probably save the psychodramatic movement from oblivion*" (1947e, p. 7).

SPONTANEITY DRAMA TO SAVE A MARRIAGE

It was within the context of the *Stegreiftheater* that Moreno first applied the techniques of spontaneity drama to the resolution of emotional problems. In this case it was a marital problem and Moreno, who liked to be the first, could easily have claimed the title of Father of Marriage Therapy. As a matter of fact, many years later, a practitioner of that discipline identified him as the unrecognized pioneer of marriage therapy (Compernolle, 1981).

One of the stars of the *Stegreiftheater* was a young woman, identified in Moreno's account as "Barbara," but whom we now know was Anna Höllering (Marineau, 1989). Young and beautiful, she was the primary portrayer of ingénue roles in the dramas. A young man, whom Moreno identifies as "George," was frequently in the audience. George was a poet and playwright and it was soon apparent to everybody that the major attraction to him was watching Barbara. A romance evolved and they were eventually married. Everything seemed fine until George sought out Moreno one day, greatly upset. It turned out that the couple was having problems. "That sweet, angel-like being whom you all admire, acts like a bedeviled creature when she is alone with me. She speaks the most abusive language and when I get angry at her, as I did last night, she hits me with her fists" (Moreno, 1946b, p. 4). George complained and asked if Moreno could do anything to help. Moreno promised to try.

That evening when Barbara came to the theater, Moreno had a little talk with her. She was doing great work, he told her, but he was afraid that she might be getting stale. He thought, he said, that people would like to see her in different kinds of roles, "roles in which you portray the nearness to the soil, the rawness of human nature, its vulgarity and stupidity, its cynical reality, people not only as they are, but worse than they are, people as they are when driven to extremes by unusual circumstances. Do you want to try it?"

Barbara was enthusiastic and only wondered if she could bring it off. Moreno expressed his confidence in her acting abilities and mentioned that news had just come in about the murder of a prostitute by a stranger, still at large. He wanted her to play the prostitute and appointed another actor to be the murderer. He asked them to prepare the scene.

A street was improvised on the stage, a café, two lights. Barbara went on. George was in his usual seat in the first row, highly excited. Richard, in the role of the apache, came out of the café with Barbara and followed her. They had an encounter, which rapidly developed into a heated argument. It was about money. Suddenly Barbara changed to a manner of acting totally unexpected from her. She swore like a trooper, punching at the man, kicking him in the leg repeatedly. I saw George half rising, anxiously raising his arm at me, but the apache got wild and began to chase Barbara. Suddenly he grabbed a knife, a prop, from his inside jacket pocket. He chased her in circles, closer and closer. She acted so well that she gave the impression of being really scared. The audience got up, roaring, "Stop it, stop it." but he did not stop until she was supposedly "murdered." After the scene, Barbara was exuberant with joy, she embraced George and they went home in ecstasy. From then on she continued to act in such roles of the lower depth. She played as domestics, lonely spinsters, revengeful wives, spiteful sweethearts, barmaids, and gun molls. (Moreno, 1946b, pp. 4–5)

George gave Moreno daily reports. Something was happening, he soon recounted. While Barbara still had her fits of temper, they had lost their intensity, and she might laugh in the middle of them, reminded of something that she had played recently on the stage. Something was happening to George, too. Watching her play on the stage was building in him a greater tolerance for her and her behavior. He was less impatient with her. Moreno assigned roles to her more carefully, according to what he assessed as her needs and George's. Eventually, he invited the two young people to act on the stage with each other, and they did so. Their "duettes" began to resemble scenes from their daily lives. Then came scenes from their respective families, scenes from their childhoods, of their dreams, and plans for the future. After every one of these performances, Moreno writes, people would come to him and ask why the Barbara–George scenes seemed to affect them so much more than the other spontaneous dramas. It was because audience members recognized that these scenes portrayed the real lives of real human beings, their hopes, their fears, their struggles, their successes, and their failures. Experiencing these dramas evoked in audience members memories of their own struggles, paralleling those of the actors. He identified this as audience therapy.

It was in this way that Moreno first experimented with the techniques of spontaneous drama to treat emotional problems. Years before the notion of marital or family therapy became commonplace in mainstream mental health practice, Moreno had demonstrated the use of spontaneity techniques to restore equilibrium to the relationship of a husband and wife. He would later be given credit as a pioneer of family therapy (Compernolle, 1981). Although Moreno applied this approach to other couples and individuals during the time of the *Stegreiftheater*, and later in America at the Hudson Training School, it was not until 1936 that the systematic development of psychodrama as a means of restoring emotional equilibrium truly began and psychodrama became the method for which Moreno was most widely known. That story is told in Chapter 10 of this book.

IMMIGRATING TO AMERICA

Although the *Stegreiftheater* developed a significant following, it was not the resounding success for which Moreno hoped. He may very well have anticipated that his new form of theater would be a true competitor of the conserve, or conventional, theater. Moreno was disappointed that his other ideas also seemed to fall on barren ground in Europe. He attributed this to the rigidity of society and wondered if he might have a better reception in a newer culture. Marineau (1989) lists several other personal reasons that motivated his desire to move, including growing anti-Semitism, increasing personal debt, and a legal controversy that had generated publicity adverse to him. The two young and vigorous cultures that attracted him were post-revolution Russia and America. Although he had friends who had immigrated to Russia, he decided that America provided a better choice.

Sometime in 1924 or 1925, Moreno had a dream that featured sounds coming from magnetic fields of steel discs. With the considerable assistance of a young and brilliant engineer, Franz Lörnitzo, a model of a machine that recorded sound on a steel disc was built and patented. An American company indicated that it was interested in the invention, called the Radio Film device, and in December 1925, Moreno took the model and sailed for New York.

Marineau's (1989) biography describes Moreno's adventures as a new immigrant in this country during the next few years. The first five years were a struggle, Marineau states. He was on a temporary visa and had no license to practice medicine. In his autobiography, Moreno says that the Radio Film device was sold to the General Phonograph Corporation in Ohio, and that the company engaged him and Lörnitzo for a period of six months to further develop the invention.

Then it was back to New York, where he knew practically nobody except his brother, William, who supported him financially and emotionally. He met Dr. Bela Schick, a doctor at Mount Sinai Hospital, who became interested in his work with children. Schick arranged for Moreno to work in the hospital's mental health clinic. Here he met Beatrice Beecher, who became interested in his spontaneity work. Learning of his visa problems, she proposed that they marry with the understanding that it was only until he obtained citizenship, after which they would divorce. And this is indeed what happened. They were married in 1928 and divorced in 1934 after he had become a naturalized citizen.

Before proceeding with his life and work in America, there is one more momentous event in Moreno's life that stands as capstone of the European or religious phase of his life. This event deserves a chapter for itself.

3 Role Reversal with God

World War I brought the Religion of Encounter to an end. Chaim Kellmer volunteered as an ambulance driver for the army despite being sick with tuberculosis, and died before the end of the war. Jan Feda returned to Prague and András Petö to Budapest, where he later won fame for his work with crippled children. Hans Brauchbar relocated to Russia and disappeared. Moreno volunteered for military service but was turned down because of the unclear status of his citizenship, he said. As an advanced medical student with considerable clinical experience, he was, however, employed by the government as a medical officer. He was first assigned to Mitterndorf and later to a camp in Hungary. He took his final medical school examination in February 1917 and was awarded his medical degree.

At the end of the war, Moreno left government service and looked for a place to practice his profession. He wanted to practice outside the city, he says, in the countryside where he could practice among plain people. He found that place in Bad Vöslau, a village where he became both the public health officer and the chief physician of the local textile factory. The factory paid him a salary and the village provided him with a house. He soon attained an outstanding reputation as a doctor.

It was in Bad Vöslau that he met and developed a relationship with Marianne Lörnitzo, a local schoolteacher. As described by Moreno, it was a complex relationship, initially one of intense spiritual intimacy. The relationship was both physically and spiritually intimate. He describes Marianne as his muse, a catalyst for his creativity. Their relationship is reported by Moreno (1989b) and at some length by Marineau (1989).

Sometime during the year 1920, Moreno had an unusual experience in which he began to hear voices:

> not in the sense of a mental patient, but in the sense of a person beginning to feel that he hears a voice which reaches all beings and which speaks to all beings in the same language, which is understood by all men, and one which gives us hope, which give our life direction, which gives our cosmos a direction and a meaning, that the universe is not just a jungle and a bundle of wild forces, that it is basically infinite

creativity which is true on all levels of existence, whether it is now physical or social or biological, whether it is in our galaxy or in other galaxies, far away from us, whether it is in the past or in the present or in the future, ties us together. We are all bound together by responsibility for all things, there is no limited, partial responsibility. And responsibility makes us automatically also creators of the world. (Moreno, 1972b, pp. 200–201)

In a state of total inspiration and with the words rushing through his mind, Moreno began to write them down—in red pencil on the walls of the house in which he was living. Copied from the walls of the house, the writings were published anonymously as *Das Testament Des Vaters* (1920). Moreno translated the work into English as *The Words of the Father* (1941d) and added a great deal of expository material.[1] Both versions were published anonymously. That was because Moreno felt that these were not his words. He did not author them. He felt as though they had passed through him just as they pass through every being, and in every language or mode of understanding. They require no priest or prophet to interpret; they come directly from God to every creature. Moreno has suggested that this is his most important production and considered it the culmination of the religious phase of his life.

Moreno s biographer writes that *Words of the Father* is the most fascinating book that Moreno ever wrote. Few would disagree. *Words of the Father* is fascinating because of its origin, fascinating because of its premise that the *Words* come directly from God, and fascinating because the *Words* reflect the major philosophical concepts upon which the Morenean methods are founded. *Words of the Father* is also the most controversial of Moreno's works.

As Marineau notes, *The Words of the Father* expresses Moreno's philosophy of co-creativity and co-responsibility and one can find in it the rudiments of all his later concepts: spontaneity, creativity, the conserve, encounter, and the moment.

THE I-GOD

The Words of the Father comprises nothing less than a new conceptualization of God. Moreno points out that although God Himself remains the same throughout time, ideas of what and who God is are subject to change. These evolutions in the concept of God tend to come in times of great crisis, when something has happened that cannot be understood in terms of the prevailing notions of God.

The mythologies that have been handed down from ancient times suggest that humankind has always pondered the meaning of existence and our place in the cosmos. Questions about how the world came to be and our relationship with both the world and the power that created and controls it seem to play a part in the culture of every tribe, nation, or race that has ever existed. The concept of the Godhead then represents the attempt to solve this puzzle. It represents the central, meaning-giving idea of the universe, and the concept of the Godhead evolves as human culture evolves. To serve its function, it must relate our experience of the outer or physical world with the inner experience of self. As our knowledge of the physical world or of ourselves increases and develops, so must the conceptualization of God.

The Godhead concept at any particular time reflects the state of development and patterns of the culture at that time in history. Moreno compares the two previous major God concepts of the Western world. The first is the God of the Hebrews, a "He-God," a God Who created the world from outside it and then created humans whom He placed in it. He, God himself, remained outside, unreachable, and unknown:

> It was a construction of the Godhead which was suitable for the time in which the Hebrews lived; it fulfilled a great function then, for them. People were then frightened and dependent upon an enormous Supreme Creator whom they could trust and who guided their lives and who gave their life a meaning. It was a God whom they never saw, it was something like a He-God, He, the God, a God who was outside their world but of whom they felt that he is the greatest help in their lives. (1972b, pp. 198–199)

With Christ, a new dimension is added. God becomes very close and personal. While the Hebrew He-God spoke to humankind through selected men, the prophets, the Christian Thou-God sends his Son to communicate to the people:

> He was brought to visibility in the form of a personal appearance of God. He was the Thou-God, the God who is near, not as much the God of power and enormous wisdom and intelligence but the God of love and sweetness and closeness. And that was the God which Christ brought into this world. (1972b, p. 199)

Now, 2,000 years later, Moreno suggests that the concept of the Christian God, "while it as not exactly failed, does not meet current needs of the day sufficiently" (1972b, p. 199). Huge numbers of people no longer believe in the existence of God. In Soviet Communism, God was essentially outlawed.

A major problem arises from the fact that:

> the concept of God—particularly in the form of the Christian God—has been the center of all our value-systems. Commendable qualities like love, charity, morality, wisdom, creativity and strength, were vested in him, the supreme arbiter of all human values. All deviations from Him,

such as hate, selfishness, license, stupidity, sterility and weakness, were held to be criminal and satanic. (1953a, p. xviii)

Because this value system was so thoroughly and deeply embedded in all aspects of culture and society, secularization of values could not occur as a gradual and peaceful process. The inability of those who defended the old value system to revise the God concept in a rapidly changing world was a fundamental cause of the worldwide upheaval that was manifested by the Second World War, by the wars, conflicts, and the atrocities associated with them that have continued ever since. Equally responsible for the current crisis are those, such as the Communists, who attacked the old system without offering a replacement for it. The world of humankind cannot maintain itself without a system of values. It is to this end that a new conceptualization of God is called for, and a new conceptualization of God is presented in *The Words of the Father*, a Godhead for these times:

> The God who is the God of love has been betrayed so many times by men that something more had to be added, a God which does not come from the Thou but who comes from within our own person through the I, through me. . . . In the old testament God is a He, in the new testament he is a Thou; but now there is a new God, a new voice of experience, a new communication with God which comes through the I itself, through me, through you, through every me, the millions of me's. (Moreno, 1972b, p. 200)

The new notion of the I-God supersedes and subsumes all previous conceptualizations of God, including those of the Hebrew "He-God" and the Christian "Thou-God," perhaps especially these two major God-concepts of Western civilizations. The I-God is first of all a God of all beings, of the whole universe, the God of Jews, Christians, Hindus, Buddhists, Zoroastrians, agnostics, atheists, the God of every living thing. This is a God who speaks without an interpreter and who speaks directly to all beings. His voice is understandable by all beings:

> I AM GOD THE FATHER,
> CREATOR OF THE UNIVERSE. (p. 5)[2]

Moreno insisted that the "voices" he heard were not like the voices the hallucinating patient hears. The "words" are not words in the usual sense of human created auditory symbols. They are more like messages, preverbal messages emanating from every being in the universe, understandable by every being in the universe:

> THEY HAVE BEEN
> BEFORE THE WORLD WAS CREATED,

THEY WILL BE
WHEN THE WORLD IS GONE. (p. 6)

The words are God's revelation of himself and his universe. They give humankind hope and direction. They tell us that the universe is basically infinite creativity.

Moreno is not presenting us with a new or different God. God does not change; the human conceptualization of God changes according to the times and the needs of humanity. Moreno presents us with a new concept of God. While there have been religions with a god and religions without a god, Moreno wrote, this is the first time that there has been a concept of a God without a religion. The Godhead depicted here needs no church to introduce him and he does not favor any particular race over any other, any system of religious belief over others, any country over another.

I AM NOT YOUR GOD,
I AM GOD.
I AM NOT THIS NATION'S GOD
NOR THAT NATION'S GOD,
I AM GOD.
I AM NOT THE GOD OF THIS CLASS
OR OF THAT CLASS,
I AM GOD. (p. 55)

And:

I AM.
WHETHER OR NOT YOU BELIEVE IN ME,
EVEN IF, IN ALL THE UNIVERSE,
THERE IS NO ONE TO RECOGNIZE ME,
I AM. (p. 58)

He communicates just as easily to those who have never been inside a church, temple, or mosque as to the devout who never miss a service, to theists and atheists alike. He needs no prophets. He interprets himself. He is not outside the universe. He is present here and now. A problem with previous notions of God, Moreno suggests, has arisen in the past when those individuals who have heard God have not understood that God passes through them. They, in turn, have deluded others into confusing them with the idea of God.

Previous conceptualizations of God have considered God from the perspective of human beings looking toward the Almighty Creator from their own little speck in the universe. The I-God, on the other hand, is pictured from God's own perspective. Here is God, perceiving and reflecting upon the whole universe that he has created, as well as upon himself. He speaks in the first person, saying "I, your God," and "I am the Father, the Creator of the universe." He is present, here, in every moment.

> THE UNIVERSE WAS FINISHED.
> I SAW ALL THINGS IN THEIR PLACES.
> I KNEW THE VERY CELL IN MY BODY
> FROM WHICH EVERY BEING,
> LARGE OR SMALL, DESCENDED. (p. 44)

Moreno wrote:

> It seems to me, that if there is a God, this is the way He would think, feel, act, create and judge. He, its Author, would see the universe as a whole. Here we have Him assuming and expressing—and rightly—complete objectivity and total knowledge of the universe. It is the Absolute speaking. (1941d, p. ix)

The God presented here is not represented as an object, an essence, or "a substance molded after the image and within the experiential limits of man." Instead, this God creates and experiences with all the subjectivity of a real being. "It is vital," Moreno says, "that God have a subjectivity of His own." Deprived of subjectivity, God would be a god who is dead. The Godhead has a subjective existence of his own, and this means that he is alive and creative in the present. "Subjectivity is an indispensable premise to the most important function of god, that of being the creator of our universe," Moreno writes. "Whereas, by his objectivity, God participates in the majesty of Nature, by His subjectivity God shares in the small miseries and sufferings of the millions of little 'subjects' who fill the world. Consequently, in addition to being a cold, distant god, He is a passionate, personal god" (1941d, p. ix).

However, God's subjectivity cannot be the same as the subjectivity we experience. It is a subjectivity that is beyond that of the human being, the subjectivity of the Absolute Creator of the world. We experience only the moment and the situation we are currently in. The moment experienced by the Godhead must include the moment of every individual being. At any moment in the existence of the universe, there are millions of these individual moments that comprise God's moment.

With respect to creative acts, there is a paradoxical situation. Although the Absolute Creator is involved in every creative act, he is perceived as sharing his creativity with his creations. His relationship with the universe is seen as one that emphasizes fellowship and coexistence, co-responsibility rather than dominance or sovereignty. Every new living thing that emerges into the universe is endowed with creative ability and becomes, with God, a co-creator of the ever-changing universe. There is thus a universal interdependence between God and the beings of the universe:

O WHO IS MORE
IN NEED OF HELP THAN I?
WHO NEEDS
SO MANY HANDS AS I?
WHO NEEDS
SO MANY SOULS AS I?
WHO NEEDS
SO MANY LANDS AS I?

IF ONE CARRIES
TOO HEAVY A BURDEN,
ONE HAND MORE
IS SUFFICIENT.
IF ONE IS LONELY,
ONE SOUL WHO LOVES HIM
IS SUFFICIENT.
IF ONE NEEDS
FOOD AND REST,
ONE SPAN OF EARTH
IS SUFFICIENT.
BUT I NEED ALL THE HANDS
THAT THERE ARE,
NONE SHALL BE MISSING.
I NEED ALL THE SOULS
THAT THERE ARE,
NONE SHALL BE MISSING.
I NEED ALL THE LANDS
THAT THERE ARE,
NONE SHALL BE MISSING
IF I AM TO CARRY
YOUR BURDEN TO THE GOAL.
HELP ME!
I, WHO GAVE BIRTH TO ALL,
MUST BE FULFILLED BY ALL. (pp. 18, 19)

God's function as creator has been neglected, Moreno maintained. His omnipotence, his omniscience, his wisdom, righteousness, goodness, charity, and love have all been discussed and explored. His creator function has been largely relegated to those few sentences depicting the initial creation of the universe at the beginning of time. This is misleading, Moreno asserted. The creation of universe was not over and done with in six days; it is *still* being created. The universe is in the process of continuously becoming. It is always being created. Furthermore every new being born is enlisted in the co-creation of the world to come.

> Therefore the world which a man finds at his birth is a world which millions of his fellow-beings have aided God in creating. It is not a world imposed by a tyrant—a God-dictator. It is a world in which each man can help to create and into which he can project his own dreams. (Moreno, 1941d, p. xii)

> I CREATED ALL
> THAT HAS BEEN CREATED
> WITH THE AID OF ALL THE BEINGS
> WHO WERE CREATED.
>
> FIRST I WAS ALONE.
> THEN I CREATED WITH MY ALONENESS.
> AND WHEN I WAS TWO,
> THEN I CREATED WITH MY TWONESS.
> AND WHEN I WAS THREE AND MORE,
> I CREATED WITH ALL MY COMPANIONS.
>
> THIS IS THE LAW OF THE UNIVERSE:
> WHOEVER IS A PART OF CREATION
> IS A PART OF THE CREATOR.
> HE IS A PART OF ME. (p. 72)

And:

> ALL MEN ARE BORN TO CREATE.
> NO ONE SHALL HAVE POWER
> WHO DOES NOT CREATE.
> NO ONE SHALL HAVE MORE POWER
> THAN HE CREATES.
>
> YOU SHALL LEARN TO CREATE.
> YOU SHALL LEARN
> TO CREATE ME. (p. 137)

Above all, this is a responsible God, responsible to all:

> I SHALL MAINTAIN THE WORLD
> I SHALL MAINTAIN THE CREATION
>
> IT SHALL NOT BE DESTROYED. (p. 66)

And:

> I HEAR UNANSWERED CALLS FOR HELP
> RESOUNDING THROUGH MY HEAD.
> NIGHT AND DAY
> DO I HEAR CALLS FOR HELP
>
> I ARISE, I LOOK, WALK
> RUN THROUGH THE STORM
> I JUDGE, SUPPORT, COMFORT, HEAL THE SICK,
> WITHOUT REST BY DAY AND BY NIGHT. (p. 80)

And:

> HAVE YOU LOST OUR FATHER?
> HAVE YOU LOST YOUR MOTHER?
> HAVE YOU LOST YOUR HUSBAND?
> HAVE YOU LOST YOUR WIFE?
> HAVE YOU LOST YOUR ONLY BROTHER?
> HAVE YOU LOST YOUR YOUNGEST SISTER?
>
> COME TO ME WITH QUICKENING PACE
> AND REST YOUR HEAD UPON MY LAP.
> TAKE YOUR PLACE AT MY RIGHT HAND
> OR AT MY LEFT.
> I AM YOUR MOST PERFECT FATHER.
> I AM YOUR MOST PERFECT MOTHER.
> I AM YOUR MOST PERFECT HUSBAND.
> I AM YOUR MOST PERFECT WIFE.
> I AM YOUR MOST PERFECT BROTHER.
> I AM YOUR MOST PERFECT SISTER. (p. 107)

THE NEED FOR A NEW CONCEPTUALIZATION OF THE GODHEAD

As the meaning-giving, central idea of the universe, the concept of God is the source of ethical principles and of a standard of values. Humankind has always been challenged by the meaning of the universe and by our presence in it. In times of crisis, Moreno contended, new concepts of God have appeared and the idea of the Supreme Being has found new strength in each new concept.

We are born to create, Moreno declared. It is the essence of our existence, this craving to create. The quintessence of this creativity is God, continuously ready to join in the course of events:

Once it is created, the universe is never separated from Him. It expands
in continuous interaction with him. . . . Due to God's co-identity with
every creative agency throughout the universe, He is not only in the
center but at every point upon the periphery of the universe as well as
at every point between.

Thus we see that God, Himself, is present in all men's struggles—in
the sense of co-existence and not as a shadow or an alter-ego. Since
God is inseparable from the universe and since the universe is inseparable from every man in it every man is inseparable from God. However remote any individual may seem from the center of existence, this
being is still a part of the Creator. Hence, it can well be said that God
does not interfere with the course of events because that would mean
interfering with His very Self, for what happens is, in essence, God
Himself. (Moreno, 1941d, p. xi)

Living a meaningful life then means that we discover our own creativity,
and our creativity is that aspect of us that connects us with the Godhead.
All creativity is God's and my creativity is that part of myself that is identical with God. By exercising our creativity, we are not only a part of creation, but also a part of the Creator. "The world becomes our world, the
world of our choice, the world of our creation—a project of ourselves."

Moreno's new conceptualization of God is an intriguing one. This is a
God who speaks for himself, not *through* prophets or priests, a God of all
individuals, whether they recognize and acknowledge him or not, a God
who is immediately present and who is present in all parts of the universe,
who is coexistent with the universe, a God who is still creating the universe
and creating it in partnership with every being that comes into existence.

Throughout *The Words of the Father* there rings the theme of Moreno's
major opus, *Who Shall Survive?*, and the answer to the question that the
title poses. Both Moreno and God insist that there is a place in the world
for every being born into it:

THIS IS MY PRAYER:
MAY EVERY BEING BE BORN
AT LEAST ONCE.
BETTER BE BORN FOR DESTRUCTION
THAN NEVER BE BORN.
BE FERTILE
AND MULTIPLY YOURSELF,
MULTIPLY ME.
THIS IS MY COMMANDMENT:
BE NOT UNBORN,
LET ME NOT BE UNBORN. (p. 24)

And:

THIS IS MY PRAYER:

MAY ALL BEINGS BE BLESSED
WITH A PLACE IN THE UNIVERSE
A PLACE IN THE SUN
OR A PLACE IN THE MOON.
IT DOES NOT MATTER WHERE,
IF IT IS ONLY A PLACE
WHERE THEY CAN CREATE
ME.

I HAVE PROVIDED FOR ALL
A PLACE IN THE UNIVERSE.
GO AND TAKE IT.

THIS IS MY HOUSE, THE UNIVERSE.
I HAVE DIVIDED IT UP.
MAY ALL BEINGS BE BLESSED
WITH A HOME,
A PLACE IN THE UNIVERSE.

MAY YOU BE BLESSED
WITH A HOME.
MY UNIVERSE BE YOUR HOUSE.
I HAVE MADE ITS SPACES
SO IMMENSE
THAT ALL SHALL FIND
A PLACE IN IT. (p. 25)

And:

EVERY MAN IS A THOUGHT OF GOD.
HE WHO KILLS A MAN
KILLS ONE OF MY THOUGHTS.

EVERY MAN IS ONE OF MY THOUGHTS.
HE EXISTS BY MY DIVINE RIGHT. (p. 116)

And:

TO DENY EXISTENCE TO ONE MAN
IS TO DENY EXISTENCE TO ME. (p. 139)

Perhaps the most radical of Moreno's ideas is the novel notion that as God creates us, we are creating God in turn. This is an aspect of *The Words of*

the Father that has not been noted by other commentators on Moreno's
ideas. The idea comes up in several verses. Here is a sampling of them:

> HOW CAN ONE THING
> CREATE ANOTHER THING
> UNLESS THE OTHER THING
> CREATES THE ONE THING?
> HOW CAN A FIRST THING
> CREATE A SECOND THING
> UNLESS THE SECOND THING
> ALSO CREATES THE FIRST? (p. 53)

And:

> WHAT WOULD YOU BE
> IF I WERE NOT?
>
> WHAT WOULD I BE
> IF YOU WERE NOT? (p. 101)

And:

> WHAT WOULD THERE BE TO CREATE
> IF THERE WERE NO GOD TO BE CREATED,
> IF YOU COULD NOT CREATE ME? (p. 108)

One of the greatest problems of our time, Moreno said, is the loss of faith in
a supreme being who symbolizes the highest value system for the way we conduct our lives and ourselves. Nietzsche proclaimed that God is dead. It makes
no difference, Moreno claimed. It doesn't matter if God is dead, as Nietzsche
maintained, or not. We don't even know if God exists or if he ever existed at
all. It makes no difference because we can give him new life simply by following the example of Christ, who embodied God. It wasn't Jesus's intellect
or scholarship that counted; it was the fact of embodiment. In the world of
psychodrama, embodiment is "central, axiomatic, and universal. Everyone
can portray his version of God through his own actions and so communicate
his own version to others. That was the simple meaning of my first book, in
which I proclaimed the *I-God*" (J. L. Moreno, 1966c, p. 156).

Moreno professed that he was amused that his proclamation of I-God
was taken as the most outrageous manifestation of his megalomania when
the I-God is characterized as humble, weak, inferior, and so in need of help.
Prophets and religious and political leaders, he says, have always tried to
play God and impose their power and superiority upon the masses. Now
psychodrama has turned the tables and every man can contribute to the
image of God through embodiment of their images.

The added commentary in the English translation makes it clear that the use of the word *father* is not meant to suggest male gender in the human sense. It is employed instead of "creator" to imply a sense of the relationship between God and denizens of the world. God is not a specific ancestor but comprises the whole chain of ancestors, human and animal, and, in fact, the whole chain of organisms preceding and including the human being. It stands for the universal concept of parenthood in the universe.

The Words of the Father are messages that we get from the world we live in, especially the messages that tell us about ourselves, who we are, and about the world we live in. They may be stimulated by words expressed in human languages, from inspirational phrases, poetry, books, and the like, but they are not those words. Rather they are the inspirations and intuitions and flashes of insight that those words or nonverbal experiences evoke. Moreno asserted that there is no scientific explanation for these experiences.

The concept of words may become a little clearer when the concept of the "voice" is considered. Moreno makes it clear that he is not talking about hallucinations here. Hallucinations always speak a human language, and we already know that the words do not occur in that form. The voice always occurs in the here and now, in the present. It is not a reflection of past events. The voice "is experienced in moments of extraordinary emergency as flashes of intuition. More than at any other time it makes itself felt in moments of bold creativity, in creative acts which seem to surpass any personal, human origin, and in moments of love" (Moreno, 1941d, p. 155). Then he mentions inspiration and the fact that very simple events can touch off profound inspiration. The voice, then, is the voice through which we perceive intuitively and that transmits inspiration. Now we have a possible grasp of the meaning of what Moreno means by the concept of words and "God's language." We are dealing here with something like Gendlin's (1981) concept of preverbal understanding. This is knowledge, information, or wisdom that we experience but that we have not yet put into words. All of us have had the experience of reading or hearing something that strikes us as unquestioningly truthful. We know immediately that we somehow knew what was presented although we, ourselves, have never put it into words. It is understanding, undoubtedly involving the emotional system, at a preverbal level.

The words as conceptualized here are transmitted instantly from "place to place, instant by instant throughout the universe" (Moreno, 1941d, p. 156). This is in direct conflict with the laws of classical physics, which hold that no signal, and it takes a signal to carry a message, can travel faster than the speed of light. The claim of instantaneous transmission is "another way of expressing the idea that every part of the universe partakes of the essence of God and that all these places and instants are parts of an indivisible unity (p. 156)," a statement of the wholeness quality of the universe.

One implication of the concept of the words is that all ideas, all knowledge, exists in the cosmos in an ineffable form until those ideas are comprehended and expressed by a human being. This notion is supported by Jonathan Moreno's statement about his father that "he always believed that ultimately all ideas derive from the same spontaneous-creative source" (J. D. Moreno, 1989, p. 4). Sociometry suggests that ideas, thought, and feeling are collective activities and reverberate in social atoms and social networks.

These ideas bring to mind the work of David Bohm and his conceptualizations of the implicate and explicate orders. Bohm, whose ideas will be more thoroughly discussed in another chapter, suggests that there exists a subtle order of energy fields, the implicate order, from which the physical world that we know, the explicate order, emerges. This implicate order, unlike the physical world, is characterized by nonlocality and holism. The implicate order might well be the "spontaneous-creative source" of all ideas. Moreno might also have found Bohm's *Thought as a System* to contain ideas kindred to his own. Nichol, in the foreword to this book, states:

> The essential relevance of Bohm's redefinition of thought is the proposal that body, emotion, intellect, reflex and artifact are now understood as one unbroken field of mutually informing thought. All of these components interpenetrate one another to such an extent, says Bohm, that we are compelled to see "thought as a system"— concrete as well as abstract, active as well as passive, collective as well as individual. (1994, p. 4)

With respect to the "creation," the expository material in *Words of the Father* indicate that the view presented in Genesis, which has God creating the universe in six days, is modeled after man's own ideas of creativity, in which it is the finished product that is the reward of the effort and energy put into creating it. God's creativity according to the *Words* has never stopped and never will as long as the universe exists. The creating continues unceasingly and that which has been created takes part in the ongoing creative process. There is also the suggestion in the *Words* that the universe may be full of intelligent beings and other planets that rival or exceed the wonders of our own. Beyond that is the notion that there may be many other universes about which we know absolutely nothing, and that "the Creator is present in every being of every universe, aware of and inseparable from every action, thought and feeling. It is no wonder that man has repeatedly tried to solve the mystery of God" (Moreno, 1941d, p. 157).

THE PERENNIAL PHILOSOPHY

Moreno's theology has some similarities with "the perennial philosophy," apparently first named by philosopher-mathematician Godfrey Leibnitz and expounded by Aldous Huxley (1944). The central theme of the perennial philosophy is the idea that God can be directly experienced and that it is possible for a human being to see deeply and directly into the nature of reality. The experience is always profound, even life changing, and characterized as an archaic, primordial, or mystical experience. Common to these experiences, which have occurred to individuals over millennia, is the notion that we come from a single ground or source, and we return after an earthly sojourn to that ground. *Perennial* refers to the fact that such experiences have apparently happened to individuals of all times, from all stations of life and cultures.

Friedman identified a common core of the perennial philosophy:

> In all the religions [considered as belonging to the perennial philosophy] the Perennial Philosophy describes an Absolute Ground, which is the reality of all things. The Absolute is not set apart as some sort of Creator separated from that which is created. Rather, as the ground of All, the Absolute is one, completely whole and indivisible. There is a tendency in the West to identify this wholeness with the philosophy of pantheism, but that is incorrect. The Absolute is not just *in* all things, all things *are* the Absolute. Nor is the absolute limited by our conception of the universe: the universe is only one manifestation of an ultimately undifferentiated and indefinable reality. (1990, p. 97)

The experience that brought about *The Words of the Father* was indeed a profound event for Moreno. He did have a sense of having seen deeply and directly into the nature of the cosmos. He will suggest later on that his understanding of the relationship between spontaneity and creativity came from this experience.

Moreno elaborated on his concept of the I-God in a presentation made at the Second International Congress of Psychodrama in 1966. He repeated his belief that humankind faces a major dilemma in the loss of faith in a supreme being, a model that serves as a guide for living one's life:

> The psychodramatic answer to the claim that God is dead is that he can easily be restored to life. Following the example of Christ, we have given him and can give him new life, but not in the form that our ancestors cherished. We have replaced the dead God by the millions of people who can embody God in their own person. (J. L. Moreno, 1966b, p. 156)

It was the fact that Christ embodied the truth, not his intellectual abilities or his scholarship, that made him different from others who claimed to possess the supreme truth, but who talked about it rather than living it, embodying it.

In the psychodramatic world the fact of embodiment is central, axiomatic and universal. Everyone can portray his version of God through his own actions and so communicate his own version to others. That was the simple meaning of my first book, in which I proclaimed the "I-God." None of my inspirations and pronouncements however, have been more severely criticized, misunderstood, and ridiculed, than the ideas that I proclaimed myself as God, as the Father of my mother and father, of my ancestors, and of everything which lives. . . . And it is the I-God with whom we are all connected. It is the *I* which becomes the *We*. (J. L. Moreno, 1966b, p. 156)

We can find a connection with God from a slightly different perspective. God represents all Spontaneity-Creativity that he has shared with all his creations. We, of course, are included. When we are in touch with our own spontaneity, we are in touch with God.

RELIGION AND PSYCHIATRY

Moreno complained that Freud, Wagner von Jauregg (chief of the Psychiatric Clinic of the University of Vienna), and other psychiatrists he knew did not impress him with the way they looked and acted:

> *I did not think that a great healer and therapist would look and act the way Wagner or Freud did.* I visualized the healer as a spontaneous-creative protagonist in the midst of the group. My concept of the physician as a healer, and that of theirs were very far apart. To my mind, persons like Jesus, Buddha, Socrates and Gandhi were doctors and healers; for Freud they were probably patients. (1953a, p. xxvii)

Of course, when he came to this country, his new psychiatric colleagues expressed much the same sentiments toward Moreno! To them, he did not look or act as they thought a psychiatrist should look and act. Mental health professionals did not quite know what to make of a psychiatrist who openly acknowledged playing God, let alone one who encouraged others to do the same thing. This history, especially when combined with Moreno's provocative and confrontational style undoubtedly was a significant factor in the rejection of his theories and philosophy, and in the rejection of psychodrama.

His attempts to broaden the concepts of both psychiatry and religion beyond their limitations and to seek rapprochement between them, Moreno wrote, were repugnant to both psychiatrists and theologians. However, since then Jung, Binswanger, and others after them have engaged the notion of spirituality in their work, and today's mental health professions include pastoral counseling as a matter of course, even if mainstream psychiatrists, psychologists, and other psychotherapists who see their methods as founded on a reductionist, positivist science still tend to shy away from religious issues.

NOTES

1. This added discussion is the source for much of the material that is not otherwise referenced in this chapter.
2. All the passages in capitalized letters that follow are from *The Words of the Father* (Moreno, 1941d). The numbers in parentheses identify the page number of the verse.

Part II
The Philosophy

4 Morenean Philosophy

J. L. Moreno always contended that his first love was philosophy. He matriculated at the University of Vienna initially as a philosophy student. Faced with the need to earn a living and at the urging of his maternal uncles, he then entered the medical school of that university. There are several different philosophical issues to be considered in this chapter. These include the ideas or hypotheses that Moreno identified as his personal philosophy, the principles that guided his life course.

Moreno insisted that the accepted philosophy of science was inadequate for a science of society. He offered his suggestions for modifying the philosophical foundation of social sciences and the practice of social research. The major issue he addressed here was the difference in subject matter between the physical and biological sciences compared with that of the social sciences.

Finally, there is the existential, phenomenological foundation upon which all his methods are based. Physics and biology, the "hard" sciences, are solidly based in a positivist philosophy. Only that which can be objectively observed and measured counts. This effectively places meaningfulness out of reach of scientific endeavor. Phenomenology and Existentialism provide the philosophical position for the systematic investigation of meaning.

Moreno was often critical if not disparaging of Sigmund Freud and Freud's psychoanalysis. This has usually been perceived as Moreno's jealousy of the popularity of psychoanalysis compared with Moreno's methods. There is a far more substantive reason. Freud and psychoanalysis are philosophically a perfect antithesis of the philosophy and approach to human nature upon which Morenean methods are based.

Moreno came to America from a culture in which Freud and his ideas were greatly marginalized. Anti-Semitism played its part, but the major source of Freud's rejection was his emphasis upon sexuality and the role it played in neurosis. Psychoanalysis theory and method had been accepted and appreciated to a far greater extent in America than it had been in Austria or the rest of Europe. Moreno may have been surprised to find psychoanalysis so deeply entrenched not only in American psychiatry, but also in the culture itself. The objectivity and reductionism of psychoanalysis was in direct contrast to Moreno's position, which was holistic and subjective. Moreno's attacks on Freud help highlight the difference between Moreno's notions and those not only of Freudian psychoanalysis, but of the conventional psychiatry of the time, as well. Psychoanalysis, it should be noted, has evolved appreciably and Moreno's criticisms are largely aimed at the original psychoanalytic theory as propounded by Freud, many philosophical features of which have remained in the various modifications.

PERSONAL PHILOSOPHY

Moreno translated his 1923 book, *Das Stegreiftheater*, into English as *The Theater of Spontaneity* in 1947. In this work, he wrote that Vienna, in addition to being a city of immense intellectual and artistic energy, was also "the display grounds of the three forms of materialism which has become since the undisputed world master of our age, the economic materialism of Marx, the psychological materialism of Freud, and the technological materialism of the steamboat, the airplane and the atomic bomb" (1947e, p. 5). Moreno saw this materialistic preoccupation of Western culture as the problem of the age. He was not alone in his concern that technology, epitomized in the concept of the robot, could eventually enslave humankind or that humankind could destroy itself, having already invented the means of doing so (Moreno, 1945a). Moreno's answer to the problem of society's overemphasis on the materialistic lay in focusing attention on the creative process itself instead of upon the products of that creativity. By understanding and mastering the creative process, Moreno maintained, humankind can create the means to govern and control the products of science and technology and at the same time reduce violence in the world. Sixty years after Moreno expressed those concerns, worry about dependence upon technology seems especially timely. Since Moreno wrote those words, the invention of the computer and advances in communications and technology have resulted in vastly increased dependency upon technology in the industrialized world.

In "Preludes of the Sociometric Movement" (1953a), Moreno lamented the fact that his methods of sociometry and psychodrama had gained the attention and a certain degree of acceptance by sociologists and psychotherapists while the philosophy of life upon which they were grounded had "been relegated to the dark corners of library shelves or entirely pushed aside" (pp. 15–16). Rather than being applied to the task of advancing peaceful cooperation in the world, his methods were being assimilated into the status quo. So that there would be no misunderstanding, he spelled out this philosophy in three hypotheses.

The first hypothesis is that Spontaneity-Creativity is the propelling force in human progress. Sigmund Freud, whose psychoanalysis was the major comprehensive theory of the human psyche, believed that libido was the ultimate driving energy in human affairs and considered human creativity to be a derivative of libido. Freud hypothesized that suppression of the sexual drive by society then had to be otherwise directed. His conclusion was that unexpressed sexuality had to be diverted (sublimated) into socially acceptable channels, such as creative activity, or had to be expressed in aggression or neurosis. From that perspective, all the great artistic, philosophical, and scientific creations of humankind, all the great ideas, inventions, and achievements of all cultures, and even cultures themselves can be construed as the result of sexual impulses deflected from their original goal of sexual intercourse.

Moreno disagreed, proposing that the ultimate force underlying all human progress, indeed all human activity, was Spontaneity-Creativity. Humankind was born to create, not simply to procreate. Procreation was merely one form of creativity. Spontaneity, Moreno proclaimed, is "the propelling force in human progress" (1953a, p. xv). Of course, spontaneity enters into sexual activity as it does into all human activities. However, for Moreno, Spontaneity-Creativity is the basic factor, not a derivative of libido as it was for Freud.

The second hypothesis in Moreno's explication of his philosophy of life is "faith in our fellowmen's intentions (1953a, p. xv)." Moreno rejects the Hobbesian (and Freudian) view of the human being as a savage animal covered by a thin veneer of civilization who will quickly revert to fierce and violent behavior if not kept under the constraints of physical and legalistic coercion. Moreno was convinced and proclaimed that man is a social animal from birth, and that human beings are basically altruistic, concerned with the welfare of fellowmen as well as with their own. It takes very little reflection to realize that humans cannot survive, let alone flourish, without support and emotional nourishment from the others around them. In some mammalian species, offspring are given support and nourishment until they reach adolescence or adulthood. Then they go off on their own. The human being goes from family of origin into other social structures that continue to fulfill the need for support, protection, and emotional companionship. "Love and mutual sharing [is] a powerful, indispensable working principle in group life," Moreno stated.

Given the prevalence and extent of conflict and violence that exists between individuals, between groups of all kinds, between regions, nations, and states, even between religions, faith in our fellowmen's intentions may seem to be very courageous or perhaps naive. However, Moreno was convinced of what he called "the organic unity of mankind (1953c, p. 1)." Not only are we social animals; we are all joined together through innumerable social atoms, connected by networks, many of which are invisible.

If we accept Moreno's concept of the organic unity of mankind, the well-being of every living person is a matter of interest to every other human being. This doesn't seem to be a very widely held notion. In searching for the causes of conflict and turbulence in the village of Mitterndorf,

Moreno developed the notion of the preferential nature of society. People have strong attractions and repulsions with regard to those with whom they live and interact and exert considerable energy to establish relationships with those to whom they are attracted and to avoid those whom they reject. He believed that this is a universal factor and that reorganizing social units by taking these preferences into account could reduce much of the conflict, turbulence, and violence in the world. Moreno advanced his ideas at the New York State Training School for Girls at Hudson.

The third element or hypothesis in Moreno's statement of his personal philosophy reflects his conviction that through sociometry and psychodrama, and their derivative methods, such as role training and sociodrama, a spontaneous-creative social order, "a superdynamic community," can be brought into existence. His vision is of a society in which an opportunity to achieve their highest potential is available to all its members, one in which human resources would be maximized and not wasted. All the methods that Moreno developed, sociometry, psychodrama, group therapy, and the related sub-methods, were created with this purpose in mind.

The reason that society had become so materialistically oriented, Moreno thought, was that fascination with the *products* of creativity, such as inventions and theories, had distracted attention from the *process* of creativity. Society had neglected to explore and understand the creative process. We look instead with awe upon the end product, the conserves, that creative individuals have brought into existence. We applaud and reward those who have invented the wonderful devices that make our lives materially easier. Yet we have failed to study the creative process itself. As a result, Moreno saw humankind in danger from its own technology. We have created the potential for our own destruction, most obviously by developing atomic energy. Less obviously we have become tremendously dependent upon technology, even when it appears to be responsible for threatening the environment that supports life. Because a conserve, once invented cannot be uninvented; the only way to control technology, Moreno declared, is to become even more creative in order to master it. There is a race between technology and creativity through which we can keep our technology under control. Moreno's concept of Spontaneity-Creativity indicates how we can systematically become more creative. Spontaneity and hence creativity can be addressed and increased by training.

Moreno summed up his philosophy by saying that his aim is to accomplish what religion without scientific methods has failed to attain, and what social revolution that suppressed religion (in the form of Russian Communism) had also failed to achieve. Moreno made it clear that he was envisioning neither a scientific religion nor a religious science. Rather, he had in mind a science of social change that went far beyond sociology by incorporating subjectivity and the cooperation of all the members of a society in the systematic, scientific exploration of society. He also believed, contradictory to sociologists, that a science of society could and should alter social conditions so that all its members benefited.

Zerka T. Moreno echoed Moreno's complaint about the neglect of his philosophy five years before Moreno's death:

> Substitute theories are false and misleading as they abrogate or abort the complete execution of the methods. Moreno's position was therefore "Take my ideas, my concepts, but do not separate them from their parent, the philosophy; do not split my children in half, like a Solomonic judgment, Love them in toto, support and respect the entire structure upon which they rest. Make them your own as completely as I do. Role reverse with me and put yourself entirely into my position." (1969a, p. 5)

She makes the point in this article that many of Moreno's techniques have been incorporated into the mainstream of psychotherapy, often without acknowledgment of their origin and without awareness of their originator's intentions with respect to bringing about cultural change.

MORENO'S CONTRIBUTIONS TO SCIENTIFIC METHOD

The perspectives of natural science have heavily influenced conventional psychology and methods of psychotherapy. The medical model of mental health and psychotherapy is informed by the philosophy of natural science. One's philosophical position greatly influences what one sees and how one perceives what is seen. Morenean methods are phenomenological and existential. To evaluate them, they need to be looked at from a phenomenological and existential perspective. In this section, the basic assumptions of natural science will be contrasted with those of Existentialism, especially Existentialism as promoted by Moreno.

The philosophy of science identifies the basic assumptions upon which the methods of scientific research are based. It also shapes the way in which the subject matter of a science is perceived and understood. Science, as the authoritative source of knowledge about the universe in which we live, began with observations of the physical world and experimentation. Experimentation was conceived of as asking questions in such a way that nature itself could answer them. John Stuart Mill expounded the logic of experimental science. The physical and biological sciences, often referred to as the natural sciences, are based upon the principles of empiricism, positivism, reductionism, and determinism. This means that science is based on objective observation and systematic intervention. Only something that can be measured is considered to be real. The ultimate goal of science is to explain all phenomena on a physical basis. That is, a conviction that when adequately understood, any phenomenon, biological, psychological, or sociological, can eventually be reduced to the basic laws of physics.

More controversial than the above principles is the doctrine of absolute determinism, the notion that this is a cause-and-effect world in which everything that happens is the result of a preceding cause. Classical physics depicts the universe as a monumentally complex machine running like clockwork. It is even thought capable of running backward as well as forward. Isaac Newton's ingenious insights into the workings of gravity and his laws of motion that, with the proper information, held the promise of allowing one to predict the movement of everything from an atom to a star certainly promoted this vision. The model of a mechanical universe based on the principle of causality still dominates our everyday thinking and much of science, despite the near-universal sense that we, individually and collectively, have the ability to make choices and decisions independently. Support for determinism has varied from strong to moderate over time, but the controversy is still alive (e.g., Sappington, 1990; Nichols, 2011). The natural sciences are dominated by the notion of cause and effect and the primary goals are prediction and control. However, the doctrine of absolute determinism leaves no room for spontaneity and creativity.

Natural science has given us a world in which humankind has the ability and knowledge to protect itself and survive in almost any environment, and the capacity, although perhaps not the collective will, to provide enough food to nourish the whole of humankind. Science and the technology that science has spawned have resulted in a near-infinite number of machines and gadgets to transform our environment for comfort, convenience, and security, as well as economies to distribute the goods that emerge. The biological sciences have led to a scientifically based medical profession that has substantially increased our understanding of diseases and appreciably increased the means of treating them. It is no wonder then that science, at the beginning of the 20th century, was surpassing religion as a cultural force. And it is not surprising that when the studies of society and the mind emerged from philosophy and became the sciences of sociology and psychology, the methods of natural science were imitated as the preferred method of scientific inquiry. If the laws of society could be discovered as effectively as physics and biology have uncovered the laws of nature, surely the problems of society could succumb to social science and improve the lot of humankind.

Educated in the medical school of one of the early universities to promote science-based medicine, Moreno was quite conversant with the experimental scientific methods and the philosophical foundation upon which science was based. He was not so indoctrinated, however, that he was unable to question the basic assumptions. His first challenge to the principles of natural science was to the doctrine of determinism. Informed by his observations of spontaneity in both the children of the *Augarten* in their creative play and the actors of the *Stegreiftheater*, his position against determinism was critical to the origination of a theory of Spontaneity-Creativity. By his rejection of absolute determinism, he stood in direct opposition to the position of Sigmund Freud. Freud (1901/1964) embraced the determinism of natural science philosophy and believed that he had proven that all mental events, even such minor ones as slips of the tongue, were causally and absolutely determined. He considered this to be a major scientific contribution. He believed that he had delivered the "third cosmic shock"[1] to humankind by demonstrating the deterministic nature of mental phenomena that denies freedom of will and choice.[2]

Moreno did not deny that there were indeed determinants to thoughts and behaviors, but he also contended that there are moments in which our actions are truly original and creative, attributable to the moment and situation in which we find ourselves. He credits Henri Bergson and Bergson's concepts of *élan vital* and *duree* as a major influence in his own thinking. At the same time, he criticizes Bergson's philosophy of total creativity in which each moment is original and free of a past. Moreno's perspective is that our past experience does enter into each situation and moment, but that our actions are not totally determined or limited by the past.

Moreno also challenged the prevailing perception of how the scientific process works. The conventional picture is of thousands of scientists toiling away in their laboratories, testing hypotheses and identifying and gathering the facts of their respective disciplines until everything becomes clear. Science does not progress by the everyday work of the scientist in the laboratory, Moreno said, but by the insights of the genius, intuited rather than garnered through empirical or experimental methods. His ideas anticipated the widely acclaimed work of Thomas Kuhn (1962). Kuhn emphasized the intuitions that bring about what he termed *paradigm changes*, while Moreno focused attention upon the genius whose creativity is responsible for the paradigm change. The examples are many but three that stand out in the history of science are Copernicus's heliocentric theory, Newton's ideas about gravity, and Einstein's notions of relativity theory. An act of creativity is actually an act of perception, of looking at something like an apple falling off a tree and seeing the similarity to the motion of the moon. The function of the laboratory scientist then is to confirm these insights and translate them so that ordinary citizens can understand them.

Moreno's most important contribution to the scientific method is his critique and suggested revision of the experimental method applied to the social sciences: "The chief methodological task of sociometry has been the revision of the experimental method so that it can be applied effectively to social phenomena" (Moreno, 1951b, p. 31). This fact has never been fully appreciated even by most of the sociologists and social psychologists who responded so enthusiastically to Moreno's first explication of sociometry in the 1934 edition of *Who Shall Survive?*

It is the nature of the subject matter, Moreno (1947a) reasoned, that calls for a different approach to the study of social phenomena. The first task of any science is to discover the conditions under which the significant facts can emerge. While these are well known in the physical and biological arenas, the problem of creating the conditions under which the significant facts of human relations emerge is far more complicated. In the natural sciences we do not expect the subject matter, whether it be planets and stars, falling bodies, or living organisms, to contribute to the study of themselves. Scientific exploration is not an activity that these entities engage in. The subject matter of the social sciences is another matter. Scientific study is a human activity and the social sciences then become a type of self-study. The structure of human society, the patterns of attractions and repulsions that bring parts of society together at one time and push them apart at another, cannot be so directly observed by a neutral and independent observer, as can the movements of the planets and stars. An external social structure may be identified, a family, a village, or a social institution, for example, and described, but sociometry has shown us that there is an inner structure that underlies and interacts with the external structure, a phenomenon that influences everything that happens and that can only be made manifest by enlisting the full cooperation of the members of the social entity under investigation. Sociometry brings together subjective and objective methods of investigation. Sociometric research differs from traditional sociological research in that the researcher eschews the artificialities of the contrived experiment and the experimenter's usual position as an outside or independent observer. The sociometric investigator becomes a member of the group. In this way the researcher gains access to subjective knowledge that is otherwise lost to social research. This is a frightening idea to one trained in traditional research methods in which great pains are taken to prevent the researcher from becoming personally involved with the subject matter in a way that could influence the outcome of the experiment. It is also frightening to share the research responsibility and researcher status with the participants in the experiment. The most important principle in sociometric research is that the sociometric experimenter must secure the genuine cooperation of all members of the group, who must be convinced that the experiment, the sociometric exploration of the group, will somehow be beneficial to each and every one of them and to the group as a whole.

A critical distinction between academic sociology and sociometry is reflected in the goals of each. Traditional social scientists accumulate demographic information on identifiable groups or collect data to test hypotheses from one or another sociometric theories. Their research offers few, if any, immediate answers to society's problems. It sometimes seems as if sociologists design their experiments to avoid influencing those social entities that they study. Sociometry, on the other hand, is a revolutionary method aimed at instigating a microscopic revolution. Unless it makes a difference, Moreno asks, how do we know that we have learned anything of real value?

HUMAN SCIENCE

The methods of natural science applied to sociology and psychology have not enthralled everybody. The problem is that so much of what is of most interest in psychology and sociology, personal experience, values, and meaning, are subjective and intangible and cannot be observed and measured as the positivistic, objective methods of natural science require. These phenomena are beyond direct observation by the researcher and therefore cannot be the subjects of natural science methods.

Since the emergence of sociology and psychology as sciences, a number of philosophers and scientists have been skeptical of a natural scientific approach to the study of human affairs. Nineteenth-century philosopher Wilhelm Dilthey is credited with distinguishing between aims of the natural sciences and of the cultural or human sciences, objecting strongly to the exclusive use of the methods of natural science in the human sciences. He argued that the goals were different, that the natural sciences were designed to explain in terms of cause and effect, while the human sciences aimed at understanding human nature, especially the holistic nature of the functions of the mind and its creative capacity. Dilthey criticized the experimental psychology of his day that had adopted the methods of natural science as incapable of dealing with the great and significant creative actions of the human mind and particularly of penetrating into the world of history. He rejected causal explanations for mental processes and emphasized the impact of the social environment on the actions and reactions of the individual (Holborn, 1950).

Despite the fact that Dilthey's ideas were highly respected, natural science methods have dominated the social and psychological sciences, although not without questions and controversy. Søren Kierkegaard emphasized subjectivity and the importance of discovering the true self and is credited as the founder of Existentialism. Edmund Husserl developed phenomenology, a philosophical method and movement that were a protest to scientism. His student, Martin Heidegger, extended existential philosophy, and phenomenology and Existentialism are often considered as linked. These two philosophies have provided alternative approaches to natural science methods in social sciences and perhaps even more so in the field of psychology.

EXISTENTIALISM

J. L. Moreno's first published works, from 1914, *Ein Ladung zu einer Begegung (Invitation to an Encounter)*, to 1920, *Das Testament des Vaters (The Words of the Father)* expressed the philosophy of the Religion of

Encounter. A reading of these works makes it obvious that Moreno and the other four members of the group had been strongly influenced by the existential philosophy of Søren Kierkegaard. They strove to embody the principles of Kierkegaard's Existentialism. The first principle was the all-inclusiveness of being and the constant effort to maintain from moment to moment the natural, spontaneous, uninterrupted flow of existence. The second principle was the notion that all existing things were good in and of themselves. Other concepts included the notion of the moment, the idea of the situation, and the conviction that conduct should be based on Spontaneity-Creativity rather than on ethical and cultural conserves. "And above all, the urgency, the urgency of their immediate experience" (Moreno, 1989a, p. 48). All Moreno's later methods and theory were based, he says, upon these ideas.

Moreno (1956a) examined Existentialism in an article that later became one of the six lectures that comprise *Psychodrama, Second Volume* (1959a). In this discussion, he suggests that there are three periods of Existentialism. The first was Søren Kierkegaard's protest against the sugarcoated religion of his day. The second was the heroic Existentialism, which Moreno claims is exemplified by the lives of Tolstoy and Charles Péguy, as well as by the members of the Religion of Encounter. Finally, there is the intellectual Existentialism of philosophers, "men like Jaspers, Heidegger and Sartre" (1959a, p. 213). Moreno was critical of the latter whom, he says, concern themselves with the philosophical problems of existence but not with existing and existence itself. "The heroic-Socratic existentialism of Kierkegaard has gradually turned into a kind of intellectual existentialism of the middle class," Moreno wrote. "Its exponents are intellectuals rather than doers" (p. 213). What motivates the intellectual existentialists, he thinks, is the desire to reconcile existentialist philosophies with those upon which scientific method is founded.

On the one hand, there are the wholly subjective and existential situations of the individual and, on the other hand, the objective requirements of the scientific method. Moreno (1956a, 1968) resolves the dilemma by separating existential validation from scientific validation. To illustrate the difference, let us consider a psychodrama in which the protagonist reenacts a past experience. The researcher who is interested in scientific validation may ask how we know that the protagonist is presenting the scene as it actually happened. The existentialist would say that genuine interaction between director and protagonist in a psychodrama session results in an existentially valid experience for both. As long as the protagonist is faithfully reenacting his here-and-now experience of the event, the psychodrama is existentially valid.

Through psychodrama, the inner subjective world of the protagonist is externalized on the psychodrama stage. The thoughts, memories, dreams, hopes, and fears of the protagonist are turned into concrete behavior. That which has been invisible and intangible is made visible and tangible, available to observation and objective evaluation. In this way, psychodrama bridges the gap between the phenomenological, the existential, and empirical science (see J. D. Moreno, 1974).

The difference between the conventional scientific and the sociometric methods is clearly seen in their respective ways of looking at human behavior. Scientific psychology began with the recognition of lawful relationships between characteristics of the environment and the perceptual response to them and this prototype has obtained since. The individual is considered an organism in an environment. Much psychological research can be categorized as S-R (stimulus-response) or S-O-R (stimulus-organism-response) research. Another more radically behaviorist approach was initiated by B. F. Skinner's concept of operant conditioning, which considers how behavior is learned by the consequences of an organism operating upon the environment. This conceptualization, it might be noted, is essentially the same for human and nonhuman subjects alike.

Where psychologists think of an organism-in-an-environment, sociometrists and psychodramatists perceive an actor in a situation. A situation consists of far more than just a physical environment. We begin life by being born into a situation over which we have little choice, it being a situation created and provided by our parents. A situation always involves the place in which we are, the here and now (the moment), an individual in a role, a demand for action, and other people with whom to interact. The place ordinarily includes things and people, both of which are meaningful to the individual, rather than stimuli that may elicit a response. A situation contains a demand, need, or desire for some kind of action (act hunger) with another person or persons. Life is a series of situations, each emerging from the one before and leading us into the next. We deal with each situation as best we can, sometimes successfully, sometimes not, and each situation leaves us a little bit different than we were.

PHILOSOPHY OF PSYCHOTHERAPY

Sigmund Freud deserves credit for recognizing the psychological basis of hysteria and establishing the first truly psychotherapeutic method to treat a psychological problem. Freud, who had begun his career as a neurological research scientist, was totally committed to the positivistic, reductionist, objective methods of natural science. He accepted the deterministic nature of mental phenomena even though it denied freedom of will and choice. His radical positivistic position is pointedly reflected in a letter to his student, friend, and colleague, Marie Bonaparte, in which he wrote:

> The moment a man questions the meaning and value of life he is sick, since objectively neither has any existence; by asking this question one is merely admitting to a store of unsatisfied libido to which something else must have happened, a kind of fermentation leading to sadness and depression. (Freud, 1975, p. 436)

Because psychotherapy was originated in the practice of a physician, it is not surprising that it developed in the framework of a medical model of illness. This has given us the concepts of mental illness, psychopathology, etiology, diagnosis, signs and symptoms, a classification of psychological disorders, and an assortment of treatments. The psychotherapist, like the physician, is seen as a source of knowledge and skills needed to repair a sick individual. Psychotherapy from this perspective can be considered one of the tinkering trades and the psychotherapist likened to an appliance repair person (see Goffman, 1956). The medical model of mental illness like the profession from which it came is based on physiological science and shares its natural science philosophy.

Although many methods and theories of psychotherapy have been proposed since the advent of psychoanalysis, including a number that are identified as existential and phenomenological, the medical model still holds sway in the field of mental health. This paradigm has had a major influence upon the development and perception of psychotherapy methods and upon the whole field of mental health. Adherence to the medical model may well be responsible for the difficulties that researchers have encountered in attempting to provide a scientific basis for psychotherapy. We still do not understand why the 250 or more different theories and methods of psychotherapy seem to have about equal success. It is unclear even just what success is and how to measure it, let alone what normality is (Wampole, 2001).

The psychotherapist, practicing a conventional method of psychotherapy, interviews the client, looking for the signs and symptoms by which the therapist can make a diagnosis. Or the therapist reflects, reframes, or interprets something that the client has expressed. The therapist may point out irrationalities in what the client has just said, or utilize any of a number of techniques that he/she has learned. The existential therapist, on the other hand, meets the client on a common plane, person-to-person. The situation is defined as two people out of whose encounter will hopefully come knowledge that allows the patient to lead a fuller, more satisfactory existence (Binswanger, 1956). Rather than assess psychopathology, the psychodramatist normalizes it. To the paranoid individual, the delusion is existentially valid. "The psychodrama stage provides for all forms of pathological behavior a world *sui generis*. . . . providing a place where it can fulfill and perhaps transform itself, unencumbered by the restrictions of the prevailing culture" (Moreno, 1959a, p. 219).

OTHER WRITERS ON MORENEAN PHILOSOPHY

Blatner, in his *Foundations of Psychodrama* (2000), and Kellermann, in *Focus on Psychodrama* (1992), have both dealt with philosophy and psychodrama to some extent. Blatner's chapter on philosophical and theoretical considerations is a broad discussion of a variety of philosophical issues. He discusses the concepts of modernism and postmodernism, existentialism and phenomenology, hermeneutics, constructionism, and narrative, finding that Moreno's work can probably be aligned with postmodernism. However, there is practically no discussion of Moreno's personal philosophy or the philosophical thought behind Moreno's work. Indeed, Blatner wrote that Moreno never articulated his underlying philosophy.

Kellermann is much more thorough and specific. He compares the view of psychodrama from a natural science perspective with that from a human science frame of reference along a number of relevant issues. The goal of his book, he states, is to improve standards of research on the psychodramatic method by presenting an analysis of the "essential therapeutic ingredients" in psychodrama (1992, p. 13). He hopes to "reduce some of the confusion which surrounds the theory of psychodramatic technique (p. 13)."

While his presentation of psychodrama from the two perspectives of natural and human science is astute and complements what I have written above, Kellerman runs into several problems. The first is his insistence that psychodrama be defined as a method of psychotherapy. As will be seen in a later chapter, I have identified psychodrama as a method of communication, one function of which is psychodramatic psychotherapy. Articles on the nontherapeutic applications of psychodrama date from the early issues of *Sociometry* (e.g., Franz, 1939, 1940, 1942; Shoobs, 1943; Lippitt, 1943). To define psychodrama by one of its uses is tantamount to defining interview as a method of psychotherapy since it is the vehicle for most psychotherapeutic methods. Many problems exist when such a restricted definition of psychodrama (or of interview) is adopted.

The next problem is that in carrying out his task to identify the therapeutic essentials of psychodrama, Kellermann approaches from the position of natural science and the medical model of psychotherapy, even while recognizing that psychodramatists are generally much more familiar with the existential approach.

Finally there is Kellermann's suggestion that there is a dearth of theory with respect to the psychodramatic method. Kellermann overlooks the fact that there is a considerable body of theory ranging from the theory of Spontaneity-Creativity, the concept of surplus reality, role theory, catharsis, the theory of action, the social atom, social networks, sociometric gravitation, the psychodynamic effect, and other sociometric theories. There is sufficient theory that what psychodrama accomplishes and how it is accomplished should cause little confusion for those who are familiar with it.

NOTES

1. The first cosmic shock, according to Freud, was the discovery by Copernicus that the earth, created by God as the home of humankind, is neither the center of the universe nor even the center of the solar system. The second was Darwin's discovery that humankind is not a special creation of God, but that we are related to the other animal life on the planet.

2. By advocating psychological determinism, Freud either relinquished any claims of creativity with respect to his originating and developing psychoanalysis or exempted himself from the doctrine he espoused. That is, either his every thought was determined by everything that had happened in the universe before or determinism did not apply to him.

5 The Canon of Creativity

MOTTO: A science of man should start with a science of the universe. A central model of the universe hovers continuously in our minds, if not consciously then unconsciously, whether magical, theological, or scientific. It influences the form the central model of man takes. An incomplete or deficient model of the universe is better than none.

—J. L. Moreno, "Canon of Creativity"

The twin concept at the heart of the Morenean system is the Doctrine of Spontaneity-Creativity (Moreno, 1953b). Creativity has always been a prime philosophical and scientific question. We stand in awe of human creativity manifested in all its forms: in the great works of art, painting, sculpture, theater, poetry, and fiction; in the profound theories of great philosophers since the days of ancient Greece; in scientific discoveries and explanations of the workings of the natural world; and in the uncountable number of technological inventions by which we have gained so much control over our natural environment.

We also wonder about creativity in the physical and biological realms. How did the universe evolve and how is it continuing to evolve? How has our planet changed from a collection of gases to the foundation of our existence? How did life emerge and how has it evolved? How have new species of all life-forms been created? As Moreno put it, "Creativity is *the* problem of the universe; it is, therefore, the problem of all existence, the problem of every religion, science, the problem of psychology, sociometry and human relations" (1956c, p. 126).

Human creativity is especially important for Moreno and for most of us. Human creativity has given us substantial control over the physical environment. It has enabled us to make use of nuclear energy, a two-edged sword that not only can be a boon for humankind, but also has the potential for the destruction of humankind. Many worry whether or not we can prevent this catastrophe from happening. Of considerable current concern is whether we can keep the pollution of the atmosphere, caused by the by-products of human creativity, from making earth an uninhabitable planet. Moreno believed that the way to contain the potential destructiveness of human creativity was to become even more creative. Understanding the creative process and applying it to the problems of society could accomplish this. Humankind needs to become more creative, creative enough to learn how to live in peace with each other and with the consequences of our own creativity.

Moreno stated that his first ideas about spontaneity came from his engagement with children in the parks of Vienna. The *Stegreiftheater* (the theater of spontaneity) later became the initial laboratory for Moreno's systematic study of Spontaneity-Creativity. The spontaneity theater was a prime setting in which to study creativity. Artists, whether painters, sculptors, poets, or playwrights, Moreno pointed out, create their works in private. We see the finished works, but we cannot observe the creative process itself. In the conventional theater, as well as in other art forms, the creating is done out of sight of the viewers. The author composes the play in the author's study; the actors learn their roles and rehearse before there is an audience; the scenery is prepared and the play is produced in its highly finished form, with a proscenium arch separating the actors from the audience. We only see the finished product, and while we may admire it greatly, and analyze or critique it, we are not privy to the creative process itself.

In the theater of spontaneity, on the other hand, there is no backstage, no script, no rehearsal, and there is minimal scenery. The spontaneous drama is created and produced at the same time. The actors create their roles and their interactions as they play them in the here and now. Spontaneously created drama made an excellent laboratory for the investigation of spontaneity and creativity. Working with the spontaneity players, making interaction diagrams, watching how different actors interacted with each other, Moreno began to identify the principles of spontaneity and spontaneity training.

Moreno's notion of Spontaneity-Creativity is the foundation stone of all his major theories and methods. To him, it was an insight into the very nature of the universe and it provided a basis for his conviction "that human beings do not behave like automatons but are endowed in various degrees of initiative and autonomy" (1955b, p. 361). Our behavior is not so totally and absolutely determined as the deterministic doctrine of natural science would have it.

Because spontaneity was an evolving concept, Moreno's discussions are sometimes inconsistent and difficult to follow, a factor that opened him to considerable criticism. Aulicino (1954) presented a cogent critique, beginning with Moreno's habit of combining metaphysical, philosophical, and scientific elements in his writing. He pointed out the difficulty of measuring the variables of spontaneity, such as novelty, adequacy, and the degree of the warming up process. He noted the ambiguity in Moreno's various attempts to clarify concepts, including spontaneity itself and the cultural conserve.

Sorokin (1949, 1955), in his earlier article, was also severely critical of what he considered unacceptable ambiguity in Moreno's discussions of Spontaneity-Creativity. He also questioned the validity and usefulness of spontaneity tests and testing. In his 1955 article, he questioned the whole idea of breaking down the creative process into two components, spontaneity and creativity. Moreno pled guilty to a lack of clarity in his discussions of spontaneity but asked for leniency, explaining "it is difficult to convey the full meaning of undeveloped concepts like spontaneity and creativity which are in transition from a pre-scientific to a scientific formulation" (1955b, pp. 361–362).

THE DOCTRINE OF SPONTANEITY-CREATIVITY

In the second edition of *Who Shall Survive?* Moreno presented a graphic depiction of his theory of creativity, calling it the Canon of Creativity.

He reprised this in the December 1955 issue of *Sociometry*, the last issue that he published before he gave that journal to the American Sociological Society. In this article, he elaborated upon his earlier discussion. Moreno's depiction of the Canon of Creativity is reproduced in Figure 5.1.

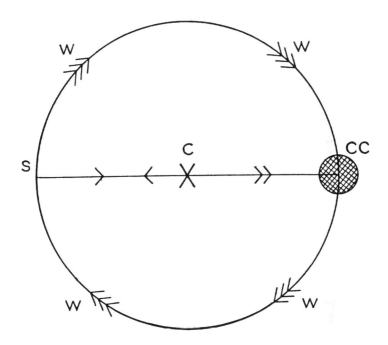

CANON OF CREATIVITY
SPONTANEITY-CREATIVITY-CONSERVE

FIELD OF ROTATING OPERATIONS BETWEEN SPONTANEITY-CREATIVITY-CULTURAL CONSERVE (S-C-CC)

S—Spontaneity, C—Creativity, CC—Cultural (or any) Conserve (for instance, a biological conserve, *i.e.*, an animal organism, or a cultural conserve, *i.e.*, a book, a motion picture, or a robot, *i.e.*, a calculating machine); W—Warming up is the "operational" expression of spontaneity. The circle represents the field of operations between S, C and CC.

Operation I: Spontaneity arouses Creativity, C. S—>C.
Operation II: Creativity is receptive to spontaneity. S<—C.
Operation III: From their interaction Cultural Conserves, CC, result. S—>C—>>CC.
Operation IV: Conserves (CC) would accumulate indefinitely and remain "in cold storage."
                  They need to be reborn, the catalyzer Spontaneity revitalizes them.
                  CC—>>>S—>>>CC.

S does not operate in a vacuum, it moves either towards Creativity or towards Conserves.

Total Operation

Spontaneity-creativity-warming up—act $\Big\langle$ actor
conserve

Figure 5.1   J. L. Moreno's Canon of Creativity.
Source: *Who Shall Survive?* with permission.

According to Moreno, the entire universe is infinite creativity and spontaneity is the catalyst that releases creative processes. On the diagram, he places creativity (C) at the center. A diameter is drawn through the center of the circle. Spontaneity (S) on the left is considered necessary to act as a catalyst of creativity, giving rise to a conserve (CC), the product of a creative act or event. The conserve can be a cultural conserve if it is the product of human creativity, or a physical or biological conserve if it occurs in one of those realms.

Spontaneity has a reciprocal interaction with creativity and the conserves. Interacting with creativity leads to the emergence of conserves that need spontaneity to be revitalized. In turn conserves can engender spontaneity. Warming up (W) is defined as the operational expression of spontaneity. It emerges in response to the situation and may be activated by existing cultural conserves, such as a piece of music, oratory, or other man-made entity. Spontaneity also serves to reactivate and revitalize established conserves. The warming up process is pictured along the perimeter of the circle, activating both conserves and spontaneity.

Moreno's presentation of the Canon of Creativity leaves a lot to be explained. It is clear that Moreno made a clear distinction between spontaneity and creativity and sees the dynamic interaction of the two as the creative process. It is not so clear, however, as how they differ and just what they are. Moreno's metaphorical explanation—"Spontaneity and creativity are thus categories of a different order; creativity belongs to the categories of substance—it is the arch substance—spontaneity to the categories of catalyzer—it is the arch catalyzer" (1953c, p. 40) doesn't help that much.

I, along with many others, have been ruminating on the Morenean concept of spontaneity and its role in the creative process since I first encountered Moreno's ideas more than 50 years ago. Although it is easy to observe behavior that seems to reflect what Moreno meant by spontaneous, both in life and on the psychodrama stage, the concept of spontaneity itself is not an easy one to define. I have long been dissatisfied with Moreno's favorite definition of spontaneity as a response reflecting novelty, adequacy, or a combination of both. A response is observable, and even Moreno said that spontaneity is, like other forms of energy, invisible. One can only observe the effects, not the form of energy itself. The following discussion is my reinterpretation of the elements in the Canon of Spontaneity-Creativity. This is how I have made sense of them.

Creativity

Usually we think of creativity either as the ability to bring into existence something new, a form, a method, an instrument, a theory, or work of art, or as the process by which something new, original, and meaningful is brought into being, as manifested in the creative activities of artists, writers, and scientists. Moreno gave the word *creativity* a new meaning and substituted

"Spontaneity-Creativity" for what is conventionally considered the creative process. Although everybody familiar with Moreno's ideas, especially the students of psychodrama and sociometry, accept the notion of Spontaneity-Creativity, the idea is not so well understood beyond Moreno's proclamation that spontaneity acting on creativity results in a new conserve.

Creativity, within the Morenean system, can be understood as potential. "The universe is infinite creativity," he said (1955b, p. 359). "Creativity is the ever nourishing maternal center," he wrote. And "creativity is the arch substance. . . . [Spontaneity] is the arch catalyzer" (1955b, p. 361). Within the context of Spontaneity-Creativity theory, creativity represents potential, both manifested and possible. It includes that which *has been* created and that which *can be* created. Whatever is possible belongs to the category of creativity.

Creativity, then, must include everything that has ever been created, the stars in space, space itself, planets, the elements of which planets are composed (plus some elements that have been created by man), all the forms of life that have ever evolved, both existing and extinct. Creativity also includes all those things humankind has created: languages, tools, methods, cultures, societies, social structures, and social institutions, all the sciences, religions, books, musical works, paintings, and so forth. These are the cultural conserves. In other words, creativity incorporates the world that we know and live in. It includes all the evolutionary stages that the world has gone through.

But this is not all. If we are willing to relinquish the doctrine of absolute determinism, as Moreno did, it is possible that there are things that might have been created but were not: life-forms that might have evolved but didn't, languages and tools that might have been invented but weren't, books that could have been written, music that might have been composed, and so forth, things that *could* have been created but for some reason (Moreno might say for a lack of spontaneity) were not. Creativity must comprise all of these things also.

It must be obvious that contrary to the biblical notion of the universe having been created in seven days, creativity in the world has not come to a halt. The universe is still being created. One does not have to be very old to remember the emergence of television, jet engines, nuclear bombs and nuclear-generating plants, and, of course, the computer and all its accouterments, peripherals, and software programs. If creativity is the arch substance, then it must also comprise all those things that will be created in the future, new life-forms, new products of human creativity, new societies and social orders, new languages, tools, works of art, scientific theories, conserves of every category.

And, finally, assuming again that determinism is partial and not absolute, then the potential for being created is not inevitable. In this case creativity subsumes all those things that *might* be created in the future—but which will not be. "The universe is infinite creativity."

The Conserve and the Cultural Conserve

Moreno devised the term *conserve* to signify the end product of a creative act. Anything that has been created, everything that can be named or identified, is a conserve. The stars, the planets, and other heavenly bodies are conserves, the results of the spontaneous-creative forces of the cosmos. Continents, oceans, and other geological features of this planet are also conserves. Every life-form is a conserve, a biological conserve. Every individual member of every life-form is also a conserve.

Moreno denoted the subset of conserves, which is the result of human creativity as cultural conserves. Every language that exists, and every language that has ever existed, is a conserve, as is every word in each of them; so is every alphabet. All the tools, instruments, appliances, and so forth, that have ever been invented and fabricated, from the stone ax to the supercomputer, from the wheel to the space shuttle, are conserves, as are all the myths of all cultures and all the religions with all their rituals, practices, hymns, sacred writings, and the like. All the laws and social institutions; all the artistic creations, stories and novels, drawings and paintings, musical compositions, dramas, poems, statues, and so on; all the scientific theories and laws, and all the technological inventions that are based on them; all the great philosophical ideas—each and every one is a cultural conserve.

A singular characteristic of the cultural conserve is that once created, it can be reproduced any number of times without relying on the kind of spontaneity that is required for creating something original. Moreno often used the book as a prime example of the cultural conserve in this respect. Once the author has created the ideas and thoughts of which it is composed, and expressed them in words, the creative result can be replicated by the printing process any number of times. Once a computer has been invented, thousands upon thousands can be manufactured without having to re-create it. The same is true of all other conserves. Once created, many copies can be made of them through technological procedures (all technologies are cultural conserves, too, of course).

Conserves can also be far less tangible, embodied by human beings. Roles are one of the more important conserves. They represent the complex organizations of behavior in which we interact with each other. Also conserves are all the tremendous variety of skills that are critical to taking the roles embedded in a culture, basic skills such as reading, writing, and arithmetical calculation, as well as the advanced skills of the surgeon, the research scientist, or aeronautical engineer, or the artistic skills of the artist, musician, novelist, or orator.

Conserves give a distinct consistency and stability to the universe. In an ever-changing universe, conserves provide a partial permanence that allows for a certain degree of predictability. Without conserves, the world as we know it is unimaginable. The universe would be a swirling mass of subatomic particles or energy without form or differentiation. Or perhaps it would resemble the end of the world that the law of entropy predicts, a uniform, undifferentiated, unmoving mass of atoms.

A casual reading of Moreno's work can lead one to believe that Moreno was against the conserve. That is not so. His concern was with an over-reliance and overemphasis on the conserve to the detriment of attending to and understanding the creative process. He was an advocate for training people, especially children, to access the spontaneity that catalyzes creativity. Spontaneity, then, would replace to a large extent the rules of living that children are now taught. In this way, people would learn to live more creative lives rather than learning to limit their creativity and live by the conserves.

It was cultural conserves, the products of human creativity, with which Moreno was most concerned and it is cultural conserves with which we need to be most interested. Cultural conserves make human culture and society possible. Moreno approved of the positive side of conserves in these words:

> Conserves represent an enormous vitality and reality, not only in our human culture but also in the universe at large. The universe is full of them. Every stone, plant and star, every animal organism is a conserve. Creativity is the universe itself, spontaneity is the key to its door and conserves are the furniture, the equipment which fills it. One cannot overemphasize the importance of the conserves which fill the store-houses of our culture. . . . The intellectual conserves, as philosophical and scientific systems, are reprinted again and again, unchanged in every generation. Nothing new is added to them because their creators are dead, but they can still arouse other thinkers to new variations of these ideas or to new ideas. (1955e, p. 386)

The conserve provides the basis for culture and society. The technological reproducibility means that the fruits of creative thinking can be shared with one's fellow human beings. Only one person needs to invent the wheel for all to make use of it. Some conserves are the result of group creativity as language must have been. In current times most significant advances in science and technology are the products of teams. Watson and Crick and their discovery of the double helix structure of the gene come to mind, or Bohr, Heisenberg, and Schrödinger and quantum theory. That which one generation creates, whether language, mythology, scientific fact, or tools and instruments, can be passed down to their children. Whether the brainstorm of a single individual or the collaborative genius of a group, the works of the creative intelligence of one era are available to members of future generations. The cultural conserve gives humankind and human society its distinctive characteristics.

The conserve is of major importance in the creative cycle. Conserves inevitably figure into new creative acts. A great new novel is expressed in words that are, of course, conserves. Words, in turn, are composed of the letters of the alphabet, another conserve. The ideas may be new and fresh and never put together in quite the same way, but the language is indispensable for the ideas to be communicated. New theories are expressed in the conserve of language, too, while musical composition makes use of previously invented musical notation. An artist creates a master painting making use of previously developed brushes, pigments, canvases, and other materials. Scientists invent tools and then use them to test their theories. It is nearly impossible to imagine a creative act that does not depend upon cultural conserves.

There is a complex relationship between cultural conserves and spontaneity. For a musician to perform a piece of music, one that has been performed a number of times, or for actors to perform a play after the first time, requires that they infuse the performance with spontaneity or run the risk that the performance will seem dull and not alive. The same is true for a familiar prayer. Each recitation requires that the individual invest it with spontaneity or it simply becomes words with little meaning to the individual. Thus spontaneity gives a freshness to conserves without which the conserve becomes mechanical and lacking in liveliness.

On the other side, conserves may serve to trigger spontaneity. A stirring speech, such as Franklin Roosevelt's address to Congress on December 8, 1941, may serve to motivate and activate a whole nation to the unwelcome task of going to war on another continent. The crisis papers of Thomas Paine are given credit for playing a part in stimulating the American Revolution. A piece of music, a painting, a novel, an essay, an instrument, a theory—any conserve may serve to inspire others to creative acts.

Paradoxically, the cultural conserve is not only the vehicle for culture and society, but it is also the source of much of the dissension and violence in the world, and, Moreno feared, contains the germ of potential destruction of the human race. Beyond the obvious fact that science and technology have deciphered secrets of atomic structure, giving us a potential means for destroying most if not all mankind and simultaneously making the planet an impossible habitat, are intellectual conserves that can be destructive in more subtle ways. Such conserves include religious convictions and beliefs, political philosophy, nationalism and racial prejudice, and scientific and unscientific theories, among others. Awareness of religious wars and the Inquisition is too widely known to belabor here. It is also pretty obvious that the other great causes for war have been attributable to differences in the conserves of political philosophy.

It must also be obvious how racial and ethnic prejudices, as well as nationalism, are conserves, deeply entrenched notions and patterns of thinking that can serve destructive ends. The events in the last decade of the 20th century in Yugoslavia, a federation of six republics and multiple nationalities that had been cobbled together at the end of World War I, offer an example. Under the totalitarian Communist regime, the various ethnic groups were able to function in relative cooperation and intergroup dissensions remained repressed. Economic problems combined with the loss of the leadership of Marshal Tito in 1980 resulted in the reemergence of national and ethnic discords. This conflicted with the attempts of Serbia to maintain and dominate the federation, resulting in war, first in Slovenia, then Croatia, and finally Bosnia. The fact that the hostilities between those national and ethnic groups can be traced back at least 1,000 years testifies that the underlying intellectual conserves, convictions of the members of one group that those of another are unworthy, untrustworthy, or dangerous, or in the case where a race is enslaved, not fully human, are incredibly tenacious. Moreno was convinced that sociometric investigation would enlighten us about how these conserves are maintained. Understanding that process could provide a means of resolving or controlling those concepts that underlie violence and war.

How scientific theories can function as a negative force as well as a positive one is worthy of further discussion. Thomas Kuhn (1962) has disabused us of the notion that science is a slow and steady process of accumulation of knowledge in and about a particular field of inquiry. He pointed out that scientists work within a certain framework of deeply imbedded beliefs, a paradigm, shared by the scientific community. A paradigm is maintained until it is no longer consistent with the results of scientific investigation. At that point, there is a revolution and features of the existing paradigm are discarded and a new one, within which scientific investigation continues, takes its place. This is not a smooth and easy process, however, and paradigms are not easily overthrown. Scientists tend to hold tenaciously to their beliefs, inculcated during their education in their particular fields of study. A major example of paradigmatic revolution occurred with Einstein's theory of relativity, which challenged the notion of an absolute space and time, concepts that had been uncontested since the time of Isaac Newton's great work.

These beliefs that are really theories, or visions as David Bohm called them, are conserves in Morenean parlance. They are conserves that are so highly valued that they often are regarded as inviolable truths and are generally safe from inspection and reflection. Therefore, a scientist doesn't often examine or even recognize these beliefs. One such conviction is that scientific work is objective. A common notion is that the scientist asks the question, designs the research that might answer it, and accepts without subjective involvement the result that is obtained. Actually the scientist is always subjectively involved, beginning with the choice of the problems he/ she chooses to investigate to the interpretation of results. Kuhn believed that these choices and interpretations are severely constrained by the prevailing paradigm.

In short, those conserves, which Kuhn labeled paradigms, result in a narrowing and rigidity of thought on the part of scientists. New ideas, even unanticipated results, are often ignored and discarded. Theories that diverge too far from paradigmatic beliefs are considered as not worth considering. It is quite possible that among the thoughts, ideas, and theories that have been overlooked and ignored because they lie outside our paradigms are some that could alleviate much of the collective misery humankind faces today.

Moreno (1953c) anticipated some of Kuhn's ideas in a discussion of the emergence of the scientific method. The real advances in science, he wrote, come from the insights of a few geniuses. The job of the scientist is to steal the ideas of the genius and make them understandable to all the nongeniuses in the world. He used the myth of Prometheus, the demigod, who stole fire from Zeus and brought it to mankind as a model. I will argue later that Moreno's work was too much at variance with the prevailing paradigms of the social sciences of his time, and that this is a significant reason, among others, for the lack of acceptance of his philosophy and theories, even while many of techniques were widely adopted.

The problems conserves get us into are not within the conserves themselves. The problem is that most of us have been guided toward living a conserved life rather than a spontaneous one. We are all dominated by conserves, Moreno said. We are awed by them. The more conserves dominate us, the greater is the probability that our behavior is consistent and predictable. If it weren't for the spontaneity that reenergizes them, renews them, much of the world would be deadened. Society would function like a machine and we would function like robots. "Spontaneity is the principle of 'unconservability' and 'unpredictability.' Conserve is the principle of 'conservability,' 'constancy' and 'predictability.' Creativity can remain unfrozen and linked to spontaneity, or it can freeze and be linked to conserves" (Moreno, 1955e, p. 388).

Perhaps it is a genetic or constitutional predilection, but it seems as if most people are looking for absolute answers, the right way to do things, the right way to behave, how to be in the world. The struggle is between living spontaneously versus living according to conserves. There is no question that today's society encourages us to comport ourselves by fairly highly prescribed rules. However, many who live spontaneously engender approval and envy from their fellow humans. Spontaneity is an appreciated value and those who are spontaneous are often perceived as more real, more trustworthy than those whose actions are calculated and planned.

Lewis Yablonsky (1972), sociologist, close friend, student, and colleague of J. L. Moreno, wrote about the dangers of the over-conserved lifestyle, coining the term *robopathology*. Yablonsky's worry was not so much focused on the rebellion of the robots as it was about the dehumanizing effects of a technological society:

> The problem of the physical machine takeover of the destiny of people is obviously a phenomenon of enormous proportion. An even greater problem, one that is more subtle and insidious, exists. This involves the growing dehumanization of people to the point where they have become the walking dead. This dehumanized level of existence places

people in roles where they are actors mouthing irrelevant platitudes, experiencing programmed emotions with little or no compassion or sympathy for other people. (p. 6)

This condition that Yablonsky called robopathology refers to people who function more like automatons than like compassionate human beings. Robopathology, he suggested, is the dominant socio-psychological pathology of our era and is a product of technocracy, which imposes excessive planning and encourages conformity to social values and standards. Technocracy represents another way in which we are endangered by the conserves of our own creation.

The notion of the conserve is one of Moreno's most important contributions. It is a single concept, a category that includes both tangible artifacts and intangible entities like hypotheses, theories, and inspirations. Conserve can be thought of as cutting the Gordian knot of Cartesian mind-body dualism. The tangible body and the intangible thought are actually on a continuum. A product of thought, a scientific theory, for example, or an idea for a new mousetrap, an invention, is at first a subjective event in the mind of its author. It is a conserve because it can be replicated in a number of ways. The theory can be articulated by lecture or by an article in a scientific journal. Plans for the mousetrap can be drawn or an actual version of it produced. The published theory is read by others in whom it stimulates thoughts both for and against it. Hypotheses, more conserves, are generated to test its validity.

Spontaneity

Spontaneity theory may be Moreno's most important and the least understood of all his theories. The seeds of the concept were sown during Moreno's interactions with children in the *Augarten* of Vienna. The principles were first expressed in *Ein Ladung zu Einer Begegnung* (*Invitation to an Encounter*), later in Das *Testament Des Vaters* (*The Words of the Father*), and first studied systematically in Das *Stegreiftheater* (*The Theater of Spontaneity*). Understanding Moreno's spontaneity theory has been significantly complicated by the fact that Moreno chose a common word that has similarities to his theoretical concept but that has a less technical definition (Kipper, 1967). Spontaneity in the vernacular also has connotations that are inaccurate with respect to the technical concept.

The idea of spontaneity evolved in Moreno's mind over time. He originally wrote about it as if it were a personal attribute of the individual. Eventually spontaneity became identified as a unique kind of energy in the universe, the energy of a universal creative process. It is spontaneity interacting with creativity that results in the emergence of something novel, new species, new machines, new works of art, new theories, new roles, new acts. Spontaneity in the Morenean sense is an essential component of the creative process.

I have spent much time attempting to grasp Moreno's concept of spontaneity, trying to understand spontaneity as more than a novel and appropriate response to a situation of varying degrees of newness. I knew from his writing that Moreno believed he had discovered an important principle of the cosmos, and I wanted to comprehend it. I found his description of spontaneity as "unconservable energy" both puzzling and intriguing. Like anyone who has ever taken a course in physics, I was aware that a basic precept was the law of conservation of energy, which holds that energy may be transformed from one form to another but that it can be neither destroyed nor created. Unconservable energy is truly an oxymoron, a contradiction in terms. What can Moreno have meant by the idea?

Moreno himself appears to have had difficulty in communicating precisely what he meant by spontaneity. He referred to, described, and characterized spontaneity in many articles—and in many different phrases. Although these comments have similar themes, one does not find the precision or consistency that typifies a scientific definition. Sorokin (1949), Aulicino (1954), and Kipper (1967), all supportive of Moreno and his ideas, have made careful critiques in attempts to identify and clarify problems in Moreno's presentations on the related concepts of spontaneity and warming up. In response to these and other criticisms, Moreno pleads for forbearance, stating "it is difficult to convey the full meaning of undeveloped concepts like spontaneity and creativity which are in transition from a pre-scientific to a scientific formulation without using all available objective and subjective resources" (1955f, p. 361). There is no question that for someone who is expecting a precise and formal presentation of scientific theory, Moreno's style of writing creates big problems. It is also true that the concept of spontaneity was evolving in Moreno's mind over some years. And it is correct that his discussions leave inconsistencies and make it difficult for us to grasp just what Moreno had in mind by the concept of spontaneity.

Moreno's preferred definition that appears in several places (and several slightly different versions) is: "Spontaneity is the variable degree of adequate response to a situation of a variable degree of novelty" (1953c, p. 722). Even this, as Kipper (1967) pointed out, presented a problem in that this definition is not congruent with the notion of spontaneity as a form of energy. Only the effects of energy can be directly observed, not the energy itself. The "variable degree of adequate response" is an effect of spontaneity, not spontaneity itself. As Aulicino pointed out, this definition also leaves unspecified how adequacy of response and degree of novelty are measured. The nature of the relationship between adequacy and novelty is also left unidentified.

To give the reader a sense of the problem, I list here a sampling of statements, which Moreno made over the years about spontaneity:

1. "Spontaneity" and "spontaneous" have finally come to mean a value—a human value. Spontaneity has become a biological as well as a social

value. It is today a frame of reference for the scientist as well as for the politician, for the artist as well as the educator (1940a, p. 212).

2. Disorderly conduct and emotionalisms resulting from impulsive action are far from being desiderata of spontaneity work. Instead, they belong more in the realm of the pathology of spontaneity (1940a, p. 218).

3. Spontaneity can be present in a person when he is thinking just as well as when he is feeling, when he is at rest just as well as when he is in action (1940a, p. 219).

4. The s factor cuts into and delimits the meaning of intelligence . . . Intelligence tests do not measure spontaneity and spontaneity tests do not measure intelligence—in its narrower sense (1946b, p. 78).

5. The individual is not endowed with a reservoir of spontaneity, in the sense of a given, stable volume or quantity. Spontaneity is (or is not) available in varying degrees of readiness, from zero to maximum, operating like a psychological catalyzer (1946b, pp. 85).

6. A type of universe that is *open*, that is, a universe in which some degree of novelty is continuously possible—and this is apparently the type of universe in which human awareness has arisen—is a favorable condition for the s factor to emerge and to develop. It could not exist in a type of universe that is closed to novelty, i.e., one which is determined by absolute laws (1946b, p. 87).

7. Spontaneity is a readiness of the subject to respond as required. It is a condition—a conditioning—of the subject; a preparation of the subject for free action (1946b, p. 111).

8. We see spontaneity on two levels: the crude, ready spontaneity during the course of any life process; and, then, the spontaneity on a higher level, occurring in situations that do not fit the patterns of a person, which are surprising and unexpected. It is useful to distinguish between instinctive and creative spontaneity (1946b, p. 111).

9. Spontaneity and creativity are thus categories of a different order; creativity belongs to the categories of substance—it is the arch substance—spontaneity to the categories of catalyzer—it is the arch catalyzer (1953c, p. 40).

10. Although the most universal and evolutionary the oldest, it is the least developed among the factors operating in man's world; it is most frequently discouraged and restrained by cultural devices. A great deal of man's psycho- and sociopathology can be ascribed to the insufficient development of spontaneity (1953c, p. 42).

11. Spontaneity operates in the present, now and here; it propels the individual towards an adequate response to a new situation or a new response to an old situation (1953c, p. 42).

12. The universe is infinite creativity. But what is spontaneity? Is it a kind of energy? If it is energy, it is *unconservable*, if the meaning of spontaneity should be kept consistent. There is an energy that is conservable. . . . There is another form of energy that emerges and that is

spent in a moment, which must emerge to be spent and that must be spent to make place for emergence (1953c, p. 47).

13. It is a truism to say that the universe cannot exist without physical and mental energy that can be preserved. But it is more important to realize that without the other kind of energy, the unconservable one—or spontaneity—the creativity of the universe could not start and could not run, it would come to a standstill (1953c, p. 59).

14. Spontaneity can be defined as the adequate response to a new situation, or the novel response to an old situation (1953c, p. 336).

15. In the course of interaction between two actors the more warmed up one is, the more warmed up the other tends to become. Spontaneity begets counter-spontaneity (1953c, p. 706).

16. Spontaneity is the variable degree of adequate response to a situation of a variable degree of novelty. Novelty of behavior by itself is not the measure of spontaneity. Novelty has to be qualified against its adequacy *in situ*. Adequacy of behavior by itself is also not the measure of spontaneity. Adequacy has to be qualified against its novelty (1953c, p. 722).

17. But I postulated that spontaneity and creativity are observable facts and can be subjected to experiments, laboratory studies, and systematic analysis (1955f, p. 363).

18. No one has ever seen spontaneity. Spontaneity is a hypothesis (1955f, p. 372).

19. It was an important advance to link spontaneity to creativity, the highest form of intelligence we know of, and to recognize them as the primary forces in human behavior (1955e, p. 392).

20. Without creativity the spontaneity of a universe would run empty and end abortive; without spontaneity the creativity of a universe would become perfectionism and lifeless (1953c, p. 336).

The word *spontaneity* first shows up in Moreno's writings in the context of spontaneity training. In *Das Stegreiftheater* (*The Theater of Spontaneity*), published in 1923, he proclaimed that spontaneity training would be the main subject in schools in future. At this point Moreno considered spontaneity to be a cerebral function, comparable to but distinctly different from intelligence. He related spontaneity to action when confronted with the unexpected. He also considered it to be a function that is susceptible to training, a point that he made many times in his writing:

> The sense for spontaneity, as a function, shows a more rudimentary development than any other important, fundamental function of the central nervous system. This may explain the astonishing inferiority of men when confronted with surprise tactics.
>
> The study of surprise tactics in the laboratory shows the flexibility or the rigidity of individuals when faced with unexpected incidents.

Taken by surprise, people act frightened or stunned. They produce false response or not at all. It seems that there is nothing for which human beings are more ill prepared and the human brain more ill-equipped than surprise. . . . When compared with many other mental functions such as intelligence and memory, the sense for spontaneity is seen to be far less developed. This may perhaps be so because in the civilization of conserves that we have developed, spontaneity is far less used and trained than, for instance, intelligence and memory. (Moreno, 1941b, p. 211)

Moreno apparently still regarded spontaneity as a mental function or a trait when he wrote in the first edition of *Who Shall Survive?* (1934) that spontaneity training provides a means of increasing "spontaneability" of the residents of the Hudson Training School for Girls.

When Moreno published the "Spontaneity Theory of Child Development" (Moreno & Moreno, 1944), the notion of spontaneity as energy began to emerge. In this paper, the Morenos emphasized the radical change in situation that birth brings about, the infant having moved from a safe, closed, protective, confining equilibrium to a world with open, unlimited space, from darkness into a kaleidoscope of shapes and colors, light and darkness:

He moves into this world with such a suddenness, that his successful adjustment is one of life's great riddles. Within a few minutes, he practically changes from one world to another.

The infant is moving, at birth, into a totally strange set of relationships. He has no model after which he can shape his acts. He is facing, more than at any time during his subsequent life, a novel situation. . . . If the infant is to live his response must be positive and unfaltering. . . . There must be a certain amount of this s (spontaneity) factor at least in crucial moments available. A minimum of spontaneity is already required in his first day of life (J. L. Moreno & F. B. Moreno, 1944, p. 92).

There must be a factor with which Nature has graciously provided the newcomer, so that he can land safely and anchor himself, at least provisionally on an uncharted universe. *This factor is more than and different from the given energy conserved in the young body of the newborn* [italics added]. It is a factor that enables him to reach beyond himself, to enter new situations as if carrying the organism, stimulating and arousing all its organs to modify their structures in order that they can meet their new responsibilities. To this factor, we apply the term spontaneity (s factor) (J. L. Moreno, 1946b, pp. 50–51).

Spontaneity, then, according to Moreno, is an energy, but it is a different kind of energy, an "unconservable" energy. Hence, it does not follow the law of conservation of energy. It is in this 1944 article that the formulation appears: "We have called this response of an individual to a new situation—and the new response to an old situation—*spontaneity* (p. 92)." This and several variations would soon become his standard definition of spontaneity.

The article "Spontaneity Theory of Child Development" is reprinted in *Psychodrama, First Volume* (1946b) and is followed by several pages of discussion entitled "General Spontaneity Theory." In it, Moreno asked two questions. The first is: "Does the s factor [spontaneity] emerge only in the human group or can the s hypothesis be extended within certain limits to sub-human groups and to the lower animals and plants? (p. 85). This question does not really get answered here, although it is obvious from later works that Moreno considered spontaneity to be a universal phenomenon. The second question is: "How can the existence of the s factor be reconciled with the idea of a mechanical law abiding universe, as, for instance, with the law of the conservation of energy?" (p. 85).

For perspective on the issue, Moreno discussed a theory of psychic energy that does follow the conventional notion of conservable energy, Sigmund Freud's concept of libido. Moreno pointed out that Freud assumed that if the flow of libido was deflected from its natural aim, sexual intercourse, that the dammed up energy must flow elsewhere, finding new outlets through aggression, substitution, projection, and sublimation. Psychological determinism in this formulation is complete and Freud was convinced that he had proven that all human behaviors, even slips of the tongue, were determined. What can't be explained in terms of the conscious in this theory can be assigned to the unconscious. There is no place for spontaneity in such a system and all human creativity can be explained as a by-product of unexpressed sexual intercourse.

Moreno was clear that spontaneity was unconservable and that spontaneity exists only in the present. It is not retrieved from past events; it cannot be carried over into future ones. An individual does not have a reservoir of spontaneity from which to draw as needed (1946a). One must access exactly as much as one needs in the moment.

Perhaps, he said, conservation of energy and the other laws of physics hold firm in the world of physical and biological conserves, but they may not rule in the realm of thought and meaning. He pointed out that quantum theory was producing other ideas and concepts that conflicted with the laws of classical physics. Perhaps it was possible that a physical basis for the unconservable energy that he called spontaneity would be found there.

Unknown to Moreno, a concept that fits the definition of spontaneity had already been proposed, and an interpretation of quantum theory that closely matches Moreno's Canon of Spontaneity-Creativity existed: David Bohm's theory of the implicate order. Bohm (1917–1992) was a productive physicist and friend and colleague of Albert Einstein. With Einstein, he became troubled with the Copenhagen interpretation of quantum theory that predicted with great accuracy the outcomes of experiments but, according to Niels Bohr, could not describe an objective reality. Bohm developed an alternative interpretation of quantum theory that did describe reality. In the next chapter, I will discuss Bohm's theory of the implicate and explicate orders and how they correlate with Moreno's understanding of creativity.

The Warming Up Process

The phrase *warming up* is used in a number of contexts in the Morenean methods. A group warms up to engaging in a psychodrama or another activity. A chosen group member warms up to the role of protagonist and then to a relationship, a feeling, a mental state, or an event to be explored on the psychodrama stage. Directors and auxiliary egos also must warm up to their respective roles. We talk about warming up to roles both within and outside psychodrama. We warm up to emotional states. We also warm up to the spontaneity state. Athletes warm up for a game both physically, through exercises, and mentally. Sometimes this is called psyching oneself up in the vernacular. Warming up is preparation for action. It is the process of accessing spontaneity.

Moreno wrote that the warming up process is a "condition that exists before and in the course of any creative act—before and during an act of sleeping, eating, sexual intercourse, walking, artistic creation or any act of self realization" (1955f, p. 367). Every act or action is initiated by spontaneity. However, there are different levels or intensities or forms of spontaneity. Moreno presented several classifications of spontaneity. In *Psychodrama, First Volume*, Moreno (1946b) gave a three-part classification. He listed (1) the spontaneity that activates conserves, in other words, the initiation of repeated actions that are adequate to the situation but generate little or no novelty; (2) another form called "originality," which pertains to individuals who add something new to existing conserves, improving them but not changing their essence; and (3) creative spontaneity, which leads to invention and production of truly new works of art, inventions, and ideas.

Spontaneity that energizes well-learned responses requires the least effort of the three types, although some actions that the individual does not like performing may take a considerable amount of effort to initiate. Originality requires more effort from the individual who is always seeking to live in a world of novelty, to make the most of his/her talents, to create him/herself. Accessing the spontaneity for truly creative endeavors is the most difficult. This level of spontaneity requires great effort and cannot be sustained indefinitely.

Moreno first studied the warming up process by observing the players of the *Stegreiftheater*. Here is how he described it:

> The Impromptu agent, poet, actor, musician, painter finds his point of departure not outside, but within himself, in the spontaneity "state."

This is not something permanent, not set and rigid as written words or melodies are, but fluent, rhythmic fluency, rising and falling, growing and fading like living acts and still different from life. It is the state of production, the essential principle of all creative experience. It is not given like words or colors. It is not conserved, or registered. The impromptu artist must warm up, he must make it climbing up the hill. Once he runs up the road to the "state," it develops in full power. (1947b, p. 44)

The spontaneity state, therefore, is the condition of being in contact with spontaneity, or the quantum potential, to a greater degree than usual. It requires effort and can be maintained only for brief periods of time. The individual, whether artist, inventor, philosopher, or scientist, who is seeking inspiration is trying to attain the spontaneity state. The warming up process is the path to that condition. It is preparation for action.

The warming up process is of special importance because it is the aspect of the creative process over which we have some voluntary control. Moreno's solution to the problems of humankind was greater spontaneity, resulting in greater creativity in living. He was convinced that we could be trained to be more spontaneous. In the present explanation of Spontaneity-Creativity that means learning to access the quantum potential at will and more easily. By learning about our own process of warming up, we can increase the possibilities of responding to situations appropriately and effectively. By understanding the dynamics of the warming up process, we can teach others to respond more appropriately and effectively.

The common elements that trigger the attempt to access spontaneity are tension and a demand for action. They may come from outside, such as finding oneself in an unexpected situation or in a situation in which a lack of action or an inappropriate act will have dire consequences. Or the tension may come from inside, as is frequently the case with the creative artist. There are two major categories of obstacles to warming up, conserves and anxiety.

The relationship between conserve and spontaneity is paradoxical. Conserves can reduce access to spontaneity and they can also stimulate access to spontaneity. The problem is not that conserves are bad, Moreno maintained, but how we make use of them. Imagine the primitive human, he pointed out, who when born is the most helpless life-form on earth. Only the capacity to create, to create means of finding or making shelter, ways of hunting, fishing, and growing edible plants, ways of protecting themselves from predators kept humankind alive and flourishing. These conserves, these ways of dealing with the exigencies of survival, also made it possible to pass these skills to fellow humans and to succeeding generations. In short, conserves made society possible through the accumulation of knowledge and skill, coming from each generation's experience and creativity and passed along to the next.

Over the several millennia of human existence a prodigious number of conserves have been created. While many of them have served their purpose and disappeared and are no longer active in today's culture, the complexity of present-day society has burdened us with an overload of conserves. Early humans had few conserves to call upon. They were forced to rely upon their spontaneity as their lives consisted of moving from one novel situation to another. Today we are conserve bound with a ready rule, skill, tool, or theory to handle almost any situation. We live in a machinelike society and have become machinelike to match. A mechanized society values living by rules and conforming behavior over spontaneous behavior and originality.

On the one hand, conserves may engender spontaneity. A poem, a patriotic song, a magnificent painting, an invention, a philosophical or scientific theory, any of these may inspire others individuals to great ideas, great works of art, or great acts. On the other hand, conserves may stand in the way of accessing spontaneity. To access spontaneity, one must put aside conserves as much as possible in order to open oneself to the potentiality of creativity enfolded in the quantum potential. It is probably not possible to escape conserves altogether, and creative endeavors today inevitably make use of some conserves, such as words, mathematical or musical notation, and so on.

There are several ways in which conserves stand in the way of accessing spontaneity. Effort is saved by relying on a conserve that may be a more or less adequate response to the situation in lieu of attempting a novel as well as adequate response. A minimum of spontaneity is called upon to activate the conserved response.

Beliefs and opinions, conserves learned from and shared by many people, are often accepted as facts. This happens in all fields of human endeavor: religion, science, philosophy, and politics. It requires considerable energy to question entities that are widely regarded as facts, but the history of science is replete with such events. And yet to get to a broader understanding of the physical world, Albert Einstein had to go beyond Isaac Newton's facts of gravity.

We take our experiences as factual without much question. Yet we know that several people sharing the same situation may experience it quite differently. We tend to understand and interpret an event primarily from one side—ours. What we understand, feel, and tell ourselves about an event is itself a conserve and easily becomes an obstacle to accessing spontaneity. Experiences in which we have been unsuccessful in some way, especially experiences in which we perceive ourselves as being unjustly treated, leave us with a loss of emotional balance and a need for completion. Situations that have some even remotely similar element can activate that need that stands in the way of accessing spontaneity. Psychodrama provides a means for reevaluating such experiences and freeing one up for easier access to spontaneity.

The other impediment to spontaneity is anxiety. Moreno considered anxiety to be loss of spontaneity. A phenomenological interpretation of the meaning of anxiety is that anxiety is a fear of loss of the self. The implication is that one must be in touch with spontaneity to experience a sense of oneself. Since the quantum potential links all beings, this suggests that a sense of oneself means being linked through spontaneity to everyone else. This supports Moreno's notion of the organic unity of humankind.

MORENO DEMONSTRATES THE WARMING UP PROCESS

Pitirim Sorokin, a Harvard professor of philosophy, was a friend and colleague of J. L. Moreno. Sorokin also shared Moreno's interest in creativity. After Moreno published *Psychodrama, First Volume*, Sorokin (1949) published a critique of Moreno's theory of Spontaneity-Creativity, based on Moreno's discussions in *Psychodrama, First Volume* and *Words of the Father*. His critique was aimed at two different aspects of Moreno's discussion of Spontaneity-Creativity. Sorokin thought that Moreno tried to cover too much ground with the concept of spontaneity, describing too many different types and different situations. He pointed out inconsistencies and contradictions in Moreno's treatment of spontaneity. He was particularly critical of Moreno's notion of spontaneity testing on the psychodramatic stage.

Sorokin also criticized what he saw as Moreno's rejection of spontaneity as energy. In his 1946 discussion of spontaneity and spontaneity training, Moreno had rejected the notion that spontaneity was a form of energy modeled after the classical concept of energy. He had used Freud's theory of libido as an example of such a hypothesis. Moreno had not yet formulated his notion of spontaneity as an unconservable energy.

Sorokin agreed wholeheartedly with Moreno in rejecting the Freudian concept of libido and with Moreno's repudiation of applying the concepts of natural science to the social sciences. "In all my works I have been combating this thoughtless, superficial, and essentially incompetent aping of the natural sciences, still fashionable among certain sociologists, psychologists, and other social scientists" (Sorokin, 1949, p. 223). Moreno, Sorokin thought, should consider a modified theory of energy rather than reject the idea that Spontaneity-Creativity was itself energy. He went on to say that in his own studies of creativity he had found that the application of a properly modified and applied principle of energy had been heuristically fruitful.

In spite of his criticisms that identify most of the issues with which others have had difficulty incorporating into an integral concept of spontaneity, Sorokin was laudatory of Moreno's theory of Spontaneity-Creativity. Any fruitful theory, Sorokin said, initially raises problems and calls for clarification. He had only pointed out the ambiguity of two aspects of Moreno's theory. His criticism was not meant to question the central and valid features of Spontaneity-Creativity theory.

Six years later, Moreno produced another article on the theory of Spontaneity-Creativity, published in the 1955 issue of *Sociometry*, the final issue under Moreno's ownership. Before publication, Moreno sent a copy of the paper to Sorokin, who responded with another paper that again questioned certain characteristics of the theory. Moreno answered with still another article, a reply to Sorokin. This last paper is of particular interest in that it begins with Moreno describing his own warming up process to the creation of the piece.

Moreno described having Sorokin's article in hand and beginning to read:

> What happened—I am trying to give a "phenomenological" description of the process—is the following: As I read it [Sorokin's article], two things happen. One is the reproduction of Sorokin's article in my mind. I lift it from the paper upon which it is typewritten, so to speak, in order to duplicate it within my own thinking . . . a second phenomenon enters into the picture—as I begin to react to it. I get, as we say, "warmed up"; all kinds of ideas come to me: "We agree on this point—creativity"; "Oh, this is not what I mean by spontaneity. . . ." But suddenly I read a sentence about creative "conserves" which alarms me. Conserves by themselves without an "intervening" factor do not become creative. We build up the conserves and try to make them look like idols. I see the ghosts of Plato and Aristotle coming back. It makes creativity look stale and makes a puppet out of God. No! No! . . . More than the creators, we admire their conserves until they become sacred, like the Bible," Beethoven's music or the "Pyramids." At this point, I come to the decision that I must answer it; and herewith I answer Sorokin's reply to my theory of creativity. It is a new phase in my warming up process which takes place. Up to this point, I am warmed up to Sorokin's comments, just reacting to them without any further plans in mind; but now that I have decided to answer the comments, my warming up is directed towards a goal of my own—the production of my (this) article. . . . The sum of it is that I am gradually getting "ready" to write. I am only uncertain as to what I should say beyond what I have said so many times, I am at a loss as to what form it should take in order to put my ideas across better. In this moment of indecision, I have an inspiration: to start my response to Sorokin's comments in the manner in which I am doing it "now" by giving an actual account of what I am going through, convinced that by such an existential mode of presentation, I can make more plausible to Sorokin and to the readers my concept of the relationships between creativity, spontaneity and the conserves. (1956c, p. 127)

It was this inspiration to begin the article with an account of his internal process while reading Sorokin's paper, Moreno said, that spurred him into action to write a response to Sorokin. This inspiration was the peak of his spontaneity, the intervening factor interacting with the conserve of Sorokin's paper that resulted in a new conserve, Moreno's paper replying to Sorokin.

Creative change seems to be a benchmark of our universe, and humankind has shown a considerable precociousness toward certain aspects of creating, primarily in the domain of dealing with our physical environment. Moreno's concern is that humankind has been spectacularly creative in the realm of science and technology but has had a tendency to overvalue the *products* of creativity. In our admiration of what we have created, we have neglected to understand and study the *process* of creating. We have thereby put all humankind in jeopardy. We have created the means by which we can destroy much if not all humankind, possibly life itself as we know it, but at the same time we seem unable to create a global society in which we can exist peacefully and in collaboration with our fellow human beings.

While a solution to these problems was his goal, Moreno came to the decision that no one person, no two people, no small group of people could bring it about. This was a task so immense that it required the cooperation of everybody, every living person. Every member of humankind is related, however distantly, to every other member. And *that* is the meaning of his oft-quoted and, he sometimes said, little understood opening statement in *Who Shall Survive?*: A truly therapeutic procedure cannot have less an objective than the whole of mankind. Mankind is a social and organic unity.

6 The Physics of Spontaneity-Creativity

I puzzled over Moreno's concept of spontaneity for many years. Like fellow psychodramatists, I observed behavior on the psychodrama stage and in life that certainly fit the definition of spontaneous behavior as a novel response to a familiar situation or an adequate response to a new situation and labeled it spontaneous. I wanted a better understanding. I could not figure out how one could measure either dimension, novelty of the situation, or adequacy of response, other than by subjective judgment. Another question was how these two criteria of spontaneity were related. Was one unit or degree of novelty equal to one unit of adequacy? Moreno's solution to measurement was subjective evaluation by observers. Other attempts at measurement of spontaneity (Keller, Treadwell. & Kumar, (2002); Kipper & Hundal, 2005) have only identified individuals who report the frequency of experiences that were considered spontaneous. Above all, I found Moreno's description of spontaneity as an unconservable energy incomprehensible.

Although my grasp of physics was limited, I was quite aware of the concept of conservation of energy, the second law of thermodynamics. This is as powerful a law of nature as any ever proposed. Energy can be transformed from one kind to another, electric energy to light energy, for example, but energy cannot be either created or destroyed. Unconservable energy is therefore absolutely an oxymoron. There can be no such thing.

Moreno, however, was not unsophisticated or naive and he was always convinced that his theory of Spontaneity-Creativity was valid. He had no doubt that this energy that he called spontaneity did exist and that it was an unconservable form of energy. He suggested that quantum research might eventually substantiate his ideas:

Atomic nuclear research seems to confirm in principle, or at least does not contradict, the picture of the universe which the theory of spontaneity-creativity has envisaged. Its structure is not permanently set but when novel situations emerge, the responses to the surrounding field take the form of creative acts. As long as the universe was visualized as dominated by eternal, rigid laws, there was no place for "uniqueness" and for "explosive" changes and with it no place for creativity as the ultimate principle, at least not for the on-going, here-and-nowness of it. But a revolution has taken place on the highest level of conceptualization. We can say with greater certainty than ever that the supreme power ruling the world is Spontaneity-Creativity. It has created a rational cosmos which coexists interdependently with man's perception of it but amenable to his intervention as long as he knows and abides by its rules. (1955f, p. 373)

I first discovered the ideas of David Bohm in *Looking Glass Universe* (Briggs & Peat, 1984). This book, subtitled *The Emerging Science of Wholeness*, suggested that a paradigm shift in the natural sciences is under way. This shift is from a Newtonian perception of a mechanical universe composed of interacting parts that can be understood by analyzing its basic units (once conceived of as atoms) to a vision of the universe that can only be comprehended as an undivided whole. Einstein's theory of relativity and the quantum theory of Bohr, Heisenberg, and Schrödinger signaled the beginning of this shift, Briggs and Peat wrote. In addition to David Bohm's theory of the implicate order, Prigogine's concept of dissipative structures, Sheldrake's morphogenetic fields, and Pribram's holographic brain are additional examples of theories from divergent scientific areas that all point toward a truly holistic universe.

I found Bohm's ideas fascinating and read some of his books: *Wholeness and the Implicate Order* (1980), *Science, Order, and Creativity* (Bohm & Peat, 2000), *The Undivided Universe* (Bohm & Hiley, 1993), *Unfolding Meaning* (1985), *Thought as a System* (1994), and *On Creativity* (1998). Although my elemental familiarity with calculus was insufficient to understand much of the mathematical reasoning in some of his works, Bohm included enough expository material to give the layman a reasonable comprehension of his ideas. Discussions of his work by other authors: *The Essential David Bohm* (Nichol, 2003). *Turbulent Mirror* (Briggs & Peat, 1989), *Bridging Science and Spirit* (Friedman, 1990), and *Infinite Potential*, a biography by David Peat (1997) increased my comprehension of Bohm's work. All of these publications serve as sources for this chapter.

I recognized immediately that there were many commonalities between Bohm and Moreno. Both proposed a holistic approach. Both rejected the doctrine of absolute determinism. Neither was limited to his respective discipline. Both exhibited an intense interest in creativity. The contributions of both tended to be ignored or rejected by colleagues of their respective disciplines. Both engendered some degree of hostility from colleagues. Bohm's concern about the mechanistic conceptualization of the universe in classical science, and its negative effect on human society seemed to echo Moreno's concern about the effect of materialism on humankind. Eventually I discovered a more important similarity: Bohm's theory of the implicate and explicate orders provided a physical basis for understanding Moreno's Canon of Spontaneity-Creativity.

David Bohm earned his Ph.D. from the University of California, Berkeley, working under the supervision of J. Robert Oppenheimer. He began work on plasma theory, became well known for his discoveries in this field. In 1951, he became a member of the Department of Physics, Princeton University. While there, he wrote a textbook on quantum theory (Bohm, 1951) in order, he said, to better understand Niels Bohr's Copenhagen interpretation. He also met Albert Einstein, who was at the Institute for Advanced Study, and the two became friends and colleagues. Einstein told Bohm that he had not really understood quantum theory until he read his, Bohm's, book.

In the same year, Bohm was called before the House Un-American Activities Committee to testify against former friends and colleagues. He refused, was indicted, tried, and cleared. However, Princeton refused to renew his appointment and he could not find another position in the United States. He held positions in Brazil and Israel, and finally was appointed as professor of theoretical physics at Birbeck College, University of London. He produced two scientific theories considered radical by his discipline during his lifetime, the causal interpretation of quantum physics and the theory of the implicate order. For Bohm, prediction and control were not the ultimate aim of science. He believed that physics was about understanding nature, and for him, as it was for J. L. Moreno, meaning and creativity were what was most important.

BOHM AND THE IMPLICATE ORDER

David Bohm and Albert Einstein shared a sense of frustration with the science in which both had made significant discoveries. The two most powerful theoretical contributions to physics in the 20th century were Einstein's theory of relativity and the development of quantum theory. Both theories add predictability and accuracy to classical Newtonian physics, a benchmark of effective theory. Both led to new advancements and discoveries in physics. Both make the observer a variable in experimentation. Both emphasize the holistic nature of the universe. In these respects, the two theories are congruent and consistent with each other. But paradoxically, there also exist irreconcilable incompatibilities. For example, Einstein's universe is a deterministic one. The universe of quantum theory is a probabilistic one in which indeterminism is inherent. Quantum mechanics requires reality to be discontinuous, noncausal, and nonlocal. Relativity theory requires reality to be continuous, causal, and local.

These contradictions bothered Einstein and Bohm (as well as many other physicists). There must be, they believed, some way to reconcile the two theories. Einstein believed strongly that there must be what he called "a hidden variable," an explanation or theory at a deeper level of reality that could account for both relativity theory and quantum theory and resolve the apparently irreconcilable differences between them.

Relativity theory deals with the macro world, the physical world that we experience. It is a world of things and beings. It has long been held that the universe is dynamic flow, always in action, as Greek philosopher Heraclites thought when he noted, "You cannot step twice into the same river." The earth turns on its axis and circles the sun while the moon circles the earth. Even inert objects are perceived as composed of atoms in constant motion. Originally considered to be indivisible bits of stuff, atoms were then discovered to consist of electrons, protons, and neutrons, arranged as tiny planetarian systems with electrons circling a nucleus of neutrons and protons. The physical world is conceived of as consisting of matter and energy.

Newton discovered that gravity tethered the moon to the earth and the planets to the sun. Einstein's theory of relativity superseded that idea with the notion that space was curved by the mass of the earth and the sun. Relativity theory also established the constant speed of light and consequently that observations were dependent upon the position and movement of the observer. This brought the observer into science in a new way. In classical physics the observer and the observed are considered as independent of each other. Now they must be considered together as aspects of the act of observation. Relativity theory deals with the same world as does classical physics, but it improves the accuracy of scientific observation in this macro world.

Quantum theory, on the other hand, deals with the micro world of subatomic particles. It is highly formal, providing a calculus that can predict with great accuracy the results of quantum experiments. In other words, it predicts rather precisely how the instruments will read in quantum experiments. What it does not do is describe an individual quantum process. The conventional interpretation of quantum theory, the Copenhagen interpretation, says nothing about reality itself, about what a quantum system or a particle is. Philosophically, this means that it does not provide an ontology of quantum processes. It is epistemological, providing knowledge about the behavior of quantum systems. While this can be very useful for prediction and control in technical processes, it fails to describe the nature of the world that underlies this knowledge.

There are several interpretations of quantum theory, the most widely accepted one being the Copenhagen interpretation associated with Niels Bohr, Werner Heisenberg, and Erwin Schrödinger. Despite the contradictions between quantum mechanics and relativity theory, Bohr remained adamantly against the notion of hidden variables, insistent that quantum theory was basic and that there could be no underlying theory that would resolve the contradictions. One physicist, John von Neumann, published a paper demonstrating that a hidden variables theory was mathematically impossible.

The search for reality, for unseen causes behind the vagaries of nature, has been a feature of human behavior perhaps forever. Spirits, mythological gods, God, the natural elements of fire, water, air, and earth, atoms, and gravity have all been called upon to explain what is hidden behind what we can perceive, a deeper theory with greater power to explain current events and to predict future ones. And always there is something left unexplained that calls for a still deeper theory. As Gödel established, no system can be completely explained from within that system.

Bohm did not allow Bohr's and von Neumann's rejections of a deeper theory deter him from developing one. He proceeded to publish just such a theory in the *Physical Review* (1952). Bohm continued to work out his ideas and published *Wholeness and the Implicate Order* (1980), a collection of papers spelling out his theory of the implicate and explicate orders.

Bohm's theory takes the view that reality is an unimaginably vast sea of energy comprising a spectrum of increasingly subtle orders. At one pole of this spectrum, the most manifest, is the explicate order, the physical universe that we know through our senses and instruments such as telescopes and microscopes and other sophisticated devices that increase the sensitivity of our senses. This explicate order, Bohm maintains, unfolds from the subtler implicate order. As a matter of fact, it is continuously unfolding from and enfolding into this implicate order. The implicate order is, in turn, unfolding and enfolding into a super-implicate order that itself unfolds and enfolds into a super-super-implicate order, and so forth, continuing through an infinite number of ever more subtle orders.

This summary of Bohm's theory requires considerable elaboration and the following discussion can only be considered as relating some of the major features of Bohm's thinking. This is my understanding of his ideas and is based on the following references: Bohm (1952, 1980, 1985, 1990). We begin with the concept of order because order is a very important notion to Bohm. He writes that the notion is so vast that it is hard to convey in words and he takes most of a chapter in *Wholeness and the Implicate Order* (1980) to discuss and illustrate the meaning of order. It is especially important because quantum theory signals a new order or paradigm in physical science.

In his exposition of order, Bohm uses the concept of subtlety. He refers to the derivation of the term from Latin, where it means "finely woven." He gives this example of subtlety with respect to order. Insurance companies use actuarial tables to predict how many people within a certain age range can be expected to die and use that information to determine life insurance rates. They do not know who among these people will die, but they can predict how many life insurance policies they will have to pay out. By collecting information on the health and life habits of the individuals in a particular pool of people, it would be possible to make predictions about which ones are likely to die. Such information would represent a more subtle order of data. We will deal with the concept of subtlety in more detail as we proceed in this discussion.

Bohm uses many analogies to illustrate his concepts. He found an analogy for the concept of enfoldment while watching a science program on television. The apparatus consisted of two cylinders, a smaller one inside a larger one. The space between was filled with a viscous fluid like glycerine.

A drop of nonsoluble ink is inserted into the fluid and the inner cylinder is rotated a number of times. The drop of ink is pulled out into a thin thread, which becomes thinner and thinner as the cylinder continues to be turned. Eventually, it becomes invisible to the eye. This represents enfoldment. The ink drop is enfolded into the glycerine. Now, if the cylinder is turned in the opposite direction, the thread reappears and eventually the drop of ink is reconstituted. It has been unfolded.

The drop of ink is stretched out so that it no longer occupies its original little space in the glycerine but is spread out over a lot of space, enfolded. When the rotation is reversed, the drop of ink is unfolded and pulled back together. Bohm further noted that if one inserted a drop of ink, rotated the cylinder a few times, then inserted a new drop of ink, rotated that a few turns, and inserted a third and maybe a fourth drop of ink, in the unfolding process, the first drop of ink would reappear and, as the cylinder continued to be rotated, would enfold again and the second drop of ink would be reconstituted. Then the third and the fourth in turn would do likewise. Bohm points out that it could look like a single drop of ink was moving from one place to the next. This suggests an explication of how electrons in an atom move from one orbit to another without occupying the space between, the so-called quantum leap.

Locality and nonlocality are important concepts in Bohm's theory. Locality is a feature of the explicate order. "No two things can occupy the same space" is a familiar expression of the notion of locality. More important is that an object can only affect another object at a distance through the action of some form of energy. Furthermore, no form of energy can travel from its source at a speed greater than light. Light from the sun has a powerful influence on what happens on earth. However, it takes light between eight and nine minutes to reach the earth. Events such as solar flares do not instantly affect the earth. The implicate order, on the other hand, is characterized by nonlocality. This means that points at a distance can instantaneously influence each other.

Bohm found that holography provided a way of explaining the concepts of enfolding and unfolding as well as locality and nonlocality. In conventional photography, the light from a scene is focused by a lens and projected onto a film plate in the camera. Although the image is reversed, objects in the scene maintain their relationship to each other. If Aunt Alice is to the right of Uncle George when the picture is taken, she will be on his right on the film. Once we have developed and printed the picture, we could cut it in half, one half containing Aunt Alice and the other showing Uncle George. This illustrates locality.

The holograph is a very different way of creating an image of an object. Typically, a half-silvered mirror divides a beam of light from a laser,. One half of the beam is so directed that it reflects off the subject toward a film plate. The other half of the beam is so aimed that it meets the light so reflected at the film plate. The two beams of light interfere with each other.

This means that the light waves combine where they meet. If two wave peaks coincide they add together. If a peak meets a trough, the result is a leveling out. The combined light hitting the film results in an interference pattern on the film. When it is developed all one sees are very fine lines on the plate. There is no image as in conventional photography. However, if the laser is then directed through this film plate, an image of the original subject appears in front of the plate. It is a three-dimensional image composed entirely of light. One can look at it from different angles and see exactly the same thing as if looking at the original subject. However, you can stick your hand into the holographic image, something you cannot do with the original. Furthermore, although the image is quite stable, the photons composing it are constantly changing at an incredible rate as they leave the laser and pass through the holographic plate at the speed of light.

Perhaps the strangest difference between the holograph and the conventional photograph, however, is this: If we cut the holographic plate in half and then shine the laser through one half of the plate, we do not get an image of half of the subject; we get the whole image. And if we cut the half into quarters, again we get the whole image. As a matter of fact, the whole image is everywhere embedded in the holographic plate. We could also say that the image is *enfolded* everywhere in the plate, and that shining the laser light through the plate unfolds the image. This aspect of holography illustrates nonlocality, a quality of quantum theory.

The world we know, the world of classical physics and of relativity theory, is a world in which there is locality. That is, things are separate from each other. No two things can occupy the same space. If an object influences another object, it is because of a flow of energy from the one to the other. For example, the picture on your television set is there because of a signal from a transmission source, a television station or studio, and, according to physical law, that signal can travel from the source to the receiver at a speed not exceeding the speed of light. In a quantum experiment, on the other hand, a change in one particle can result in an *instantaneous* change in another particle at some distance from the first. This experimentally demonstrable fact establishes nonlocality in the quantum world.

With those illustrations in place, we are ready to return to Bohm's conceptualization of physical reality. He began with a new interpretation of quantum mechanics. A central element of quantum theory is the Schrödinger equation, which is necessary to arrive at the probabilistic solution of a quantum problem. Bohm mathematically transformed this equation into two terms, one of which describes a subatomic particle in the classical scientific sense. The other describes a wavelike term that Bohm called the quantum potential. *Potential* is a common term in classical physics, where it refers to the capacity of energy to move matter. Matter may be an automobile or train, or it may be atomic or subatomic particles moved by electromagnetic energy. We can illustrate with an easily pictured example. Imagine that we drop a stone into a pond. Gravity is the source of kinetic energy that is transferred to the water when the stone enters the water. This energy moves the molecules of the water, creating a series of waves, ripples in the water that spread out in all directions from where the stone enters the pond. These ripples describe a sine wave with troughs and peaks, and as they spread farther from where the stone entered the water, they become smaller and smaller. The potential is represented by the height of the wave and is proportional to the distance from the source of energy.

The quantum potential is quite different from the classical potential in that it does not have a source in the physical world, nor does it force the particle to move. Instead the quantum potential provides information to the electron, information that links it to the whole universe. It is sometimes referred to as a pilot wave in that it guides the particle. Bohm uses the example of a ship guided by radio waves to illustrate the nature of the quantum potential. The radio waves, by which information on how fast or slow to move, or when to turn left or right, provide no power to propel the ship. Instead they provide information to guide the ship, which moves under its own powerful engines. A more familiar current example is the drone plane of the military. It flies under the power of its own engine but is controlled from thousands of miles away by radio waves. In a similar manner, Bohm considers the quantum particle to move under its own energy, guided by the quantum potential. The quantum potential accounts for the wave-particle dual nature of particles and is responsible for the strange phenomena of quantum theory, including the nonlocal character of quantum reality, according to Bohm.

The quantum potential arises from the quantum field. We have envisioned what happens when a stone is dropped into a body of water. Now we will drop two stones in, a few feet apart. Waves go out from each. Some of them intersect with the waves from the other stone. When two peaks or two troughs come together, the wave doubles in amplitude. But if a trough and a peak coincide in the same space, they cancel each other out and the amplitude is zero. This is an example of interference and occurs with other energy waves, such as electromagnetic waves, as well. Now, if we drop a bunch of stones into our pond, many waves are created and they intersect each other in numerous ways, forming very complicated interference patterns. In holography, light waves reflected off the subject meeting the light beam from the laser create a similar complex interference pattern, which is captured on the holographic film plate. In the implicate order, all the quantum potentials intersect with each other, forming what Bohm labels the "quantum field." In this quantum field, *the quantum potential of every particle interacts with the quantum potential of every other particle. This means the quantum potential of any particle is interdependent upon all the particles in the universe.* Everything is thus interconnected with everything else. As a result, we have Bohm's concept of unbroken wholeness. "This view calls into question the validity of a space-time continuum as being the foundation of reality" (Friedman, 1993, p.47).

As we have noted, Bohm hypothesizes that the ultimate reality is a vast sea of energy. Quantum theory indicates that such an energy exists. It is derived from the concept of zero-point energy, the lowest possible energy that a quantum system possesses. Calculations indicate that there is more energy in a cubic centimeter of empty space than there is in the known physical universe. This energy is undetectable by today's instruments because it is of a wavelength too small to be measured by today's instruments. We can only detect wavelengths longer than 10^{-16} cm, although wavelengths as small as 10^{-33} can have meaning. This provides a very wide range of scale in which an immense amount of structure may be waiting to be discovered, Bohm says.

The holograph gave Bohm the concept of enfolding and unfolding. The holographic image roughly corresponds to the explicate order, the holographic plate to the implicate order, and the laser to the implicate order that is necessary for the image to unfold. He paints a picture of an enormous amount of activity as the explicate order unfolds and enfolds from and back into the implicate order continuously while the implicate order unfolds and enfolds into the super-implicate order, the super-implicate similarly interacting with the super-super-implicate order, and so on, for an infinite number of orders. An article by Will Keepin (2008), posted on the Internet by Alex Paterson, offers an analogy that helps depict these relationships. He writes:

> To clarify these concepts with an analogy, consider a video game. The first implicate order corresponds to the screen, which is capable of producing an infinite variety of explicate forms or images. The images on the screen, which constitute the explicate order, can be regarded as manifestations of the first implicate order. The second implicate order corresponds to the computer, which provides the information that organizes the various forms in the screen, or first implicate order. Finally, the player of the game represents a third implicate order [the super-implicate order], whose actions and inputs organize the second implicate order. This creates a closed loop, and creative possibilities can emerge over time.

Bohm summarized his theory of the implicate order in an article on the relationship of mind and matter:

> In this work [*Wholeness and the Implicate Order*], which was originally aimed at understanding relativity and quantum theory on a basis common to both, I developed the notion of the enfolded or implicate order. The essential feature of this idea was that the whole universe is in some way enfolded in everything and that each thing is enfolded in the whole. From this it follows that in some way, and to some degree everything enfolds or implicates everything, but in such a manner that under typical conditions of ordinary experience, there is a great deal

of relative independence of things. The basic proposal is then that this enfoldment relationship is not merely passive or superficial. Rather, it is active and essential to what each thing is. It follows that each thing, is internally related to the whole, and therefore, to everything else. The external relationships are then displayed in the unfolded or explicate order in which each thing is seen, as has already indeed been indicated, as relatively separate and extended, and related only externally to other things. The explicate order, which dominates ordinary experience as well as classical (Newtonian) physics, thus appears to stand by itself. But actually, it cannot be understood properly apart from its ground in the primary reality of the implicate order. (1990, p. 273)

SOMA-SIGNIFICANCE

In *Unfolding Meaning*, Bohm seeks to mend the "Cartesian split," the separation of mind and body initiated by René Descartes in the 17th century, which has pretty much been a doctrine of natural science since. Descartes concluded that mind and body (matter) were different substances that could have no interaction. Although that proclamation seems to defy common sense, materialistic science has widely considered mind and mental activity to be an epiphenomenon of neurological activity, a by-product that does not actually influence the body or matter.

The problem of the relationship of the mental and the physical is further complicated by relativity theory and quantum theory, both of which involve the observer with the observed, eliminating the classical science's position of independence of the observer from the observed. A number of thinkers have been convinced that Descartes was wrong (e.g., Penrose, 1989; Damasio, 1994). Bohm believes that his approach to quantum theory provides a way to understand the relationship between mind and matter that does not reduce one to a function of the other. For him, they are two aspects of the same reality.

Bohm rejected the terminology of mind and body, which he feels fragments what actually is holistic, for the term "soma-significance." *Soma* refers, of course, to the body and by extension to matter, and *significance* is a broader concept that includes meaning as well as substance. Everything, Bohm insisted, from a particle to a galaxy, has both matter and significance.

Bohm introduces the terms *soma-significance* and *signa-somatic* as substitutes for mind and body. Every kind of significance is carried by some kind of somatic arrangement and organization of distinguishable elements. That is to say that meaning is anchored in matter. The words that involve the arrangement and organization of distinguishable letters of the alphabet carry a meaning to the reader just as electrical signals in a television set carry a meaning to a viewer. These meanings are carried somatically by electrochemical processes into the brain, where they are apprehended and unfolded as meanings on a higher level. These in turn generate wider neurological activity, which enfolds and caries meaning to higher intellectual and emotional levels of meaning.

> As this process takes place these meanings, along with their somatic concomitants, become ever more subtle. The world subtle is derived from the Latin sub-texere, signifying woven from underneath, finely woven. The meaning is rarefied, delicate, highly refined, elusive, indefinable, intangible. The subtle may be contrasted with the manifest (which latter means literally what can be held in the hand). The next proposal is then that reality has two further key aspects, the subtle and the manifest, which are closely related to soma and significance. Thus, as has already been pointed out, each somatic form (such as a printed page) carries a meaning. This meaning is clearly more subtle than the form itself. But in turn, such a meaning can be grasped in yet another somatic form; electrical—chemical and other activity in the brain and the rest of the nervous system—which is evidently more subtle than the original somatic form that gave rise to it. This distinction of subtle and manifest is clearly only relative, since what is manifest in one level may be subtle on another. (Bohm, 1985, pp. 74–75)

A television broadcast offers an example. The camera picks up the physical scene and transforms it into more subtle electrical signals. These give form to a still more subtle radio wave that is spread out into space. The wave is detected by an antenna, which converts it back into electrical signals, which go into the receiver and are projected onto a tube to be transformed into a manifest picture. Here we see a content being transformed again and again into ever more subtle levels and then back into more manifest levels. Seen by a viewer, the picture carries a meaning that goes through all the transformations described above.

Both somatic and significance aspects are present in every experience. One does not have meaning unless it is associated with some physical process nor does one have a physical situation that does not have meaning for anyone who experiences it. So far the emphasis has been upon the soma-significance relationship as we have traced changing levels of significance through levels of increasingly subtle soma. Bohm also points out that meaning at a given level actively affects the soma at a more manifest level.

An example is a shadow seen at night. If this suggests an assailant to the one who perceives it, the soma is immediately and directly affected as adrenaline flows; the heartbeat increases and other bodily changes take place. The body prepares to take appropriate action. If, on the other hand, the shadow is seen simply as a shadow, the somatic response is very different. Whatever the meaning of a physical situation is to an individual, that meaning eventually turns into a response that alters some physical aspect of the situation. That may result in alteration of the position of the perceiving individual or some aspect of the situation outside the perceiver.

> From each level of somatic unfoldment of meaning, there is then a further movement leading to activity on to a yet more manifestly somatic level, until the action finally emerges as a physical movement of the body that affects the environment. So one can say that there is a two- way movement of energy, in which each level of significance acts on the next more manifestly somatic level and so on, while perception carries the meaning of the action back in the other direction. (Bohm, 1985, p. 77)
>
> You can see that ultimately the soma-significant and signa-somatic process extends even into the environment. Thus, meaning may be conveyed from one person to another and back through sound waves, through gestures carried by light, through books and newspapers, through telephone, radio, television, etc., linking up the whole of society in one vast web of soma- significant and signa- somatic activity. And similarly, even simple physical action may be said to communicate motion and form to inanimate objects. Most of the material environment in which we live (houses, cities, factories, farms, highways, etc). can thus be described as the somatic result of the ever-changing meaning that material objects have had for human beings over the ages. Going on from here, even relationships with Nature and with the Cosmos are evidently deeply affected by what these mean to us. In turn, such meanings fundamentally affect our actions towards them, and thus indirectly their actions back on us are influenced in a similar way. Indeed, insofar as we know it, are aware of it, and can act in it, the whole of Nature, including our civilization which has evolved from Nature and is still a part of Nature, is one movement that is both soma-significant and signa- somatic. (p. 78)

This back-and-forth movement, enfoldment of significance into the somatic and unfoldment of significance from the somatic, with each continually changing the other, parallels the enfoldment and unfoldment of the implicate and explicate orders. Meaning is unfolded from the somatic and enfolded back into it just as the matter of the explicate order unfolds from the implicate and enfolds back into it. Just as the implicate and explicate order are in continual enfolding and unfolding, so are the somatic and significant.

PARALLELS: IMPLICATE ORDER AND CANON
OF SPONTANEITY-CREATIVITY

We are now ready to look at some of the parallels between Bohm's concepts of the explicate, the implicate and the super-implicate orders, and Moreno's Canon of Spontaneity-Creativity.

For Bohm, the basis of reality is the immense body of energy that includes the implicate order, which is, in Bohm's terms, a generative order. From this is unfolded the universe, the world that we live in and of which we are a part, the explicate order. And, of course, the explicate order includes not only the galaxies, the stars, the planets, and especially planet Earth, but everything on the earth, the continents, the oceans, the plants and animals, and the human species with all its inventions and discoveries, its thoughts, theories, hopes, fears, and dreams. All of these unfold from the implicate order.

In the earlier discussion of the Canon of Spontaneity-Creativity, I pointed out that Moreno's concept of the conserve includes everything that has ever come into existence and everything that will eventually come into being. That includes both things and mental products, such as alphabets, languages, theories, and whatever can be imagined. Moreno's concept of conserve is very much like, if not identical to, Bohm's concept of the explicate order.

The implicate order itself, in which every thing is enfolded in every other thing, is the quantum field from which the explicate order unfolds. It carries the potential for everything that we find in the explicate order, everything that has been unfolded, and everything that will eventually be unfolded.

I have interpreted Moreno's concept of creativity as the potential for becoming. Included are all the conserves that have ever existed plus everything that could have come into existence but didn't or hasn't. Creativity seems to me to be very like Bohm's implicate order.

This leaves the important notion of spontaneity in Moreno's scheme of Spontaneity-Creativity and the super-implicate order from Bohm's theory. And just as the conserve is the result of spontaneity, an "unconservable energy" serving as a catalyst to creativity in the Canon of Spontaneity-Creativity, it is the enfoldment and unfoldment movement between the implicate order and the super-implicate order that results in the explicate order unfolding and enfolding into the implicate order.

This correspondence of the major elements of Moreno's Canon of Spontaneity-Creativity and Bohm's theory of the implicate order is impressive. It suggests that these two scholars, starting from very different points of origin, have discovered essentially an identical theory of reality. Moreno seems to have "received" the Canon of Spontaneity-Creativity during the experience that gave rise to *Words of the Father*. Bohm worked out the notion of the explicate, implicate, and super-implicate orders in a very strict scientific process. And both suggest amazingly parallel systems for understanding how the universe works.

The fact that Bohm's work provides a solid scientific foundation for Moreno's concepts of Spontaneity-Creativity probably makes very little difference to most practitioners of the Morenean methods. For some, however, especially those who come to psychodrama with a strong research background, it is comforting to know that basic Morenean theory can be supported with a theory based on quantum theory—just as Moreno predicted.

HOSTILITY FROM COLLEAGUES

There is another similarity between the work of Bohm and Moreno. Although David Bohm had made significant contributions to physics from the time of his Ph.D. dissertation research, he felt that his identification of the quantum potential was by far his major contribution. He anticipated that the scientific community would receive it with considerable excitement. At the same time, he worried that the major figures of quantum physics might react unfavorably since he had, in fact, defied some of their dictums and had produced something that they had said was impossible, a hidden variables theory. Bohm's fears were realized. His work was variously called "juvenile deviationism," "ingenious, but basically wrong," and "foolish simplicity" by the giants of quantum theory. J. Robert Oppenheimer, who had been Bohm's mentor at one time, is even reported to have said, "if we cannot disprove Bohm, then we must agree to ignore him" (Peat, 1997, p. 133). Not all reactions to Bohm's work were negative, of course. His ideas, especially about thought and its place in the universe, may have gotten more attention from nonphysicists than from his colleagues.

In a recent book, Huston Smith (2001), highly regarded philosopher, relates a revealing experience concerning Bohm and physicist colleagues. A professor of philosophy at Syracuse University, Smith had occasion to invite a distinguished visitor to the campus. His choice was David Bohm. As was politic, he checked with the Physics Department to see if they would approve of him, a philosopher, inviting a physicist to campus. The department declared itself delighted with his choice and only asked that Bohm attend a Physics Department colloquia. Smith relates the following tale of Bohm's visit.

Bohm first gave a presentation for the general public, a presentation that was heavily attended by members of the physics department. The colloquium was two days later. As Smith and Bohm arrived, the chairman of the department pulled Smith aside and told him that he expected that Bohm would not have a very warm reception. It seems that things he had said in the prior presentation had not sat well with the members of the physics department.

There was a huge turnout for the colloquium. After being introduced, Bohm talked, Smith writes, for an hour and a quarter, all the time covering blackboards with what to Smith were "incomprehensible equations." At last he stopped and the chairman asked for questions:

> Instantly the arm of a senior professor in the front row shot up. "Professor Bohm," the questioner said, "this is all very interesting philosophy. But what does it have to do with physics?" I glanced at the solid bank of equations that stared out at us from the blackboards, with not a single *word* in sight. Without batting an eye, Bohm replied, "I do not make that distinction."
>
> A pall fell over the hall. With one or two polite questions, the afternoon ended. (2001, p. 191)

It is curious that the contributions of two extraordinarily creative minds meet with as much rejection as did the theories of Bohm and Moreno. We are accustomed to thinking that people of science are unusually rational and objective. We would expect them to examine novel ideas with skepticism, perhaps, but not hostility.

Moreno provided a sociometric analysis of the development of a science that provides at least a partial answer. Advances in science come from the intuitions of the rare genius. "These men of inspiration do not provide tangible proof for the correctness of their intuitions, they are all based on their authority" (Moreno, 1953c, p. 23). Confirmation is the task of the scientific collective. Moreno developed a kind of sociogram by examining quoting behavior of scientific writers. He selected a group of individuals deemed pioneers in their fields of endeavor. Then he inspected their bibliographies and reference lists and noted all the people that they had quoted. Next he searched the bibliographies and reference lists of these people to see whom they had and had not quoted. Then he constructed sociograms where being quoted equaled attraction, unquoted equaled indifference, and unfavorable or critical reference equaled rejection. He found mutual quotations and chain structures, just as in sociometric testing.

Moreno found that there were positive and negative pair relations with respect to the pioneer. The rest of the individuals fell into two groups, one of which was attracted to the pioneer either directly or more often indirectly through key individuals positively related to the pioneer. Moreno called this creator love. The second group was rejecting of the pioneer, either directly or indirectly through key individuals who were negative toward the pioneer or in the pioneer's disfavor. "A chain reaction produced a social network of negation which might be called antipathy for the pioneer or *creator envy*" (1953c, p. 27). Psychodramatic production, Moreno writes, revealed profound hostility reinforced by key individuals. This hostility resorts in creating a distorted picture of the pioneer and his contributions.

Moreno's depiction is reminiscent of Kuhn's (1962) description of scientific progress. Introduction of a new paradigm is a threat to the existing state of affairs. The initial reaction is rejection and even hostility toward the originator. The new vision slowly gains acceptance as key individuals support it and demonstrate its value.

Part III
The Morenean Methods

7 Group Psychotherapy

J. L. Moreno considered himself the "father" of sociometry, psycho-drama, and group psychotherapy. There have been no serious contend-ers for that honor with respect to sociometry and psychodrama, but Moreno shares the title of originator of group psychotherapy with sev-eral others. The most frequently mentioned in this respect is Joseph H. Pratt, MD, based on his work with tuberculosis patients in 1905 (1917/1963). Moreno's claim has to do with his group work with the prostitutes of Vienna in 1913. It is also widely accepted that Moreno coined the terms *group therapy* and *group psychotherapy*. Curiously, neither man was involved with psychiatric patients or psychiatry when they conducted the work for which they are credited with originating group psychotherapy.

Pratt was a compassionate Boston physician who was concerned about poor tuberculosis patients who could not afford hospital treatment, the standard at that time. Pratt developed a home treatment plan for these patients in 1905. The program that Pratt (1917/1963) called "the tuber-culosis class" was based on a strict rest cure. This meant that patients were to spend their entire day in the recumbent position until their symptoms went away. The patient's bed or cot was preferably placed outside. In reporting on his program, Pratt notes that patients without fever were allowed to get up for meals. The treatment plan also included home visits by a nurse, a record of daily life details maintained by the patient, and attendance by the patients at a weekly meeting, the one time that patients were allowed to break their strict rest. It was the weekly meeting component of the program that gave rise to the claim that Dr. Pratt was a pioneer in group therapy. At this meeting, each patient was weighed, temperature and pulse recorded, and gains in weight posted on a blackboard. A notable feature of the meet-ing was that patients who had made great gains in the program often testi-fied to the effectiveness of the rest treatment. Pratt noted that the meetings uplifted and maintained the morale of his patients. He believed that the class meetings were responsible for helping the patients stick to the strict demands of his rest treatment. Later Pratt became interested in psychiatry and an article by him on treatment of psychosomatic disease was published in *Sociometry* in 1945.

The story of Moreno and the prostitutes of Vienna has already been related in Chapter 2 of this book. In his encounter on the street with a prostitute who was arrested, Moreno found himself confronted with the fact that there was a whole class of people who were socially ostracized because of their profession, even though that same culture created a strong demand for their services. He was angry at what he witnessed, he said, and he may have been especially moved by his new acquaintance's uncontested acceptance of the injustice that had just been handed to her by the policeman who arrested her. She apparently submitted to the judgment of society that she was unworthy of social acceptance and of being treated fairly.

Touched by the unfairness of how prostitutes were treated, Moreno reacted in a typically Morenean way (that some have called megalomaniacal) and took it upon himself do something about the situation. He persuaded his new acquaintance to call together a group of her fellow prostitutes to meet with him, a sympathetic doctor, and newspaper editor to seek answers to the many problems they faced because of their profession. With the help of Moreno, the doctor, and the editor, the group members focused at first on the practical problems of being prostitutes. Lawyers who would represent them and doctors who would treat them were found. Eventually Moreno was able to establish many small groups of 8 to 10 women in which they discussed their problems and solutions to them. Eventually, Moreno tells us, they realized that they could help each other. They started a common relief fund to deal with emergencies that one of their members might encounter. Most importantly, meeting with each other and discussing their problems and experiences ameliorated the feelings of worthlessness and helplessness that they experienced. Morale was tremendously improved among the women.

The small groups interacted with each other so that information and assistance spread through the entire community. In due course they developed a real organization with elected officers. At the end of 1913, the prostitutes held a mass meeting in one of the largest halls in Vienna. "It was one of my early efforts at applying group therapy to one of the most difficult of human problems, that of prostitution," Moreno wrote (1989a, p. 49).

Moreno's concept of group therapy was the treatment of a group of people, marginalized or excluded, and unfairly treated in society. His position was that in addition to improving the conditions of the target population, treatment of these groups was therapeutic for society at large. The superdynamic community that he envisioned in his statement of his personal philosophy was one in which all members were given an opportunity to make the best of what they were capable. One of his mantras was "every man the therapist of every other man; every group the therapist of every other group."

APPLICATION OF THE GROUP METHOD TO CLASSIFICATION

It is a well-established fact that Moreno coined the terms *group therapy* and *group psychotherapy* in 1931 and 1932, in conjunction with a project aimed at devising a method for the therapeutic organization of a prison population. The project was conducted at Sing Sing, a federal penitentiary, and resulted in a monograph entitled *Application of the Group Method to Classification* (Moreno & Whitin, 1932). Moreno later republished this work in *The First Book on Group Psychotherapy* (1957a). The story of this event is of interest not only because it was the occasion when the terms *group therapy* and *group psychotherapy* were first used, but because the project can be viewed as both a success and a failure. It was a success in that the project gave Moreno a chance to express many of his ideas about the nature of human interaction and the importance of the group on its members' actions. The project was also successful in stimulating interest in group psychotherapy. This was attributable in large part to the wide publicity that the project received because two influential organizations, the American Psychiatric Association and the National Committee on Prisons and Prison Labor, were involved in the project. It can be considered a failure because the plan for organization of a prison population was never implemented, probably for practical reasons that we will discuss later.

The story begins in 1931 when the American Psychiatric Association invited the National Committee on Prisons and Prison Labor to present a roundtable discussion in conjunction with the association's annual meeting. The National Committee on Prisons and Prison Labor was an organization dedicated to introducing innovations in penology and criminology. The invitation reflected a growing interest among psychiatrists in the problems in these fields. Moreno's work with the prostitutes in Vienna and with the dysfunctional Mitterndorf community had come to the attention of certain National Committee officials and he was asked to present his ideas at this roundtable conference.

The problems of classification and assignment, how to organize a prison's population, were the specific issues that the penologists presented in the hope that psychiatry could provide better ways than the ones they were practicing. The prevailing stratagems were usually based on homogeneity and involved classifying and assigning prisoners on some individual category, such as the seriousness of the crime, race, age, and so on. One widely applied approach, for example, called for identifying inmates as psychopathic delinquent, insane delinquent, defective delinquent, or normal prisoner. Prisoners were then placed together with those of the same diagnosis, either in a section of a prison or in different institutions. The penologists thought that there must be more effective means for the organization of inmates.

In his presentation at the roundtable conference, Moreno suggested that it would be possible to transform a prison system into a socialized community by the assignment of inmates into small groups based on interpersonal characteristics. These small groups, he maintained, would have a positive socializing effect on the inmates, would reduce recidivism, and would also decrease administrative problems for the prison staff. He had in mind creating in the prison community something similar to what he had accomplished in the community of prostitutes in Vienna.

Moreno's plan was received with much interest. As a result of his suggestions, and with the collaboration of E. Stagg Whitin, chairman of the executive council of the National Committee on Prisons and Prison Labor, Moreno was invited by the New York State Department of Corrections to conduct research on his ideas at Sing Sing prison. The results were to be presented at the following year's annual meeting of the American Psychiatric Association.

With the assistance of Helen Jennings, a graduate student of social psychology at Columbia University, Moreno set out to develop the plan that he envisioned. Their research resulted in the monograph entitled *Application of the Group Method of Classification* (Moreno & Whitin, 1932). Moreno added Whitin's name to the paper as a political move even though Whitin apparently had taken little part in the research or in writing the report. The monograph was published and sent to a number of psychiatrists, psychologists, and prominent figures in the field of corrections for their reactions. It was then presented at a second roundtable discussion at the 1932 annual meeting of the American Psychiatric Association.

The monograph begins with a reiteration of the plan that Moreno presented to the first roundtable discussion in 1931. The objective, he states, "is to suggest how it would be possible to transform the promiscuous, unorganized prison system into a socialized community through a method of assignment of prisoners to social groups" (1957a, p. 7). These groups or units were to be formed on the basis of a social analysis and are distinct unities. That is, all the activities, such as housekeeping, labor, recreation, and other social activities, were carried out together by the group members. The units were organized by first designating a leader. Characteristics to be sought in the leader were father qualities, intellectual maturity, experience, and character development. Successful performance in open society and being socially minded were also important in the leader. After the leader was selected, men who were best fitted to him were assigned to the leader's group. How those men were fitted to one another was then given consideration. "Mental type, sexual characteristics, social kinship, racial traits, former performances, criminal record, [and] actual observations of behavior in prison" (p. 8) were among the items to be examined in making assignments. Although they functioned as entities, group membership was not rigid and a group member could be transferred to another group if that turned out to be desirable.

The major part of the monograph describes a remarkably complicated system to form the groups. It began with gathering the information on the prisoners in the penitentiary files of which there was a considerable amount. Moreno selected 21 items to use for assignment and arranged them into four categories called "complexes." These were: the Nationality and Social Complex; the Educational and Vocational Complex; the Intelligence and Personality Complex; and the Delinquency and Criminal Complex. In addition to the information in the files, Moreno conducted a spontaneity test with each individual involved in the research and classified each as either "spontaneous reaction type" or "conserving reaction type." Forty-seven men comprised the initial pool of candidates for the project. From these, the monograph reports on the formation of a single group, Group I, of seven inmates.

The information from the files was entered into a chart for each person. The charts were then compared with each other to ascertain the "fit" of the individuals to each other. Although it is not specifically specified in the monograph, it seems likely that one inmate was selected to be the leader of Group I, and that his chart was compared with the remaining 46 individuals from which six were picked to make up the group. The charts for each member of Group I are included in the monograph.

Moreno identified eight forms of interrelationship: full, partial, complementary, discordant, similar, contrasting, active, and indifferent. Next, the charts were compared with each other and the 22 items in each chart scored in terms of the form of relationship indicated. Table XI in the monograph is reproduced in Table 7.1 and shows the comparison of the charts of Man 1 and Man 2, with the identification of the form of interrelationship between them.

In the Nationality and Social Complex we find that the age of Man 1 is 35 and the age of Man 2 is 25. This is scored as both "complementary" and "contrasting." Sex and race are scored as both "full" and "indifferent." Since both men are heterosexual males and of the white race, it is anticipated that these characteristics will not play an active role in how they relate to each other. The nationality item is considered "contrasting" as one is Jewish and the other Irish-Scotch, but the fact that both are sons of immigrants gets identified as "similar." At the bottom of the complex, there is a tally of the scores and the complex is scored "contrasting" since there are more contrasts than other forms of interrelationships.

Table 7.1   Table XI from *The First Book on Group Psychotherapy*

MAN 1.	Full	Partial	Complementary	Discordant	Similar	Contrasting	Active	Indifferent	MAN 2.
Data NS									Data NS
Age, 35		x				x			Age, 25
Male heterosexual	x							x	Male heterosexual
White	x							x	White
Hebrew						x			Irish-Scotch
American born									American born
Son of Rus. immigrants			x						Son of Irish-Scotch immigrants
Oldest son of seven children									One of six children; at five,
Lived with parents up to									Father died; at ten, step-father.
Offense, supports them						x			See juvenile data in DC Complex
Neighborhood, Jewish					x				Syracuse, N. Y.; Brooklyn,
									Irish Neighborhood.
	2	1	1		4			2	NS—Contrasting
Data EV									Data EV
Language, English					x				Language, English
Religion, Jewish						x			Religion, Catholic
Education, grad. 8th Gr.					x				Junior High School, 1 year
Vocation, mechanic, machines					x				Baker
Occupation, U. S. Army									
and Marine Service									U. S. Army
Manager, cashier, poolroom					x				Animal trainer
In Service 9 years, hon. disc.									In Service 1½ years
In first position 4 years					x				In one position 4 years
									Single, quarrels with step-
Home—single, with parents					x				father
Associates, gamblers, marines						x			Show people
					6	2			EV—Similar
Data IP									Data IP
Mental Age, 14½					x				Mental Age, 14½
Cooperative, responsive									Quiet, shy
Good mixer, energetic									Poor mixer
Sympathetic									Solitaire
Spontaneous reaction type			x						Conserving reaction type
Social habits, moderate									
alcoholic, gambler					x				Gambling on horse races
			1		2				IP—Complementary
Data DC									Data DC
									At 11, Industrial School;
Delinquency record up to									At 15, House of Refuge
offense, clear									(2 yrs.)
First offender						x			First offender
Offense, forgery						x			Burglary, 3rd degree
Sentence, 2½-5 years									Sentence, 5-10 years
Parole case					x				Parole case
Behavior in prison, no									Behavior in prison, no com-
complaints recorded					x				plaint recorded
					2	2			DC—Contrasting

The process calls for each person to be compared with each of the others. For the seven men of the group, this would require 21 such comparisons. The monograph, however, includes only the interrelationship comparisons of Man 1 with the six other men chosen to be Group I. It appears that Man 1 is the individual selected to be the leader of Group I.

The information in the charts is now analyzed to predict the possible influences that each item in the chart might have on the relationship between the two men. Only one analysis is presented in the monograph, probably for the purpose of economy, as the analysis is eight pages long. That analysis is called a double analysis, and Moreno indicates that triple analyses and group analyses are possible. It is implied that such multiple comparisons may have been made.

The analysis of the charts of Man 1 with Man 2 indicate that this is a comparatively subjective process heavily dependent upon the experience, knowledge, and assumptions of the analyst. With respect to the age difference between Man I and Man 2, for example, Moreno anticipates that because other attributes in the relationship are complementary, the age difference will push the younger man to regard the older as a leader and a model of behavior. But, he adds, "this holds only if discordant relations between two persons are not marked" (1957a, p. 47). Moreno also opined that the contrasting nationalities of the two men should be advantageous rather than disparaging for their relationship. His rationale is that "contrast of nationality, if it is sufficiently wide (as between Irish and Jews or between Irish and Italians, but not too wide as between Italian and Japanese, or too narrow as between English and Irish) stimulates curiosity and reciprocal enrichment if a sufficient number of other factors are similar or complementary" (p. 49). And so it goes for each of the 22 items in the chart. Sometimes they received only a line. Education is dealt with by a score of similar and the sentence: "Both received public school training" (p. 53). Others, like family situation, get several paragraphs of discussion.

Moreno was in all probability overly optimistic when he wrote that the process of grouping and coordination had been simplified to such an extent that a psychiatrist could economically implement it with a small staff especially trained for that purpose. The procedures required to carry out the plan appear to require many hours of meticulous work and someone with incredible insight into human nature to establish each group. It is hard to imagine how much effort would be required to fulfill Moreno's vision of a prison organized into these small groups that were expected to have a positive socializing effect upon the members.

REACTION TO APPLICATION OF THE GROUP METHOD TO CLASSIFICATION

Application of the Group Method of Classification was then disseminated to a number of professionals interested in prisons and corrections for their comments. This group included many of the people who had attended the initial roundtable conference. Their reactions were largely positive although many of them could be described as cautiously positive. They expressed praise for the ideas upon which the plan was based and expressed hope that it could be implemented. Some liked the approach but wondered if it was workable and if it would cost too much in terms of the services of psychiatrists and psychologists. Others found that existing conditions, such as the architecture of prisons and the huge numbers of prisoners, would present major problems in utilization of the method. There were recommendations that it should first be tried out in institutions that made use of cottage structures.

The second roundtable discussion was held on May 31,1932, during the meeting of the American Psychiatric Association. It was entitled "A Conference on the Group Method" and was moderated by Dr. William Allison White, the highly respected superintendent of St. Elizabeth Hospital. One of White's characteristics was that of discovering and promoting new ideas in the field of psychiatry. He was a strong supporter of J. L. Moreno and Moreno's contributions to the field. Some 85 people were in attendance at the conference.

Dr. White called on 14 participants to comment on the *Application of the Group Method of Classification*. Most of the speakers expressed positive feelings about the intention of the method—and then added serious reservations about practicality of implementation. Dr. White himself was favorable in his introductory comments and sometimes reframed and softened comments by participants when they were unfavorable toward the report. There was one absolutely negative reaction from Dr. Benjamin Karpman, a well-known psychiatrist and prolific author in the field of psychiatry. He began his comments by saying:

> How can a physician have come to the group notion? I do not understand. The group method arises as a compromise as we cannot afford the other, the individual method. The only way to secure results is by a complete individual study and if we have that then we will not need the group method. Also it is known that prisoners get along very well with other prisoners anyway. (Moreno, 1957a, p. 122)

The moderator finally called upon Moreno to respond to the discussion. "I am confident that he will be able to answer all questions and to wind up the discussion to the satisfaction of all" (p. 125). Moreno responded by conducting a sociometric analysis of the roundtable discussion. He suggested that the situation could be construed as a spontaneity test with those participating in the discussion not knowing what others would say, yet influenced by the attitudes of other speakers. He commented on how the personality of a speaker guided what that speaker said but was simultaneously influenced by the role the speaker played in the overall event. He credited White with being a good and strong leader whose role as moderator of the conference was responsible for the large number of attendees of the roundtable. He praised White for maintaining the dignity and moderation of attitude that was necessary for the discussion of such a difficult subject as group therapy. "He prevented ridicule which so often finishes attempts of pioneering" (p. 127). White, he said, was the center of sympathy. But, Moreno added, there was another center toward which feelings were directed, only in the opposite direction:

> He is also a center, but he may be the center of resentments and repulsions, not a center of attractions. He is undesired like a solitaire, but he has a certain distinction: he is the prototype of the unwanted individual who attempts to impose something upon a group that is by its very nature critical and suspicious towards him as towards anyone who assumes authority before the reason for it is fully demonstrated. This person is, you may have guessed, myself. (p. 129)

It is clear from Moreno's words that he felt much stronger rejection from the contributors to the roundtable than the printed words of the discussants communicate. He was obviously discouraged and felt that his ideas had not been truly understood or accepted. Moreno writes that it was after this meeting that Dr. White told him that he would first attract sociologists, then social psychologists. After that, White said, the general physicians and plain people would come along. But, White added, Moreno would not live to see group psychotherapy accepted by psychiatrists.

Moreno gives us no indication that the group method was ever put into effect in a prison setting. We can believe, however, that if it were and if it were successful, we would have heard about it and it might be in use today. The only follow-up to the Sing Sing project that I have found is in a book by Helen Hall Jennings, published in 1943, 11 years after the second roundtable conference. Jennings, referring to the Sing Sing project, wrote, "it became apparent that adult institutional groups could not be made therapeutically effective as functional units on the basis of attributes of individual members" (1943, pp. 9–10). No matter how much personal attributes were complementary or similar to those of another, they did not act that way when the two individuals who possessed them were placed together, Jennings said. In his classification work, Moreno had left out the important ingredient for people to get along together: subjective attraction to each other. Perhaps the most important result of the group method of assignment was that Moreno was introduced to Fanny French Morse, superintendent of the New York State Training School for Girls at Hudson. Impressed by his ideas, she invited him to use the institution she led as his research site.

THE FIRST BOOK ON GROUP PSYCHOTHERAPY

In 1957, the 25th anniversary of the second roundtable discussion, Moreno republished *Application of the Group Method to Classification* as part of a book entitled *The First Book on Group Psychotherapy, 1932.* The title page also lists it as "3rd Edition, 1957." It was dedicated to the International Committee of Group Psychotherapy, an organization that he had initiated six years earlier. This book is composed of several parts: the original proposal presented by Moreno at the 1931 roundtable; the monograph *Application of the Group Method to Classification*; the comments of reviewers to whom the monograph was sent; and the comments of speakers at the second roundtable in 1932. This material is bracketed between an Introduction presented in the form of an interview of Moreno by an instructor who has supposedly discussed the monograph in a seminar. The tome closes with a postscript that continues the dialogue initiated in the Introduction. It is my opinion that Moreno played the roles both of interviewer and himself in these pages, using the format of interview as a device to share his thoughts about group psychotherapy issues. The 32 questions cover a wide range of topics and provide an opportunity for Moreno to opine on many issues.

In this introduction, Moreno established that *Application of the Group Method to Classification* is the first book on group psychotherapy and the first publication of the terms *group therapy* and *group psychotherapy*. When he came to America, he explains, "therapy of the group was uppermost in my mind as the next step towards moving psychotherapy forward" (1957, p. viii). The rapid success of group psychotherapy, he proposes, was because of a favorable mental climate, unlike in Europe, where it failed to take root. A second factor, he claims, was that his proposal was based on scientific grounds. A third factor was ascribed to the National Committee on Prison and Prison Labor, along with the New York State Department of Correction and the American Psychiatric Association: "These forces spread the idea among strategic people and stimulated experiments in many places. They established the first high point in the organized development of group psychotherapy" (p. x).

The most important ideas in this introduction are Moreno's answers to questions that give him an opportunity to express his basic ideas about group psychotherapy. Every group has a unique structure and varies with respect to cohesion and depth, and that structure can be explored scientifically. Psychodrama can reveal depth dimensions and allow group members to recognize the invisible interactions going on between group members. Effective therapy is based on the therapist being aware of group members' interactions with each other as well as with him. And "the locus of the therapeutic influence is in the *group* rather than in the *therapist*" (p. xi). He underscores this principle, pointing out that in individual therapy, patient and therapist roles are fixed. The patient is always the patient; the therapist is the only therapist. In group psychotherapy, on the other hand, the group members can function as "auxiliary therapists" for each other. "It is the relationship among the individuals of the group, the *principle of therapeutic interaction,* in which the autonomy of the participating individual is not lost" (p. xii). Of course, Moreno notes, interaction may be contra-therapeutic as well as therapeutic. The task for the group leader is to create the therapeutically organized group.

In response to a question about the extent to which this principle is accepted, Moreno answers that it has become the common denominator of all varieties of group therapy, either openly or tacitly. This answer seems to be overly optimistic. Although it was certainly true at the time that some entities, such as the National Training Laboratories, were indeed involved with interactions of members of small groups, much of group psychotherapy in clinical settings and the mental health field in 1957 revolved around the interaction of the therapist with the individuals in the group. As Moreno sometimes said, they were conducting individual psychotherapy in a group setting rather than group psychotherapy. In the postscript with which Moreno concludes this book, he offers a justification of his position by an analysis of the group psychotherapy literature.

Moreno also minimizes differences among the many different orientations in the group psychotherapy field. He states that many of the apparent differences of different methods are merely semantic, caused by group workers using different terms for the same operations or the same terms with different meanings. Too much emphasis is placed on differences and too little on what is common to the various methods. He lists as some of these commonalities: free spontaneous interaction among the members; the extemporaneous character of a production; the emphasis on natural dialogue; interaction analysis and measurement; the importance of composition of groups; the cathartic value of acting out and interacting out among members; and the treatment of conflict through analysis and role playing. These, of course, are characteristics of psychodramatic group psychotherapy, but few other group modalities make use of all of them. Moreno may be expressing what he would like to be true to a greater extent than the situation that actually existed.

Toward the end of this introduction to *The First Book on Group Psychotherapy*, Moreno lays out what he considers "some general principles of group psychotherapy." These are:

1. The principle of therapeutic interaction.
2. The principle of production in the here and now, "the moment not a part of history but history part of the moment" (p. xx).
3. The principle of spontaneity and improvisation.
4. The principle of acting out, "therapeutic acting out in contrast to irrational acting out" (p. xx).
5. Actional communication is learned prior to verbal communication and often more dependable.
6. Analysis is based upon the ongoing production, not upon anything that has happened before the session took place.
7. The principle of the family situation and family catharsis in the genesis of group structure.

8. The principle of "working out" in contrast with the "working through" of the psychoanalyst.
9. The principle of integrated catharsis in contrast with abreaction catharsis.
10. Tape-recording and playback and their value in objectifying and conserving group process.
11. Interaction diagrams of therapeutic groups enabling the systematic analysis and measurement of spontaneous interaction.

Finally Moreno writes that republication of the monograph gives him the opportunity to clarify the relations between group psychotherapy and psychoanalysis:

> Freudianism represented the strongest obstacle to group psychotherapy [in 1932]. Within the last 25 years a growing reorientation and interstimulation of group theory and psychoanalysis theory has taken place. Many workers who have come to group psychotherapy from psychoanalysis, for instance Sergei Libovici (1956a, 1956b) and Nathan Ackerman (1949), symbolize a constructive mediation of the two positions. It appears quite clear that sociometry and psychodrama have been instrumental in facilitating the critical rapprochement. (p. xxiv)

Furthermore, republication gives Moreno a chance to compare his position in 1931 with his position in 1956. "It has changed radically. In 1932, as a pioneer must, I was over involved with my own ideas." Today, he says, he is concerned with the entire field of psychotherapy in all its forms. "Therapeutic thinking is spreading all over the globe: therapeutic society is the common goal, reverberating the opening sentence of *Who Shall Survive?* 'A truly therapeutic procedure cannot have less an objective than the whole of mankind'" (p. xxiv).

After the presentation of the material from 1931 and 1932, Moreno concludes *The First Book on Group Psychotherapy* with a brief section entitled "Postscript 1956." The format of this section continues the interaction with the instructor/interviewer from the introduction. The postscript is largely an analysis of publications on group psychotherapy listed in a bibliography compiled by Corsini and Putzey (1956), published in Moreno's journal, *Group Psychotherapy*. Several categories are discussed and conclusions drawn. For example, there are three times as many articles on interactive methods (psychodrama, Adlerian therapy, family therapy, therapeutic clubs, milieu therapy, and roundtable methods) as there are noninteractional approaches (client centered, bibliotherapy, psychoanalytic group psychotherapy). The types of institutions in which group psychotherapy is mentioned in the literature include mental hospitals, military institutions, schools, religious groups, and industry. There are, however, no listings for prisons, the kind of institution that is the subject of *The First Book on Group Psychotherapy*. The analysis of the bibliography also reveals that group psychotherapy has, by this time, been applied to many problems: psychosis, delinquency, psychosomatic ailments, alcoholism, neurosis, speech disorders, mental deficiency, obesity, geriatrics, marriage, tuberculosis, and physical handicaps.

Any active psychodramatist or group psychotherapist can probably confirm Moreno's final comments. As important as the literature is, Moreno claims, it has not played as important a role in the expansion of group psychotherapy as another factor:

> The greatest forces, especially in the therapeutic arts, are not writings but personal influence, example and demonstration. . . . The thousands of seminars and sessions demonstrating group psychotherapy and group psychodrama which my associates and I have run in the course of 40 years have had more to do with the present success of these ideas than all our writings put together. It is very difficult to put in written form the group experiences which take place in actual sessions. (p. 136)

There is an epilogue. After publishing *The First Book on Group Psychotherapy*, Moreno sent copies of it to members of the 1932 roundtable discussion and asked them for their comments. Moreno then published eight responses that he had received in an article entitled "Twenty-Fifth Anniversary of Group Psychotherapy Meeting in Philadelphia in 1932." The responses were quite positive and congratulatory. Moreno's originality and creativity were noted and many confirmed that group psychotherapy has proven itself as a valuable instrument in schools, correctional institutions, in work with adolescents, and with mental health. Their comments clearly documented that group psychotherapy had arrived.

By the time that the second roundtable discussion was held, Moreno had been appointed as research director at the New York Training School for Girls at Hudson, where he conducted the work that became the empirical basis of sociometry, the subject of the next chapter of this book. His publications for the next several years have to do with sociometric issues. At the training school, he continued to make use of assignment as a means of group therapy. The aims were the same, the improvement of the situation for both individual and group, but with the addition of sociometric techniques, assignments were much more finely tuned than had been possible in his original attempts at assignment therapy.

EMBRACING THE GROUP PSYCHOTHERAPY MOVEMENT

The other men, in addition to Pratt and Moreno, who are usually identified as originators of group psychotherapy include E. W. Lazell, L. Cody Marsh, and Trigant Burrow. Rosenbaum and Berger (1963) discuss their contributions at length, as does Zerka Moreno (1966a). The work of these men with respect to group therapy took place before 1930. However, it was not until World War II that the practice of group psychotherapy became common. Group work burgeoned then because of the many psychiatric casualties that occurred among servicemen during the war. The numbers were far too great for psychiatrists in the services and those in the Veterans Administration Hospitals to treat individually. Group psychotherapy seemed to offer the only economic solution and it was adopted mainly for economic reasons. For many years and even today many individual practitioners consider individual psychotherapy to be superior to group psychotherapy, and group psychotherapy to be a second choice necessary for economic reasons.

In the years following World War II, several other important changes took place in the mental health field. The number of clinical psychologists and psychiatric social workers grew markedly. At the same time as these non-physician-trained practitioners entered the field, and perhaps because of them, new psychotherapeutic methods began to develop. An enterprising compiler published a survey of more than 250 "newer methods" of psychotherapy (Herink, 1980). Many of the established methods developed group adaptations of the theories upon which they were constructed.

Moreno's concept of group therapy differed from the earlier approaches as well as from those emerging in the postwar world. Moreno's idea of group psychotherapy meant treating the group; other group therapists remained focused on the individual, and their methods could often be better described as treating individuals in a group setting. Individual psychotherapy, Moreno pointed out, is based on the psychodynamics of the individual. The treatment of a group is based on the sociodynamics that involve the interrelationships and interactions of the members of the group, not just the collection of individuals and their personal dynamics. According to Moreno, treatment of groups became possible only after the development of sociometry, which allows the group therapist to identify and characterize the constellation of relationships existing within a group.

Moreno differentiated between natural groups and synthetic ones. By natural groups, he meant groups as they are found naturally in society. Families, neighborhoods, religious and civic organizations, or a community are examples of natural groups. Most group psychotherapy, however, involves synthetic groups, groups that are formed especially for the purpose of group therapy. They are composed of members whose life paths would otherwise not be likely to cross. Moreno preferred to work with natural groups, although much of his group work actually involved synthetic groups.

Beacon Hill Sanitarium, later renamed the Moreno Institute, came into existence in 1936, and Moreno began the systematic development of psychodrama with psychiatric patients, many of whom were psychotic. Initially, he treated patients in individual sessions—although his use of sanitarium staff members as auxiliary egos made these sessions technically group sessions. He soon discovered the value of psychodrama sessions with groups of patients, even those who were psychotic. The psychodramatic method was added to Moreno's credentials and before long professional mental health workers began coming to training seminars at the Moreno Institute.

As Moreno's fame spread and the need for group psychotherapy became recognized, Moreno made use of the prestige that he had acquired to become a leading figure in the field of group psychotherapy. As the demand for group psychotherapy grew, he received many invitations from the Veterans Administration and state psychiatric hospitals to lecture and demonstrate his methods. Moreno was also invited to conduct seminars at a number of universities. In 1945, Moreno published *Group Psychotherapy: A Symposium.* Thirty-one papers by 34 authors were included (1945b). The articles were classified in 10 categories and, in addition to the headings of Analytic Group Methods, Psychodramatic Methods, and Sociodrama, these included Lecture Methods, Musical Methods, Dance Methods, and Motion Picture Methods. Among the authors were E. W. Lazell and J. H. Pratt, representing class methods.

The group psychotherapy movement spread to other countries, and Moreno was invited by the Tavistock Clinic in England to introduce his new methods in 1951. In the next few years, Moreno, in his role as an international leader in group psychotherapy and accompanied by his wife and collaborator, Zerka T. Moreno, visited many other countries, including France, Germany, Austria, the Netherlands, and Russia. Moreno instigated the establishment of the International Committee of Group Psychotherapy in France in 1951. An advisory board listed physicians from England, Strasbourg, France, and the United States and included group pioneers E. W. Lazell and J. H. Pratt. The committee was assigned with three objectives. The first was to define the professional standards of group psychotherapy and to work toward a consensus of terms, operations, and facts. In addition, the committee was to prepare for the First International Congress of Group Psychotherapy, to be conducted in 1952, and to establish an International Journal of Group Psychotherapy. The committee held its first meeting in France but the First International Congress was not held until 1954, in Toronto.

In 1957, the International Committee became the International Council of Group Psychotherapy during the Second International Congress of Group Psychotherapy in Zürich (Moreno, 1966b) and a proposal was made to establish an International Society of Group Psychotherapy. Although the council readily adopted the proposal, it was not until 1973 that the International Association of Group Psychotherapy (IAGP) came into being with J. L. Moreno and S. H. Foulkes the cofounders, and J. L. Moreno as the first president. Today the IAGP has 55 organizational affiliates from 28 countries (IAGP Affiliates, 2013).

The International Handbook of Group Psychotherapy (Moreno, 1966b) promises to provide a "complete and unique guide" to the present status of the group psychotherapy movement in 51 countries. The book contains 124 contributions by more than 150 authors in four languages. It addresses the practice of group psychotherapy "in mental hospitals, prisons and reformatories, family and marriage, in the treatment of alcoholics and drug addicts, delinquents, and sexual offenders," according to the cover flap. It is a massive tome of more than 700 pages and certainly lives up to the promises of the cover and then some. The contributions are distributed among 21 different sections, each covering a different aspect of group psychotherapy.

THE AMERICAN SOCIETY OF GROUP PSYCHOTHERAPY AND PSYCHODRAMA

In 1942, Moreno thought that there was enough interest and enthusiasm to organize the Society for Psychodrama and Group Psychotherapy, later renamed the American Society of Group Psychotherapy and Psychodrama (and referred to as the ASGPP). It may be that Moreno had hoped to attract practitioners of methods of group psychotherapy other than psychodrama. Regardless, the society has always centered predominantly on psychodrama and is the professional organization for psychodramatists. Of course, by the time that the society was established, psychodrama was practiced and considered primarily as a group method. Membership in the society was open to anyone and everyone who was interested in the psychodrama method and in supporting the aims of the society. No professional credentials or training were required for membership and membership was not required to attend the annual meetings of the ASGPP. These yearly events featured papers on method and theory as well as demonstrations of psychodrama and psychodramatic techniques.

With a few exceptions, the annual meetings of the society were held in New York City. By the 1960s, when the Human Potential Movement was at its highest level of activity, a large group of New Yorkers who displayed no other interest in psychodrama looked forward to attending these annual events, often contending for the privilege of becoming protagonists in demonstration sessions.

Another group, the American Group Therapy Association, was established in 1943, a year after Moreno founded the Society for Psychodrama and Group Psychotherapy, and was incorporated in 1952 as the American Group Psychotherapy Association (AGPA). S. R. Slavson, who was interested in progressive education and had persuaded the Jewish Board of Guardians to establish creative activity groups for maladjusted children, initiated the association. The project became referred to as group therapy and Slavson was appointed as Chairman of the Department of Group Therapy for the Jewish Board of Guardians. Unlike the ASGPP, the AGPA stressed professional credentials. Eligible for membership were psychiatrists with three years of psychotherapeutic experience and psychologists and psychiatric social workers with three years of psychotherapeutic experience. Qualifications for membership were a frequent issue for discussion (Historical Committee, 1971).

The founders of the two organizations, Moreno and Slavson, engaged in an undignified mudslinging feud for several years. Among the issues was Moreno's contention that Slavson had not recognized his pioneering work in group therapy despite the fact that Slavson had attended Moreno's presentations of Impromptu at Carnegie Hall and had indeed been a protagonist in a spontaneity test. Slavson suggested that Moreno was not the true creator of psychodrama but had taken the work of a Danish psychiatrist and presented it as Moreno's own. Both organizations are active at the writing of this book. Attempts over the years at bringing them closer together have not had much success.

TREATMENT OF A NATURAL GROUP

A case study that Moreno published in an early issue of *Sociometry* illustrates many of Moreno's ideas about group therapy and the treatment of a natural group—even though he does not refer to it as group psychotherapy (Moreno, 1937a). A woman sought Moreno's help, "suffering from hysterical attacks, suicidal ideas, and insomnia (p. 11)." Her complaint was that her husband had lost affection for her and had a new lover. It became clear, Moreno states, that if her husband would give up the lover and restore his affections for the patient, most of her symptoms would disappear. She asked Moreno to see the husband and persuade him to return to her. The husband agreed to see Moreno, who discovered that he also was disturbed by the situation, so worried that he found it hard to do his work, was afraid of losing his job, and had even made a suicide attempt. Moreno was able to give the husband information about his wife of which he was unaware. Upon seeing the wife again, Moreno was able to give her new information about him. He continued to have alternating appointments with the two and then saw them together. In the meantime, the wife had asked Moreno to see the husband's lover and persuade her to give up the relationship with the husband. Again Moreno found the third person of the little group to be suffering emotionally from the situation. The woman was depressed, had withdrawn from social activities, and exhibited some phobias. Working with the husband and wife, Moreno was able to help them reach an amicable agreement to divorce and the husband married the lover. The psychiatric symptoms of all three of the people involved in the triangle were ameliorated.

THE THIRD PSYCHIATRIC REVOLUTION

The 1940s turned out to be a fertile seedbed for group psychotherapy. The Moreno training programs in both Beacon and New York were active. The psychiatric needs of American soldiers in the World War II stimulated an extensive need for group psychotherapy. Students of Kurt Lewin established the National Training Laboratory for Group Development, all of whom had attended sociometry and psychodrama training seminars at the Moreno Institute. Carl Rogers and his students were applying the techniques of Carl Rogers's nondirective counseling to groups. Alcoholics Anonymous, begun in 1935 by Bill Wilson, employed Moreno's goal of every person as the therapist of every other person. Fritz Perls, who had attended psychodrama sessions in New York conducted by Moreno, developed Gestalt Therapy. Eric Berne, an admirer of Moreno, created Transactional Analysis. Albert Ellis devised Rational Emotive Behavioral Therapy. All three were practiced as group methods. Since then many other approaches have been devised. Yalom (1985) lists brief therapy groups, supportive-expressive, cognitive-behavioral, psychoanalytic, psycho-educational, and dynamic-interactional groups in addition to Gestalt and psychodrama. Yalom writes:

> The multiplicity of forms is so evident today that it is best not to speak of group therapy but of the many group therapies. Eating-disorders groups. Cancer support groups, groups for victims of sexual abuse, for AIDS patients, for the confused elderly, for individuals disabled by panic disorders or obsessive-compulsive symptoms, for patients with chronic schizophrenia, for adult children of alcoholics, for parents of sexually abused children, for male batterers, for the divorced, for the bereaved, for disturbed families, for married couples, for patients with myocardial infarct paraplegia, diabetic blindness, renal failure, bone marrow transplant—all of these are forms of group therapy. (1985, p. xi)

There is general agreement that there have been three psychiatric revolutions. The first psychiatric revolution refers to rejection of cruel treatment and punishment of the mentally ill. Pinel's humanistic treatment of patients in the psychiatric Salpêtrière Hospital in Paris is often cited as the signal that this revolution had taken place. Freud's identification of the psychological rather than neurological basis of the symptoms of his patients marks the second psychiatric revolution. Dreikurs (1955) states that J. L. Moreno first spoke of the third psychiatric revolution in an address to the ASGPP in 1952. Moreno considered group psychotherapy to be that revolution. He wrote:

> We can no longer maintain the patient–physician relationship as the cornerstone of psychotherapy. The crucial participants in the psychotherapeutic situation are increasingly the *patient-in-the-group*; the therapist is only a member of the group although he has a *special* and important function with it. (1956b, p. 26)

The Encounter Group Movement, also called the Human Potential Movement, emerged in the 1950s. The movement was inspired by the principles of humanistic psychology, a reaction against the mechanical and deterministic psychologies of Freud and Skinner. Like Moreno's philosophy, humanistic psychology emphasized the positive and creative potential rather than pathology and limitations. Encounter groups blended techniques from psychotherapeutic methods with those emerging from the studies of group dynamics. The aims were to bring about greater self-understanding and self-actualization, as well as an understanding of group behavior for participants.

The movement embraced a vast spectrum of activities offered by group leaders with an equally wide assortment of credentials with many groups conducted by traditional mental health professionals and many by leaders who had no formal education. The theories, to the extent that a method was based on a theory, also differed greatly, ranging from those based on scientific or quasi-scientific personality theories to others based on spiritual ideas. The movement peaked during the 1970s. Three of many books about the movement are Howard, *Please Touch* (1970); Siroka, Siroka, and Schloss, *Sensitivity Training and Group Encounter* (1971); and Schutz, *Here Comes Everybody* (1972).

Although many of these groups borrowed theory and techniques from established methods of psychotherapy, they were more often referred to as personal growth and development groups than as psychotherapy groups. Many mental health professionals, committed to the medical model, did not consider them to be group psychotherapy. No diagnosis was made of the participants. Psychopathology was not a consideration. Many unorthodox methods and techniques were involved, and many group leaders had no training or credentials in one of the mental health professions. However, these groups and support groups, such as Alcoholics Anonymous, fit Moreno's basic concept of group therapy: each person the therapist of every other person.

The term *personal growth and development* was defined in many ways, usually to fit the theory and techniques of the method to which a group leader subscribed. Most groups stressed self-awareness and this usually meant greater understanding of one's emotional reactions to others. Learning how others saw one was also a means to increased self-understanding. The psychodrama groups that could be considered as belonging to the Encounter Group Movement were generally called psychodrama training groups. Moreno often called them therapy groups for normal people, a notion that could well define the encounter group movement.

Although interest in the Human Potential Movement and encounter groups peaked in the 1970s, one can still find these groups in many parts of the country. There are opportunities to attend psychodrama training groups, many of which are listed on the website www.psychodramacertification.org. The National Training Institute is still offering human interaction laboratories. Gestalt institutes and Transactional Analysis training can be found in many localities.

Group psychotherapy flourishes today, although it has not replaced individual psychotherapy as the term revolution might suggest. Moreno considered himself authorized to define group psychotherapy by virtue of having introduced the term. He wrote: "The real issue was and is the difference between individual and group psychotherapy. In individual psychotherapy the patient is a single individual. In group psychotherapy the patient is a group of individuals" (1966a, p. 18). That definition has not been widely adopted except by family therapists and leaders of organizational development groups. Many present-day psychotherapy groups can be more accurately described as conducting individual psychotherapy in a group setting.

Students of the Moreno Institute often questioned why psychotherapeutic modalities such as Transactional Analysis and Gestalt Therapy seemed to have garnered so much more interest and so many more adherents than psychodrama. Those who had attended training events in other methods and, like this author, felt that psychodrama was so much more effective were particularly perturbed. Moreno appeared quite calm about it. "They are preparing the way for us," was his usual answer. I understand his answer more completely now than I did at the time. Moreno recognized that the notion that psychological problems belonged to the individual who voiced them was a powerful conserve. It was not going to be easily replaced. For the mental health field to recognize the extent to which psychological problems were social, primarily the result of unsuccessful interpersonal interactions, would take a long time. There is still true today.

8 Sociometry, a New Model for Social Science

Sociometric tests show in a dramatic and precise fashion that every group has beneath its superficial, tangible, readable structure an underlying intangible, invisible, unofficial structure, but one which is more real, alive and dynamic than the other. (Moreno, 1947c, p. 268)

The true sociometric test as we planned it is a revolutionary category of investigation. It upsets the group from within. It produces a social revolution on a microscopic scale. If it does not produce an upheaval in some degree it may arouse suspicion that the investigator has modified it so—in respect for an existing social order—that it becomes a harmless, poverty stricken instrument. (Moreno, 1947c, p. 270)

Sociology was a relatively new science in America in the 1930s and 1940s, when "Moreno's approach bludgeoned its way into even the drowsiest library and classroom and compelled attention," in Gardner Murphy's (1951, p. 1) evocative words. Sociology had not become the unified science the pioneers of the discipline sought. Instead, it seemed composed of many separate disciplines, philosophical doctrines, and competing epistemologies. Florian Znaniecki, well-known sociologist, wrote in 1945 that sociology "seems to be heading toward total disintegration" (p. 514).

A major concern was developing methods and techniques of research that would match the precision of the natural sciences, physics and biology. Sociological studies dealt primarily with aggregates of individuals. The techniques of measurement and statistical manipulation of data received concentrated attention. Reliability and validity of research instruments were of great interest in the evaluation of a method or technique of measurement. Objectivity was seen as a major problem. How the researcher keeps personal values and opinions from influencing the method of gathering data and from the interpretation of that material was a big issue.

With sociometry, Moreno presented the world with a revolutionary new approach to research in the science of society: "The chief methodological task of sociometry has been the revision of the experimental method so that it can be applied effectively to social phenomena" (1951b, p. 31). This fact has never been fully appreciated even by most of the social scientists who responded so enthusiastically to sociometry when *Who Shall Survive?* was published.

There have always been philosophers and thinkers who have questioned the principles and methods of natural science. Edmund Husserl, founder of phenomenology, provided one of the more enduring critiques of positivism. Husserl pointed out that the objective scientist is not actually dealing with the object itself, but with the scientist's experience of the object. Meanwhile, American sociologists have consistently looked to the physical sciences as providing the scientific model of choice. Moreno, as usual, had a new idea. It is the nature of the subject matter, Moreno said, that calls for a different approach to the study of social phenomena. The first task of any science is to discover the conditions under which the significant facts can emerge. While these conditions are well known in the physical and biological arenas, the problem of creating the conditions under which the significant facts of human relations emerge is far more complicated. In the natural sciences we do not expect the subject matter, whether it is planets and stars, falling bodies, or living organisms, to contribute to the study of itself. Scientific exploration is not an activity that these entities engage in. The subject matter of the social sciences is quite a different matter. Scientific study is a human activity and the social sciences are thus a type of self-study. The structure of human society, the patterns of attractions and repulsions that bring parts of society together at one time and push them apart at another, cannot be directly observed by a neutral and independent observer, as can the movements of the planets and stars. An external social structure may be identified, a family, a village, or a social institution, for example, and described, but sociometry has shown us that there is an inner structure that underlies and interacts with the external structure, a phenomenon that influences everything that happens and that can only be made manifest by enlisting the full cooperation of the members of the social entity under investigation:

> Sociometric methods are a synthesis of subjective with objective methods of investigation. A sociometric experiment in situ brings into realization in an unprecedented degree (a) the autonomy of the individual characters, (b) their observation and evaluation by others, (c) measurement of the subjective *and* objective aspects of their behavior, (d) the autonomy of individual groups and the interactions between them. (Moreno, 1951b, p. 36)

Sociometric exploration differs from traditional sociological research in that the researcher rejects the artificialities of the contrived experiment and the experimenter's usual position as an outside or independent observer. The research investigator becomes a member of the group, a part of that which is to be examined. In this way the researcher gains access to subjective knowledge that is otherwise lost to traditional social research. This is a frightening idea to one trained in the traditional positivistic research methods, in which great pains are taken to prevent the researcher from becoming personally involved with the subject matter in a way that could influence the outcome of the experiment. It is also frightening to share the research responsibility and researcher status with the participants in the experiment. Moreno, however, promises that there will be a trade-off:

> But by becoming a member of the group you are robbed of your role of the investigator who is to be outside of it, projecting, creating, and manipulating the experiment. You cannot be a member and simultaneously a "secret agent" of the experimental method. The way out is to give every member of the group research status, to make them all experimenter and to agree with them in the carrying out of a social experiment. If a group has a hundred persons there are now a hundred experimenters and as each is carrying on his "own experiment" there are a hundred experiments and a co-ordination of each single experiment with every other is required. Sociometry is the sociology of the people, by the people, and for the people; here this axiom is applied to social research itself. (1951b, p. 38)

The most important research principle for the sociometric researcher is securing the genuine cooperation of all members of the group who must be convinced that the "experiment," the sociometric exploration of the group, will somehow be beneficial to each and every one of them and to the group as a whole. In contrast to a sociological laboratory study, where volunteer subjects are thrown into an artificial situation created by the researcher, the sociometric experiment takes place in a real-life situation. The problem is to uncover the sociometric structure of the group, whether it be a training group of seven individuals or a community of thousands. The results are then utilized to organize or reorganize the group so that it is in better accordance with the revealed structure. It is this feature, the act of reorganization that makes sociometry an experimental science rather than just a descriptive one.

Sociometry is composed of three parts: it is a theory of the structure of society; it is a research method for revealing that structure; and it is a strategy for reorganizing groups to function more harmoniously. The first seeds of sociometry were sown in the refugee village of Mitterndorf, where J. L. Moreno first recognized the importance of personal preference in the functioning of a community. Moreno defined or described sociometry in many different ways. One of the simplest and most direct is: "Sociometry is a study of the actual psychological structure of human society. The structure is rarely visible on the surface of social processes; it consists of complex inter-personal patterns studied by quantitative and qualitative procedures" (1946b, footnote, p. 242). Sociometric testing revealed this psychological structure and, Moreno claimed, is seldom identical with the formal or official organization of a group. The ultimate goal of sociometry, reorganization, is to bring the sociometric structure and the formal structure closer together. In the words of Helen Jennings, the task is "transforming society to fit man, rather than transforming man to fit society as it is now constituted" (1941b, p. 512).

Here is a thought experiment that will help reveal the basic ideas of sociometry: Imagine that you enter a room together with 50 other people, none of whom you have previously met and none of whom have previously met each other. Perhaps each of you has been hired to compose a new team for some business and you are together for your first meeting. Or perhaps the 50 of you have enrolled in a psychodrama training workshop. As you look around at the people sharing this space with you, you will react to them in various ways, even though you have never met them before. There will be individuals toward whom you will have a feeling that, if put into words, would be something like: "I think I will like that person," or "I want to get to know him/her," or some similar feeling of attraction. Toward others, you may have a feeling of avoidance: "I hope I don't have to work closely with him/her." Or, "That person looks very angry. I don't think I want to get very close to him/her." And then there will be many to whom you have very little or no significant emotional reaction, toward whom you feel neutral. You may be keenly aware of your reactions or you may be minimally aware of them. But it is very likely that you will have them.

And so will the other 49 individuals who are sharing space with you. We can predict a number of things that will happen over the life of this group. Whatever else happens group members will look for an opportunity to make contact with those toward whom they have positive feelings. They will also attempt to avoid interaction with those toward whom they have negative feelings. The patterns of attractions and avoidances (called "rejections") that develop very early, even in a group of strangers, serve as a kind of infrastructure of a group and influence everything else that happens in the group. In Moreno's words, "there is tele already operating between the members of a group from the first meeting" (1972a, p. xx).

Individuals will find that many of their initial impressions are reinforced over time and with interaction. Some initial reactions will change over time and some positive feelings will be replaced by negative ones and vice versa. People will also find that the feelings they have for other individuals, whether positive, negative, or neutral, will be reciprocated with similar feelings to an extent that goes well beyond chance. Some people will "click," that is, recognize emotional mutuality, almost immediately.

A sociometric test made of your group at this time might ask every individual to answer a question such as "With whom in this room would you like to spend 30 minutes to get better acquainted? List them in order, the person you would like best to get to know, then whom you would like second best to know, etc." The sociometrist would then use that information to construct a sociogram that would display the data in a graphic form. The sociogram would have every individual in the group represented by a symbol, a circle for females and a triangle for males. Red lines would then be drawn between these circles and triangles to indicate positive feelings, and black lines would be drawn to indicate negative feelings. The sociogram is a diagram that depicts the emotional structure of a group. From it, the experienced sociometrist can make a number of predictions about how a group will function.

Some individuals will receive a larger than average number of attractions. They will have considerable influence in the group and in decisions made by the group. They will find themselves taking leadership roles. An even larger number will receive few or no attractions. These people will not receive a fair share of the attention of the group. Their ideas will not be readily accepted. Their social needs will likely go without sufficient satisfaction. The red lines on a sociogram depict the flow of communications. If a piece of important information is given to one member of the group, the sociometrist can predict which members will learn about it most quickly by following the network of positive attractions.

It was Moreno's contention that every group had this structure of interpersonal affinities and disaffinities, which often differed from the official structure of the group. He further insisted that this sociometric structure could only be ascertained by the sociometric test. Observation was not enough. Many of these emotional bonds will remain indiscernible to an observer, identified only when reported by the individuals.

Moreno first used a basic sociometric principle, the importance of personal preference in the functioning of a group, in attempts to reduce dissension among the inhabitants of Mitterndorf. However, it was not until years later, after he had come to the United States, that he conducted the research that confirmed his earlier hypotheses. Sociometric exploration with public school children and in the community of a correctional institution resulted in a systematic scientific sociometry. This research, along with philosophical principles associated with sociometry, comprises the content of Moreno's major opus, *Who Shall Survive?* It should be recognized that Moreno considered psychodrama and group psychotherapy to be aspects of sociometry.

Moreno's first sociometric research took place in 1931 and involved the student body of an elementary school, Public School 181, in Brooklyn, New York. This study was augmented with data from a college preparatory high school for boys. The aim was to investigate the evolution of social organization as the students grew older. The results of these investigations are reported in *Who Shall Survive?* (1934; Moreno, 1953c) and by Moreno (1957a) and Jennings (1943).

The public school project provided valuable information and allowed Moreno to propose a theory that he called the sociogenetic law. He was able to document that at each grade level, there was evidence of more and more complex social organization. His hypothesis was: "Just as the higher animals have evolved from the simplest forms of life, so, it seems, the highest forms of group organization have evolved from simple ones" (1934, p. 65).

The public school project left Moreno far short of his sociometric goal, which was to conduct a sociometric experiment with an entire community. The school was just one small sector of a community. The children spent only a few hours a day there. Their true community consisted of their parents and siblings. But it also consisted of their parents' friends, work relationships, family relationships, and on and on. Obviously a sociometric exploration of this community was far beyond feasibility. He needed some kind of more limited, more constrained community, perhaps a closed community like the refugee village of Mitterndorf.

THE NEW YORK STATE TRAINING
SCHOOL FOR GIRLS AT HUDSON

His opportunity came when Fannie French Morse, Superintendent of the New York State Training School for Girls at Hudson, New York, invited him to become the director of research for the institution she headed. Mrs. Morse had been part of the roundtable discussions of 1931 and 1932 (see Chapter 7, this volume) that resulted in the *Application of Group Method to Classification* publication. She was a compassionate and forward-looking superintendent of a corrections institution who was substantially impressed by Moreno's ideas. She believed that his theories could further the aims of the Hudson training school that she ran, and she gave him a free hand to carry out his research there. Bringing his bright young helper, Helen Jennings, along, he set out to organize the community of the school through sociometric methods.

Moreno was aware that the school was not representative of a spontaneous open community. The administration was not completely involved and economic dynamics were not a part of the community. The community consisted of between 500 and 600 members, partly staff and partly students. The latter were all girls between the ages of 12 and 17. It was a synthetic community, in Morenean terms, rather than a spontaneous one. It was a single-gender community. The students were not living with their parents in a family setting. They had been adjudicated as juvenile delinquents by the courts of the state. The major cause of commitment was listed as "sexual delinquency, early manifestation of precocious interest in the opposite sex" (Jennings, 1943, p. 27), and they are described as a cross section of nationality and social groups of the state. Rather than in their families of origin, the students lived in 16 cottages, each headed by a housemother. Rather than siblings, they lived with other girls assigned to the school. The school was racially segregated with African-American girls assigned to two of the cottages.

Despite these limitations, Moreno thought that he might be able to develop principles of social functioning that would apply to groups in a general way. He had the opportunity. He had the backing of the superintendent. He was sure that he would learn from the experiment.

Who Shall Survive? provides a highly detailed account of the massive research investigation into the psychological structure and functioning of a community composed of between 500 and 600 people, the staff and students of the Hudson training school. The research was both wide and penetrating, and it was conducted as Moreno preferred, in the midst of life itself rather than in the laboratory. The first edition, published in 1934, more than 400 pages, was succeeded by the significantly expanded 1953 second edition, more than 700 pages. The 1953 edition also featured a foldout figure entitled "Sociometric Geography of a Community—Map III" pasted inside the back cover. The map shows all the choices of the school's students, indicating the cottages in which they lived and the cottages in which they would have liked to live.

Moreno tells us that he had certain goals in mind as he started the research. At the same time, he was determined to let the direction of research grow out of the situation and to not be fixed in advance on how the study proceeded. After every step in the investigation, the results were carefully analyzed and utilized in determining the next logical step.

The first task that Moreno and Jennings undertook in their exploration of the social structure of the Hudson school was one that involved all the residents. It dealt with the residents' assignments to the cottages in which they lived. As was common practice in institutions like the Hudson training school, when a new girl came into the community, an administrator would assign her to one of the 16 cottages. The criterion for assignment was based on vacancies in the cottages and possibly the housemother's ability to deal with problematic residents. The girl herself was not consulted about which cottage she would like to live in or with whom she would like to live.

This was about to change. The population of the school, at that time 505 girls, was called together and given the following instructions by Superintendent Morse:

> You live now in a certain house with certain other persons according to the directions the administration has given you. The persons who live with you in the same house are not ones chosen by you and you are not one chosen by them. You are now given the opportunity to choose the persons whom you would like to live with in the same house. You can choose without restraint any individuals of this community whether they happen to live in the same house with you or not. Write down whom you would like first best, second best, third best, fourth best and fifth best. Remember that the ones you have chosen will probably be assigned to live with you in the same house. (1934, p. 13)

These instructions given to the inhabitants of the Hudson school are the model for a sociometric criterion. A specific activity is given and choices are rank ordered. A question like "Who is your best friend?" or "Whom do you like best?" will not give the information that is desired in a sociometric test. The girls were also asked to give reasons for their choices.

A total of 505 students took part. Each student was given five choices to make and so a possible 2,525 choices could have been expressed. The first discovery was that only 2,285 choices had actually been made. Just fewer than 10 percent of the choices had gone unused. Examination of the data indicated that there was a gradual decline in emotional expansiveness, the number of choices actually used. At each level of choice, more of them went unused.

The next feature of the data that demanded attention was a phenomenon that has since shown up in practically every sociometric test ever made. One might expect that the distribution of choices would create a normal probability curve, as do the scores on most psychological and sociological tests. A few subjects would receive a greater than average number of choices, a few would receive fewer than average, and most subjects would receive about an average number of choices. That was not the case. The choices were far from equally distributed among the students. A few girls attracted a lot of choices; a larger number were unchosen or greatly underchosen, while the rest received roughly an average number of choices. This distribution has proven to be a consistent character of sociometric explorations. Attempts to ameliorate the effect by giving group members more choices don't work. The additional choices go to the already highly chosen. Moreno called the process of leaving a number of persons unchosen the *sociodynamic effect*.

The primary plan was to test the community and then reconstruct the membership of the various cottages on the results. However, in analyzing the choices, "we found the outcome so contradicting that we could not reconstruct the home groups in the community upon their basis" (1953c, p. 241). The problem was that the data showed little mutuality. That is to say that few choices that the girls made were reciprocated by those who received those choices. Assignment is based on mutuality of choice. If student A chooses student B as someone they want in their cottage and B does not indicate a choice, either positive or negative, it is impossible to predict how they will interact if placed in a cottage together.

Moreno was sure that there was more mutuality in the cottage groups than had shown up in the sociometric test. To ascertain this, all the girls who had received a choice were interviewed and asked about each girl who had chosen them: "How do you feel about living in the same cottage with this person who chose you? Answer yes, no, or indifferent" (Moreno, 1934, p. 77). This provided the data that made the analyses of the cottages and the community possible.

The next step was a very careful analysis of the sociometry of each cottage. A sociogram was first constructed for each cottage. These are depicted in *Who Shall Survive?* along with Moreno's interpretation of the cottages' structures. He frequently suggested further actions that could be taken that he thought would improve cottage life. Figure 8.2, page 214, is a redrawing of the sociogram for Cottage C 16 constructed from the data of the first sociometric test. In the original, a red line represented positive choice. In the reproduction here, it is a solid black line. A black line showed negative choice in the original. Here it is shown by a dotted line. Neutral choice in both is the absence of a connecting line.

Each of the 16 cottages had a unique social organization revealed by a sociogram of the choices that the residents made. One of the first factors that Moreno considered was whether the choices of the members of a cottage group were mostly for each other or for residents of other cottages. Do the members want to stay in the cottage with each other, or do they want to be with those living in other cottages? If the majority of the members of an organization, in this case a cottage, want to remain within it, the group is considered introverted. On the other hand, if the majority chooses outsiders, the organization is extroverted. If the choices for inside are about the same as those for outside, the organization is balanced. This use of the terms *introverted* and *extroverted* for groups must be distinguished from the Jungian psychological classification of individuals. An introverted group may consist entirely of extroverted individuals who prefer each other's company to that of girls in other cottages. The introverted group organization, according to Moreno, tends to be warm and full of emotion. The extroverted group organization tends toward coldness as little emotion is expended within it.

The sociometric concept that is somewhat similar to the Jungian attribute of introversion–extroversion is an individual's emotional expansiveness. *Expansiveness* refers to the capacity for relationships. An individual who is emotionally expansive will connect to more people than someone with limited emotional expansiveness. Emotionally expansive people are likely to be extroverted in the Jungian sense.

The research team calculated for each cottage the percentage of positive choices which were given inside the cottage group. This was called the Ratio of Interest for Home Group, and ranged from 31 percent to 71 percent. It was found that the standard of conduct of cottages when this measure was below 35 percent was lower than the average standard of conduct in the community. In these low-ratio-of-interest cottages, the members lacked interest in increasing house morale, displayed more bad behavior, and were more prone to runaways and members asking for transfer to other cottages.

Negative choices were next considered. The girls had been limited to five positive choices but given no limit to negative ones. Moreno does not indicate why this difference in procedure occurred, but it may be that there is generally a greater reluctance to express negative choices and so no limit was considered necessary to keep the number of choices within manageable limits. In any event, considering the total number of choices made *within* a cottage, the percentage of positive choices was compared with the percentage of negative ones. Again there was great variation from cottage to cottage. For Cottage C 2, with the highest percent of positives and lowest percent of negatives, 85 percent of the choices were positive and 15 percent negative. At the other extreme, Cottage C 4, 48 percent were positive and 52 percent negative. It is obvious that C 4 would not be a very happy home, one full of dissension and hostility. Cottages in which the students made many negative choices were classified as aggressive. If the negative choices went to individuals inside the cottage, the classification was inwardly aggressive, and if they were directed to girls in other cottages, the cottage was considered outwardly aggressive.

So far, attention has been focused on the emotional choices within the cottages. The next step was to explore the emotional choices between cottages.

A score, Ratio of Attraction, expressed in percentages was calculated for each cottage in the following way. The actual number of choices that a cottage received from girls living in other cottages was compared with the maximum possible number of choices that might have been made if every girl from every other cottage had sent a positive choice to the cottage. Calculated this way these percentages are naturally low, ranging from 4% for Cottage C 2 to .9% for Cottage C 9.

The percentages were added together for a total of 41 percent. This was compared with the average percentage derived from the Ratios of Interest for Home Group, 51 percent. Despite the questionable mathematics of adding and averaging percentages, Moreno used these figures to determine that "the cohesive forces at work in this community were stronger than the forces drawing the girls away from their cottage groupings" (1953c, p. 253).

SOCIAL ATOMS

We all have, in a given moment, a large number of people with whom we are acquainted, people that we can recognize as individuals that we have met at some time or another, at some place or another. The sum total of our acquaintances is called our acquaintance volume by Moreno. A majority of those who make up our acquaintance volume mean little to us. They simply are other human beings living in the world around us whom we recognize. They don't have any specific personal meaning to us and we don't have any personal meaning to them. We are not in frequent communication with them. We do not engage in activities together.

However, there is a relatively small group of our acquaintances that *do* mean something personal to us. We either have positive feelings and are attracted to them, or we have negative feelings and try to avoid or reject them, always with reference to some activity in which we wish to engage. Reciprocally, we are meaningful to most, but not necessarily all, of these persons. In addition, there are often individuals who are either attracted to us or who reject us without our knowledge. Meaningful, here, indicates that there is an emotional connection between an individual and another person. This can be any one of the emotions that "bind or separate people, like love and hate, pity and compassion, jealousy and envy, gaiety and joy, anger and hate" (Moreno, 1960a, p. 52). This pattern of attractions and rejections of which a person is the center identifies that person's social atom.

Although there tends to be a clear line between acquaintance and member of a social atom, the boundary is permeable. Most of those in our social atom were originally acquaintances. As soon as we desire to enter a relationship with an acquaintance, that person has entered our social atom. And, likewise, whenever another person wishes to establish a relationship with us, that individual has become a part of our social atom just as we have entered theirs. To quote Moreno, "To my social atom evidently would belong all individual to who I am bound by an invisible desire which may be little or not at all manifest; also those individuals to whom I am tied in actual overt relationships" (1960a, p. 55).

Every social group is composed of a number of interlocking social atoms. The social atom is the smallest functional unit of any social organization. Although the complete social atom of an individual includes all of those who are meaningful to that person and all of those to whom that person is meaningful, we often are interested in a part of a person's social atom in reference to some specific group. Thus Moreno recognized that the students of the Hudson training school undoubtedly had meaningful relationships beyond those in the institution. However, his interest was limited to the school. Hence, he constructed social atoms for the students with respect to the cottages in which they lived and with respect to the entire population of the community. Social atoms are graphically constructed just like group sociograms except that they show the choices given and received by only the one individual (see Figure 8.1).

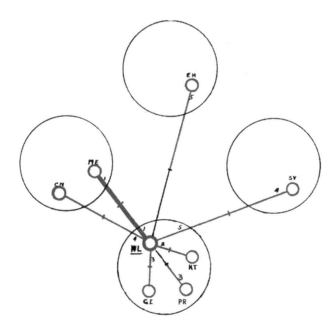

SOCIAL ATOM OF INDIVIDUAL WL
FROM THE POINT OF VIEW OF THE INDIVIDUAL (CENTRIFUGAL ASPECT)
CRITERION: LIVING IN PROXIMITY
The chart illustrates the method of tracing further the social atom of WL in respect to the criterion of living in proximity. The responses to the choices which appeared unreciprocated are ascertained. KT, GE, and CN respond with attraction to WL. WL responds with repulsion to EH and to PR.
This sociogram portrays the individual-oriented psychosocial version of the social atom.

Figure 8.1   Construction of a social atom.
Source: Who Shall Survive? with permission.

SOCIOMETRIC ASSIGNMENT

Sociometric reorganization of the Hudson training school began with newly admitted residents. This was an immediate need because the population of the training school was in continual flux with new members of the community arriving and others leaving every week. Prior to the sociometric research, newcomers were assigned on an essentially random basis to cottages where vacancies existed. A new procedure was established for the Hudson school. All new residents were temporarily assigned to a receiving cottage. During their stay there, they underwent the Parent Test and the Family Test. The Parent Test was a social event in which the new girls met and got acquainted with all the housemothers who had vacancies. Then both the new student and the housemothers expressed choices. The girls indicated which housemothers they felt they could best confide in and whose advice they believed they could best accept. The housemothers were asked to choose on two criteria, the girls to whom they were most attracted and those whom they felt could best fit into their cottage group.

The Family Test was similar except that rather than the housemother, a resident of each available cottage met with each incoming resident. The cottage representatives were chosen as girls who were well adjusted to their respective cottages. They would then also serve to introduce any newcomers assigned to their cottages.

Assignment to the cottage in which a new student would live was very carefully done and took into account more than just the choices made in the Parent and Family Tests. In addition to that information, the organization of the prospective cottages and the predominant psychological currents in each were taken into consideration. Follow-up studies on the success of placement of newcomers indicated that the best risks were when there was agreement among the various factors. Residents whose assignments showed the highest degree of *mutuality* of choice were found to be the most successful in achieving integration into both their cottages and in the training school community.

Reassignment of the girls who were already residents of the school required care and thoroughgoing consideration of the needs of the individual as well as the effect upon the cottage of removing or adding a person. The reassignment of one girl could also have repercussions for the entire school. It is obvious that Moreno paid equal attention to the individual and to the group. He clearly recognized that reassignment could have a considerable impact upon both individuals and groups. There was the effect upon the cottage *from* which a girl was moved, upon the one *into* which she was moved, upon the resident herself, and, to some degree, upon the community as a whole. Because of the impact of these effects, efforts were made to improve the individual's sociometric status and adjustment to her current cottage in lieu of reassignment. The ultimate goal was to achieve balance in the emotional currents both within the cottages and the entire community.

It took Moreno and his research team 18 months to complete the reassignment project. Sociometric analysis of the entire community was made every
four weeks. The residents who were initially considered for reassignment were
those who appeared to be in vulnerable sociometric positions in their cottages
and who were having problems in adjusting to the school. These were the girls
who were generally isolated, unchosen, or infrequently chosen, and those who
had received mostly negative choices from their existing cottage mates.

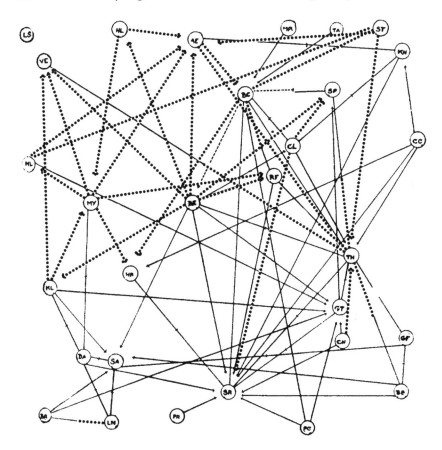

STRUCTURE OF A COTTAGE FAMILY—C16
Criterion: Living in proximity, sharing the same house; 5 choices; no limit placed on rejections.
30 girls. *Isolated* 1; *Unchosen* 6; *Unchosen and Rejected* 5; *Not Choosing* 1; *Pairs* 18; *Mutual*
Rejections 2; *Incompatible Pairs* 7; *Chains* 6; *Triangles* 2; *Squares* 0; *Circles* 0; *Stars* (of
attraction) 5; *Stars* (of rejection) 1.
    Classification: Extroverted. Special Feature—Large Number of Unchosen and Rejected.
Note for the Group Psychotherapist: In a sociodrama let the pro-group (the 19 members who
choose and are chosen) face the con-group (the 13 members who neglect the group or are
themselves neglected).

Figure 8.2   Sociogram of Cottage C 16 before reconstruction.
Source: *Who Shall Survive?* with permission.

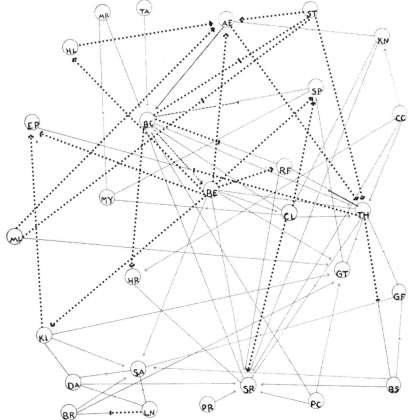

Figure 8.3   Sociogram of Cottage C 16 after reconstruction.
Source: *Who Shall Survive?* with permission.

Figure 8.2 is the sociogram of Cottage C 16 from the first sociometric test.
Figure 8.3 is the reconstructed sociogram of C 16 after three girls had been
reassigned to other cottages and one girl added to C 16. Those moved to other
cottages were designated LS, VE, and CN. The first two are in the upper-
left part of the first sociogram, and CN is in the lower-right area. Moreno

noted that there was no significant change in the attraction–rejection patterns after the reassignments but that the housemother reported that problematic behavior like temper tantrums and stolen articles had decreased by half. The new sociogram showed that the distribution of lines of communication had changed. Where there had previously been a fragmentation of the group into cliques centered on the several leaders, the new sociogram showed increased connectedness among the girls.

Reassignment involved not only sociometric data, but also spontaneity tests and role-playing tests. Carried out with cottage mates or with girls from other cottages, these tests helped add information about how a student could be expected to interact in different situations and with different people.

Moreno described in considerable detail the relocation process for several students. He includes a student who must have been one of the most difficult to place. Her name was Elsa. Her first social atom is shown as Figure 5. Elsa was rejected by 16 of her cottage mates in Cottage C 8, as well as by 15 girls from other cottages. Four of her five positive choices go to girls who live in C 8 and are all met by rejections. Her other choice, to a girl outside her cottage, receives no response. Elsa rejects three inside her group and one outside. She is rejected heavily both within her own group and by the community at large.

Attempts to better her situation in Cottage C 8 included spontaneity tests, situation tests, and role-playing sessions. The attempts to help Elsa adjust to her group did not succeed in changing the behavior that evoked rejection. She unquestionably needed a new setting. The question was where to place her and with whom. Her acquaintance volume within the school and beyond her cottage was small and the first step was to enlarge it. She was placed in role-playing groups, where she met more members of the community. As a result of new acquaintances, in another sociometric test, Elsa chose three others as girls with whom she wanted to live, and was herself chosen by four. These girls, who chose Elsa or were chosen by her, were then engaged with Elsa in more role-playing groups. "A comparison of a series of 82 situation records indicated that only two of the seven girls [Jeanette and Florence] Elsa had chosen, released from her spontaneous expressions which, in articulation of emotion and judgment, contrasted favorable with her daily behavior, or which overcame certain petty habitual trends which she had demonstrated in speech and action when interacting in these situations with the other girls" (1953c, p. 375). Elsa was eventually placed in Cottage C 13 with these two girls.

THE REORGANIZED COMMUNITY

The first result of sociometric reorganization of the Hudson school was a marked reduction in elopements, the institutional term for runaways. Both girls who were sent to the Hudson school by juvenile courts, and the staff who worked with them, were under considerable official pressure to see that they remained there until they were discharged. Girls who made the effort to elope obviously experienced even stronger social pressures to leave the school community. They were usually residents who were isolated or rejected, who had low sociometric status. They had not been able to make a place for themselves in the community. After only four months, Moreno noted, the number of runaways had dropped significantly, and by the end of a year after sociometric assignment was initiated, there was less than one elopement per month, a remarkably low figure for such institutions. This indicated, Moreno declared, that almost all admissions had achieved a minimum level of adjustment. They did not run away. In other words, most of the girls, who had been sent to the training school by the action of courts, had found an acceptable home. This is an unusual occurrence at institutions like the Hudson training school.

Sociometric testing 18 months after the initial test revealed significant changes in the social structure of the cottages. The positive choices for other girls living in the same cottage had increased in 15 of the 16 cottages. As promised in the test instructions for the criterion for living in proximity, residents were now domiciled with more of their own choices. Another measure compared the percentage of positive choices to negative choices within each cottage. For example, in Cottage C16, 67 percent of the choices for each other were positive in the original testing, while 33 percent were negative. In the sociometric test after 18 months, 73 percent of their choices for each other were positive, 27 percent negative. Twelve cottages exhibited such an increase in the percentage of attractions over rejections. Furthermore, the two cottages in which rejections were greater than attractions in the original testing had changed. After 18 months rejections no longer outnumbered attractions.

The popularity, or group attraction, score of a cottage reflects the number of residents in the whole community who would prefer to live in that cottage rather than the one in which they currently resided. The sociometry shows that this measure had increased for 4 cottages, decreased for 10, and remained the same for 2. The interpretation was that there was less difference in popularity among the 16 cottages. It was another indication that more residents were satisfied with their living assignments.

These results were achieved with assignment of newcomers and reassignment of existing members of only 102 girls, about one-fifth of the school population. A relatively small shift in the living spaces of the residents had a noteworthy impact upon the community.

In his discussion of sociometric reconstruction methods, Moreno said that his methods had been criticized as running the danger of creating too harmonious a setting. Communities so organized might be made so harmonious so that when the residents returned to the world at large they would be in danger of failing again. That was not a problem, Moreno declared, because his methods were not aimed at a harmony based solely upon positive feelings but a harmony in which there is a balance of emotional currents. No attempt was made to create cottage groups in which all choices were positive, but rather to create groups in which there was a balance of positive and negative choices. Furthermore, he proclaimed:

It may be said that the danger of too happy homes and too happy communities is very small. Unmixed harmony and love are rarely evidenced. This very study has certified the frightening truth that our social universe is overwhelmingly filled with aggressiveness, cruelties and jealousies of all sorts, and that these are deeply imbedded, not only within the individual but particularly within the complex structure of social interaction. (1953c, p. 527)

All in all, the New York State Training School for Girls at Hudson sociometric experiment was an astonishing project. It clearly demonstrated Moreno's skill in conducting empirical research. It provided the empirical data to generate and support Moreno's ideas about the preferential nature of the structure of society. It also generated an impressive group of theories about interpersonal behavior and the structure of society. It gave great impetus to small group and group dynamics research. Moreno openly recognized the shortcomings of the study and the need for further research to confirm his findings and expand his results. At the end of the second edition of *Who Shall Survive?*, Moreno lists 107 "General Hypotheses and Recommendations for Further Research" (1953c, pp. 696–717). They are worthy of further exploration and offer subject matter for hundreds of theses and dissertations.

ROLE TRAINING

It was one thing to help girls who were admitted to the Hudson training school adjust to the institution itself. However, the school was charged with not only taking care of the adolescent girls assigned to it, but also with educating them and providing training that would enable them to survive and function autonomously and productively in society at large. They were expected to be discharged from the school at about age 18, prepared to enter open society and make their way independently and successfully. The social and work situations available to the residents within the school were limited and relatively simple compared with those in the larger world.

The task of changing delinquent adolescent girls into productive citizens seemed to be quite a tall order. The outside world was vastly more complex and flexible than the more regimented and simplified world of the institution. Satisfactory adjustment to the school did not guarantee satisfactory adjustment to the plurality of social environments into which the students might go. What was called for, Moreno thought, was a method for training social spontaneity. His solution was spontaneity training and role training, which provided the students with realistic situations in which they might uncover and express aspects of their personalities that remained otherwise hidden in the routine activities of the school.

Spontaneity training involved creating situations that could be expected to happen in life outside the institutions. This included situations from home life, from work, or from community life. These situations could be chosen by the girls themselves or by the instructor. The members of the training group then played them out. Moreno gives an example of how a spontaneity training sequence might go. The subject is given instructions to warm up to an attitude of sympathy toward another girl and express it. In the next stage, she is to produce sympathy in a role that involves some function, such as a salesclerk in a dress store. After that, she is to produce the attitude while waiting on a businesslike customer. In still another stage, she is to maintain the attitude while waiting on a demanding and argumentative customer. This is done in a group and the other group members play the auxiliary roles and critique the performance of the subject.

The situations varied from simply acting out an emotional state, such as anger, sympathy, or joy, much as described above as spontaneity testing, to more complex interpersonal situations, such as helping a friend who is in trouble. The emphasis, of course, was placed on how realistic and true to life the performance was as opposed to how dramatic it may have been.

In addition to increasing spontaneity, the ability to meet the unexpected with adequate and novel responses, spontaneity training reveals personality and character traits. In the process, the girls often became aware of how certain habitual ways of responding to situations or to others were creating problems for them. Spontaneity training provided them with new and more effective ways of acting in those situations.

The role training sessions were similar to the spontaneity training sessions, except that the situations were focused on specific occupations, such as waitress, nurse, or store clerk. Situations were constructed in which the girls enacted these occupational roles, learning ways of interacting with customers, patients, supervisors, employers, or fellow workers. Students were allowed to choose the occupations in which they wished to act, and often made decisions about jobs they would seek upon discharge from the school. Moreno taped some of these training sessions and Marineau, his biographer, discovered them in his research. They are now available on DVD and can be ordered online.[1]

Moreno's work at the New York State Training School for Girls at Hudson demonstrated what could be accomplished by the use of sociometry in a closed society. Moreno was convinced that sociometry held great promise for the reorganization of society at large. He knew that this would be a far, far more demanding task than the Hudson training school posed and that it would require a Herculean effort to raise sociometric consciousness. Sociometry, he believed, would have to proceed slowly, one group at a time. As remarkable as the Hudson school study was, it has never been replicated.

SOCIOMETRY ATTRACTS THE SOCIOLOGISTS

Moreno exhibited a number of sociograms from the Hudson school study at a meeting of the Medical Society of the State of New York in April 1933. They caught the attention of not only the physicians attending the meeting, but of news reporters, as well. Articles featuring Moreno's work appeared in the newspapers of the day. An April 3, 1933 *New York Times* article was headlined "Emotions Mapped by New Geography," and it discussed "a new science named psychological geography, which aims to chart the emotional currents, the cross-currents and the under currents of human relationships in a community, was introduced here yesterday" at the 127th meeting of the Medical Society. The term *sociometry* does not appear, although Moreno is quoted and obviously gave an interview in which he described the invisible structure underlying society, the structure that sociograms depicted:

> "If we ever get to the point of charting a whole city or a whole nation," Dr. Moreno added, "we would have an intricate maze of psychological reactions that would present a picture of a vast solar system of intangible structures, powerfully influencing conduct, as gravitation does bodies in space. Such an invisible structure underlies society and has its influence in determining the conduct of society as a whole."

Always the champion of the downtrodden, Moreno emphasized the number of rejected, isolated, and underchosen individuals revealed by sociometric tests. On the basis of his findings at the Hudson school, he estimated that there could be 10 to 15 million people in the United States who were rejected by the groups in which they lived. He suggested that with sociometric methods, it would be possible to find for them other environments where they may become happy human beings. The last paragraph of the article states that "Dr. Moreno added that plans have been completed to chart a map of the psychological geography of New York City." This sentence suggests that either the reporter misunderstood Moreno or that Moreno was displaying his customary boldness.

Moreno published the first account of the work he and Helen Jennings had carried out at the Hudson training school in *Who Shall Survive? A New Approach to the Problems of Human Relations* in 1934. The book created quite a stir among sociologists and social psychologists, many of whom began to conduct research applying some of Moreno's techniques. The *Sociometric Review*, a report of the research staff to the advisory research board, was published at the Hudson training school in 1936. The following year, Moreno decided that there was enough work being carried out in the name of sociometry that he inaugurated *Sociometry, a Journal of Interpersonal Relations* with Gardner Murphy as the editor. The stated aim of the journal was to publish articles on sociometry. Moreno and Jennings contributed further articles based on their work at the Hudson training school, and Moreno also produced his first articles on the psychodramatic method in *Sociometry*. By this time, a number of sociologists and researchers from other disciplines who were experimenting with Moreno's unique techniques submitted papers to the new journal. Obviously, Moreno's *Who Shall Survive?* had stimulated a profusion of small group research.

The articles published in *Sociometry* were not by any means all related to sociometry, either in the narrow sense in which Moreno used the term or in an inclusive definition of the word. Sanderson (1943) estimated that in the first five years, about half of the articles dealt with sociometric issues. The other half, Sanderson wrote, dealt with broader-based social psychological measurement, sociological theory, personality, and "other miscellaneous topics from visceral motivation to population statistics" (p. 217). That proportion remained about the same during the entire time that Moreno owned the journal.

There were problems, however, with many of the sociometric studies. Henry J. Meyer (1952) noted that for Moreno, sociometry was a philosophy of life as well as a theory of society and a method of social research. A full sociometric experiment engendered a change in the group being studied. The sociologists and social psychologists who were excited by Moreno's sociograms and his novel approach of obtaining social data directly from the members of the group under study did not buy into the whole package. They were mesmerized by the new source of data and by the data itself. Many did not understand the nature or purpose of a sociometric study as conceived by Moreno. Their researches fell short in a number of ways of meeting the criteria for a sociometric experiment. A common failing was interpreting a sociometric test as a test of popularity. The members of a group were asked to identify their best friends or whom they liked the best rather than being presented with an action criterion: With whom do you choose to engage in this activity? Moreno designated those studies that did not meet all the criteria of a sociometric experiment as quasi-sociometric.

Failure to recognize the importance of preparation, the warming up process, was another shortcoming in many studies. The warming up process emphasizes Moreno's revision of the scientific method for social research. Sociometry is an action method and the first step is to warm the members of the group or community to the role of co-researchers. In some situations it may be enough to invite group members to choose the other members with whom to share living quarters or a table in the dining room, as Moreno and Jennings did in the Hudson training school. The importance of the criterion for group members generates a quick warming up. For an open community, on the other hand, the notion of identifying positive and negative choices among the members of one's group is a very threatening proposition to most people. It requires a very careful and delicate preparation if it is to succeed.

A sociometric experiment is composed of a number of steps: a warming up process; a sociometric test based on an action criterion; an analysis of the data; organizing or reorganizing the group based on the data; and engaging in the activity of the criterion. The sociometric test criterion must be based on an activity and it should be an activity in which the group can normally be expected to engage. It should be an activity that the group will carry out with or without sociometric intervention. The choices, both positive and negative, revealed by the test need to be compiled and presented either as a sociogram or a sociomatrix (Moreno, 1934, 1946d).

Because the sociodynamic effect causes such an uneven distribution of choices and rejections, organization or reorganization of a group is not an automatic or mechanical process. Rather, careful thought and consideration are required, especially placement of the isolate and unchosen group members. It is seldom if ever possible to give every group member their first choice, and in some situations there may be a group member who can't be assigned any of their choices. If the entire process of analysis and assignment is conducted openly, the individuals deprived of choices can usually understand the rationale and are usually mollified by a promise to give their choices priority in the next sociometric experiment.

Moreno considered the final step of the sociometric experiment to be critical to the integrity of sociometry. Group members need to be assured in the warming up phase that the group will engage in the criterion activity and that their choices will be conscientiously considered in the organization of that activity. This assurance makes the test not seem like a test in the usual sense, but rather an opportunity to express one's desires for companionship during an activity. Knowing that one's choices will have an effect ensures that the group members will make honest choices. This ensures the validity of the sociometric test. Moreno also contended that only the complete sociometric experiment could confirm or extend the sociometric laws and hypotheses that had come out of his Hudson training school project.

Some of the hundreds of reports of sociometric research in *Sociometry* and other journals did indeed follow Moreno's rules. Numerous others failed in one or more respects. Moreno called attention to these deficiencies periodically. For example, he wrote as early as 1942:

A full understanding of sociometric terms and methods requires that the underlying philosophy of social relations which gave them motivation and scope be studied hand in hand with them. Sociometric tests, for instance, have been described as a new sort of questionnaire, as a method of interviewing, as a study of verbal responses and of likes and dislikes. These are only partial descriptions of the test. A sociometric test is first of all an action and behavior test of individuals in a group. (p. 301)

In another article, Moreno (1947c) expresses disapproval of several violations of his rules for sociometric research. He criticizes the use of observations in the place of sociometric testing. He points specifically to Roethlisberger and Dickson's (1939) famous Hawthorne studies as an example. By observing workers rather than including them directly in the research as he, Moreno, would have done, Moreno said, they treat them like animals in a maze instead of like the mature adults that they are.

He finds fault with researchers who fail to utilize adequate criteria in the research they consider to be sociometric. "Who are your best friends and who are your enemies" is not even a criterion, Moreno contends. The sociometric test is not intended to simply obtain a verbal response from the subject. The objective is to stir the subject up to an action response. "Every sociometric test attempts to warm up the subject to act in behalf and in accord with his subjective reality level. It encourages him to act out, to be himself; it permits him to have . . . a goal for himself" (1947c, p. 269).

Finally in this article, Moreno criticizes those whom he calls "halfway sociometrists":

> The halfway sociometrists . . . coming from general and abstract sociological schools, preferred broad and vast sounding questionnaires of interpersonal relations with a flair for sociometric concepts to the sociometric test itself. These questionnaires fell more easily into practicable academic methods of research but they diluted and deflated the sociometric method. The true sociometric test as we planned it is a revolutionary category of investigation. It upsets the group from within. It produces a social revolution on a microscopic scale. If it does not produce an upheaval in some degree it may arouse suspicion that the investigator has modified it so—in respect for an existing social order—that it becomes a harmless, poverty stricken instrument. (p. 270)

Controversy over the meaning of the term *sociometry* in sociology developed in the early 1940s. It began with the organization of presentations at the annual conferences of the American Sociological Society. A section entitled "Sociometry" had been established in 1940 but was not repeated for the 1942 program. The program committee had planned to include sociometric papers under a section entitled "Measurement." This led Moreno to petition for the addition of a section on sociometry to the conference. Signed by 25 leading members of the association, the petition was successful. However, the question about the meaning of sociometry had been raised: Should the term, sociometry, refer to all quantitative sociological research, or should it apply only to the methods that Moreno had conceived? Some sociologists felt that Moreno had preempted the word and that it should be applied generically to all kinds of measurements, including population studies, questionnaires, attitude studies, and statistics. Others agreed with Moreno that it should refer solely to the system that he had originated.

Moreno used the controversy to clarify the mission of *Sociometry* and to narrow the range of articles in the journal. When he started the journal, he wrote in an open letter to readers and contributors, the journal was a place for sociometrists to publish their studies. Not knowing if sociometrists would be able to contribute enough to keep the journal going, he opened its pages to all comers. They came, he said, "sociologists, anthropologists, social psychologists, psychiatrists, clinical psychologists, economists," but "only a few among them were sociometrists" (1943b, p. 197). Questions have been raised, he went on to write: "What is sociometry? Is everything that the journal contains 'sociometry'? What is the relationship of social measurement to sociometry? What is the relationship of sociometry to psychodrama? What is the policy of this journal?" (p. 197). The time had come to answer those questions and establish policy for the journal, he wrote. However, he did not want to arbitrarily make the decision from his position of authority as the publisher of the journal. He wanted to be more inclusive, to consider the thoughts of those who had contributed to *Sociometry*. Therefore, he had invited a number of individuals from several fields to submit brief statements on the meaning of the term *sociometry*. The question to be answered was: What is sociometry? The contributors included sociologists, anthropologists, social psychologists, educators, psychiatrists, and others, and their statements were published as a symposium in *Sociometry* in 1943. The 22 participants, not including Moreno, included some of the more prestigious sociologists of the day, five of whom (Dwight Sanderson, E. W. Burgess, F. Stuart Chapin, Stuart Queen, and George Lundberg) were, at one time or another, presidents of the American Sociological Society. Other contributors included well-known psychologists Gardner Murphy and Theodore Sarbin and philosopher Pitirim Sorokin.

Several of the sociologists were of the opinion that all forms of social measurement should be subsumed under the sociometry section of the American Sociological Society. There was agreement that Morenean sociometry belonged to the discipline of sociology. They advocated the broad interpretation of the term *sociometry*. They expressed concern with the narrower, that is, Morenean interpretation, on two major points. Moreno's sociometry included the application of sociometric methods to real groups in life situations. Thus sociometry mixed science and technology. Sociology, they insisted, should be kept a pure science and not include applications of research. Another profession such as social work, not sociology, should handle any applications of the results of research in real life. The second reservation was the concern that restricting sociometry to Moreno's approach ran the danger of sociometry becoming a cult.

The majority of the contributors to the symposium, however, supported the use of the term sociometry to refer to the interpersonal research and theoretical orientation that had been initiated by Moreno. Moreno concluded the symposium with a 35-page article that addressed a number of issues, including the accusation of heading a cult. This paper, "Sociometry and the Cultural Order" (1943c), is probably the most concise and complete synopses of sociometry that Moreno offered. In it, he defends his definition of the method and theory that he originated under the name *sociometry*: "The term sociometry is to be reserved for the meaning which has been widely accepted and which I originally gave to it as a science" (p. 321). Excluded would be "all studies of populations in which the individual parts are considered only in a summary, symbolic or mechanical fashion, as for instance, the studies of Thorndike (1942) and Stewart (1942); all public opinion research such as the studies of Gallup (1941); and studies dealing with measurement of social attitude (Sewell, 1942). *Sociometry* would continue its editorial policy "with greater emphasis upon the role which sociometry is playing within a system of social sciences, as its core" (p. 323). All of these studies had appeared in *Sociometry*.

Moreno continued to publish the journal through the year 1955. Many of the articles continued to have a tangential connection with sociometry, and some had no connection at all. After publishing *Sociometry* for 18 years, Moreno made a decision to give the journal to the American Sociological Society. He announced his decision by publishing the correspondence between himself and Donald Young, the president of the American Sociological Society, regarding the transfer (Young & Moreno, 1955). In the first letter, he offered "to tender to the American Sociological Society the journal *Sociometry* without stipulations or conditions (177–178)." Young replied that the executive committee and the council of the society had accepted the offer and would continue "Founded in 1937 by J. L. Moreno (178)" on the title page, and he stipulated that if "the Society for any reason decides to discontinue this publication, the Journal will be returned to you or to Beacon House " (Young & Moreno, 1955, pp. 178–179)).

The December 1955 *Sociometry*, the last under Moreno's editorship, was a mammoth issue of 474 pages. The first article is Moreno's explanation of why he is giving away this journal that he founded. He acknowledged possessing ambivalence about his decision and the article itself seems to reflect this. He gave several reasons for the move, the first one being that the best way to spread a novel idea is to give it away, even though that means the originator of the idea may not be remembered for it. A second reason given was that he wanted to turn his attention to the development of sociometry in other countries. Moreno did indeed start a new journal, the *International Journal of Sociometry and Sociatry*, in 1956. Furthermore, "After having founded and nurtured *Sociometry* for twenty years, I had the itch to see how the journal would fare without me" (Moreno, 1955a, p. 265). He can see, he wrote, how his friends and enemies behave. He can enjoy the journal if it is well run and he can get angry if others make a mess of it. He gives one more reason:

I have a well developed ego and self-concern; a good part of my dreams have been preoccupied with an intensive drive for recognition. On the other hand, however, a contrary force towards self-denial is prompting me to liberate and separate my work from my own ego and aspirations and giving it to the world without any strings attached. It is creating the position which every man will be in after he has departed from this world when he can look at himself with the most objective eyes, from where nothing matters. The great difference is only that I wanted to establish this position for myself during my lifetime, gaining this objectivity towards myself by an act of free will. (p. 267)

In 1956 and 1957, the first two years in which *Sociometry* was published by the American Sociological Society (which later became the American Sociological Association), the journal contained a total of 52 articles. Only one of those (Harary & Ross, 1957) dealt with a sociometric subject. Another on role taking dealt with that subject from the alternative definition of role taking of G. H. Mead. That article listed two of Moreno's articles in its references. The association published *Sociometry* until 1977. The name of the journal was then changed first to *Social Psychology* in 1978 and again to *Social Psychology Quarterly* the following year.

Although Moreno never said so, there may have been yet another reason for turning over *Sociometry* to the American Sociological Society. He may have recognized from the nature of the research that was being offered to the journal that the world was not ready for the full impact of sociometry. Little beyond the principles of social interaction that he had discovered in his work at the Hudson training school had yet been added to the science of society that he had originated. These had not been tested, confirmed, or disconfirmed, as he had wished. No new studies matching the magnitude of that work had been attempted, nor was there any indication that they would be forthcoming in the foreseeable future. A great increase in sociometric consciousness in the population would have to occur before sociometry could come into its own.

SOCIOMETRY TODAY

There appear to have been few sociometric studies published since Moreno turned over *Sociometry* to the American Sociological Society. Moreno, with a number of other editors, published the *Sociometry Reader* (1960d), a collection largely of previously published papers. Moreno added some newly written selections but a majority of the papers had first appeared in

Sociometry. The latest date for any of these articles was 1957. The articles selected for this volume covered a number of areas. Only a minority of them contained the classical sociometric exploration as described by Moreno. Few attempts have been made to confirm or expand upon the sociometric principles that Moreno hypothesized from his Hudson training school studies.

The psychodramatists and psychodrama trainers who subscribe to Moreno's triadic system of psychodrama, sociometry, and group psychotherapy, keep sociometry and sociometric concepts alive in a practical way. These practitioners make use of sociometric principles in the selection of protagonists and auxiliary egos. They pay attention to attractions and rejections in their groups, identifying underchosen and isolated group members, taking steps to help them become more included in the group. When mutual rejection threatens the functioning of the group, encounters are facilitated to air out differences and reduce destructive tensions in the group. Some psychodrama trainers conduct classical sociometric explorations in order to teach their trainees about sociometry through direct experience and to raise sociometric consciousness.

One of the most active advocates for sociometry is Ann E. Hale, who has been conducting training workshops in sociometry for a number of years. Hale was a staff member of the Moreno Institute during the 1970s and worked with J. L. Moreno on a student version of *Who Shall Survive?* (1993). She has been an active trainer of psychodrama and sociometry. In 1981, she published a manual on sociometry that contains detailed instructions and guidelines for conducting sociometric explorations in small groups.

Hale established a website entitled "International Sociometry Training Network" in 2005. The objective of the website is to help people find publications, research, and training activities related to sociometry. Several dozen papers, many of them authored by Hale, can be found on the website and can be downloaded or printed from the website.

NOTES

1. They can be ordered from www.psychotherapy.net.

9 Sociometric Theory

A SOCIOMETRIC PERSPECTIVE

As I write, the world population is a little more than seven billion people. If we could see them all at once we would see a prodigious amount of activity, people engaged in building, walking, running, driving, buying, selling, planning, counting, watching, talking, listening, making love, eating, cleaning, carrying, and involved in the thousands of other actions in which people take part. And if you could observe a large number of individuals from afar, you would see that they are connecting first with this person and then with another. Humankind is a relentlessly active, ever-changing, ceaseless mass of billions of actions and interactions every second. We interact with others to accomplish things that we cannot realize by ourselves.

Moreno was convinced that all of humankind was interconnected, an "organic unity" in his words. The acts and actions of any person have some influence, even if infinitely small, upon every other person. Moreno was not the first to suggest the organic unity of humankind. In an early issue of the *American Journal of Sociology*, I found this statement: "It is evident that normal humanity may in some way resemble an organic whole, and its development the growth of an organism" (Mathews, 1895, p. 182). Moreno was six years old when that statement appeared in print.

The preferences that people have for others with whom they participate in specific activities occupy a singularly important place in human life. The extent to which one obtains one's preferences can affect one's well-being and health to a far greater extent than is generally recognized. The degree to which the members of a group secure their preferences for partners in the activities of the group has a significant impact upon how effectively that group functions and whether or not it thrives. It was Moreno's insight that the choices that individuals have for each other provide a structure of society. He devised the sociometric test to uncover this structure, and the sociogram and sociomatrix to display that structure visibly. These instruments generate information that can not only guide the organization of groups, but also generate hypotheses, theories, and laws about the functioning of society.

It is important to recognize that sociometric structure is an active process and not a static entity. Sociometric structure is constantly changing. There is a different sociometric structure of a group for each of the activities in which the group engages. In most groups, membership changes from time to time and some individuals leave while others enter. With each change of membership, the structure of the group is altered. Conducting a sociometric experiment, itself, can be expected to change the sociometric structure of the group. A sociometric test is totally accurate only for the moment in which it occurs.

Act vs. Response

It is the difference between perceiving the individual as an organism-in-environment and perceiving the individual as an actor *in situ* (situated in its natural place) that distinguishes sociometry from academic psychology and sociology. The organism-in-environment is a behavioral system; the actor *in situ* is an actorial system, and, Moreno (1953b) states, it is important to distinguish between the two. A collectivity of actors is a different entity from a collectivity of organisms and has a different meaning.

Warner (1954) points out that from Moreno's perspective, when one tries to understand behavior by separating an action into components, as the psychologist does, one ends up ignoring the most important characteristics of human behavior, social interaction. Acts, actions, and interactions are complex behaviors that are intended to gain a desired goal. They occur within a cultural context. There is a reciprocal relationship between the members of a group and the group's culture. On the one hand, it is the actions of the members that create the culture of the group and on the other hand the culture of the group shapes the actions of its members.

Meyer writes, "The heart of Dr. Moreno's sociometric method is *action*. Time and again in the writings of this book and elsewhere, he insists that sociometric methods require that individuals cease to be subjects for research, patients in the clinic, or objects of reform. They must become participants" (1952, p. 360). Sociometric research, Moreno insisted, is for the benefit of the people involved, not for the benefit of the researcher. Therefore, the subjects should be included in the design of the research, in the selection of criteria, for example. Sociometry should take place in life, in the real situation of the individuals, not in the laboratory of the scientist. Unless the sociometric experiment includes an activity in which the group members partake, it is, at best, "near sociometric." Sociometry is an action method.

Descriptive Sociometry

Moreno called sociograms, the graphic displays of the data garnered from a sociometric test, descriptive sociometry. He considered the lines of choice and rejection as representing sociometric facts: A red line indicates the fact that person A chose person B. He suggested that these and the other socio-metric structures of descriptive sociometry were facts in the same way that the veins and arteries of the circulatory system are physiological facts.

The first step in a sociometric exploration of the psychosocial structure of a group is administration of a sociometric test. The sociometric test, which was introduced in Chapter 8, doesn't seem like a test from the sub-ject's point of view. Instead, it simply asks for one's choices of someone with whom the subject wants to engage in an activity. To those taking a sociometric test, it seems to be in their best interest. They are being allowed to choose those with whom to engage in some task or activity instead of being assigned by an authority or by chance.

The activity for which group members are being asked to name their choices for companions is known as the criterion of the test. Moreno was clear that the criterion should be an activity appropriate to the group being tested and that is going to occur or at least very likely to occur, and that the subjects should be assured that their choices will be respected. Under those conditions, Moreno (1955d) contended, the responses of the subjects can be considered valid provided that the subjects of the test have been appropriately prepared and warmed up to take the test. Moreno labeled this definition of validity "existential validity.". Existential validity refers to the honesty with which the subjects indicate their choices. This is in con-trast to the traditional definition of validity, which seeks to establish that a test measures what it purports to measure.

Many of the researchers who tried to use the sociometric methods misun-derstood the ideas upon which sociometry was based as well as its purpose. They interpreted preference for others with whom to engage in an activity as a measure of friendship. Instead of Moreno's definition of a criterion, they asked questions such as "Who is your best friend?" or "Whom do you like best?" Moreno (1947c) rejected such questions as not valid sociometric criteria. They are too vague and do not identify a specific activity, so there is no way to assess the validity of the answers to them.

The Sociogram

Moreno devised the sociogram, introduced in the previous chapter, as a method of depicting the structure of a group in a graphic mode. Individuals are represented symbolically; males by triangles and females by circles, and lines are drawn between them to denote choices and rejections. In the origi-nal sociograms, red was used to indicate positive choice, black for negative choice, and usually no line to show indifference or neutrality. If there was a reason to include indifference in the sociogram, a dotted line could be drawn. The sociogram was intended to be a flexible instrument, alterable to meet the purposes of the sociometrist. Sociograms have been constructed to show only first choices, to show only positive choices, to show all choices, or to show mutual choices. Many other modifications have been made.

Constructing a sociogram is partly art and partly engineering. Moreno's instructions were to draw it with as few crossing lines as possible. This allows one to see the various structures quicker and more clearly. Moreno acknowledges that most of the sociograms in *Who Shall Survive?* are poorly constructed. Mary Northway (1940), an early user of sociometry in an educational setting, developed the target sociogram. Beginning with four concentric circles, Northway places the most highly chosen individuals in the center of the target. The rest are located according to their places on a distribution curve.

Forsyth and Katz (1946) suggested that a matrix provides a better way to display the data from a sociometric test. The matrix is formed by listing the names of the individuals horizontally across the top and, in the same order, vertically along the right side of the sheet of paper. Horizontal and vertical lines are then drawn to create a matrix of squares. For each person in the vertical list, a plus sign is placed in the square under the names in the horizontal list of those chosen and a minus sign for those rejected. Moreno (1946c) responded to their article, acknowledging some advantages to the matrix form and pointing out that the sociogram was superior in identifying structures like triangles, squares, and chains. He suggested that sociogram and sociomatrix complement each other, each offering good points. Toeman (1948b) wrote an article that included instructions for constructing sociograms. Hale (1981) recommends first entering the sociometric test data in a matrix and then drawing the sociogram. She has expanded the sociomatrix so that one can tally for each individual the positive and negative choices made and received, mutual choices, and incongruities. Having these readily available helps greatly in constructing the sociogram.

The Social Atom

Social scientists tend to utilize a mass approach to the study of communities, ethnic groups, nationalities, or gender. They calculate trends, attitudes, and personality characteristics of groups, and analyze these features with statistical instruments. A social group or collectivity is treated as a collection of individuals. However, society only exists with the interpersonal interactions of the members. Moreno's sociometry conceives of society as the complex interlinking of innumerable social atoms.

> The social atom is that peculiar pattern of inter-personal relations which develops from the time of human birth. It first contains mother and child. As times goes on, it adds from the persons who come into child's orbit such persons as are unpleasant or pleasant to him, and vice-versa, those to whom he unpleasant or pleasant. (Moreno, 1939, p. 3)

And:

> The hypothesis of the social atom states that a) an individual is tied to his social atom as closely as to his body; b) as he moves from an old to

a new community it changes its membership but its constellation tends to be constant. Notwithstanding that it is a novel social structure into which he has entered, the social atom has a tendency to repeat its former constellation; its concrete, individual members have changed but the pattern persists. (Moreno, 1953c, p. 703)

Social atoms are the first structures of interest to the sociometrist. A social atom consists of an individual and all the other individuals with whom he/she is meaningfully related. *Meaningful* indicates that there is an emotional connection between the individual and each person in that special group, one of any of the emotions that "bind or separate people, like love and hate, pity and compassion, jealousy and envy, gaiety and joy, anger and hate" (Moreno et al., 1960, p. 52). This pattern of attractions and rejections of which one is the center identifies that person's social atom. "It is the smallest functional unit within the social group" (Moreno, 1953c, p. 69). Jennings (1943, p. 3) wrote, "The concept of the social atom appears likely to remain among the most important contributions Moreno has made to the study of inter-personal phenomena."

We all have, in a given moment, a large number of people with whom we are acquainted, people that we can recognize as individuals that we have met at some time or another, at some place or another. The sum total of our acquaintances is called our acquaintance volume by Moreno (1947b). A majority of those who make up our acquaintance volume mean little to us. They simply are other human beings living in the world around us. They don't have any specific personal meaning to us and we don't have any personal meaning to them. We are not in frequent communication with them. We do not engage in activities together.

And then, on the other hand, there is a relatively small group of our acquaintances that *do* mean something personal to us. We have either positive feelings and are attracted to them or we have negative feelings and avoid or reject them, always with reference to some activity in which we wish to engage. Reciprocally, we are meaningful to most, but not necessarily all, of these persons. In other words, some of those to whom we are attracted are indifferent to us. Also, we may be attracted to individuals who we have not met, who do not know of our existence. By the same token, there may well be individuals who are either attracted to us or who reject us without our knowledge. They, too, become a part of our social atom. To quote Moreno (1947b), "To my social atom evidently would belong all individuals to who I am bound by an invisible desire which may be little or not at all manifest; also those individuals to whom I am tied in actual overt relationships" (p. 287). Although there tends to be a clear line between acquaintance and member of a social atom, the boundary is permeable. Most of those in our social atom were originally acquaintances. As soon as we desire to enter a relationship with an acquaintance, that person has entered our social atom.

The complete social atom of an individual includes all those who are meaningful to that person and all those to whom that person is meaningful.

To discover such an atom, one would have to test sociometrically all the groups to which the person belonged. First the family, then the community, and so forth, until we include the whole of humankind. A Morenean ambition, a sociometric testing of humankind is unlikely to occur. Nonetheless, the sociometrist can learn a great deal about social functioning by examining that part of an individual's social atom that falls within the boundaries of one of the groups to which that person belongs. Jennings (1939, 1941a, 1941b, 1942) has reported such research in a series of articles. Her research at the Hudson training school revealed not only a relatively consistency between the results of sociometric testing done at time intervals, but a consistency in social atom patterns.

Moreno (1947c) hypothesizes that the social atom of an individual develops a consistent pattern of relationships. The goal is a balance of emotions given and received, and when this is achieved, sociostasis, a social balance, is the result. A lack of sociostasis results in tensions and uneasiness that affects conduct and the sense of well-being. As we go through life, however, we sometimes lose the significant others who occupy certain positions in our social atoms. A person dies. Another moves away. Roles change. When these things happen, Moreno says, and we lose someone from our social atom, another individual is soon found who takes the place of the one lost and sociostasis is reestablished. This reparative process is almost automatic since there are numerous other social atoms around us also seeking to establish balance.

The social atom is regarded as a social structure, but it is a very active social structure and constantly undergoing change. The vast majority of one's social interactions occur with members of one's social atom. It is in these interactions that social creativity takes place. Roles are created, altered, and expanded. Since the ego or self is conceived of as one's role repertoire, it is the spontaneity within the social atom that is responsible for who one is.

Every member of a social atom is also the center of another social atom. Any two social atoms may contain a lot or a little overlap. Through the social atoms of the members of one's social atom, one is linked to others. Every social group, then, is composed of a number of interlocking social atoms, and, likewise, every group is interlocked with numerous other groups through social atoms. This is what Moreno meant when he defined the social atom as the smallest functional unit, the common denominator, of any social organization. Influence travels through this vast complex of interpersonal connections, creating extensive social networks.

The Cultural Atom

Moreno (1953c) wrote:

> Every individual, in addition to being the center of a number of attractions and repulsions, is also the center of numerous rôles that

relate one to the rôles of other individuals. Just as he has at all times a set of friends and a set of enemies, he also has a range of rôles and a range of counter-rôles. They are in various stages of development. . . . the focal pattern of rôle-relations around an individual is called his *cultural atom*. (p. 70)

If we construct a social atom and then add lines to reflect the relationships existing between all the individuals depicted in it, we have constructed what Moreno called the cultural atom. Just as the social atom is the smallest functional unit of society, the cultural atom is considered the smallest functional unit within a cultural pattern. Both constructs, the social atom and the cultural atom, reflect characteristics of the same social reality.

Other Social Structures

A number of substructures are found in group sociograms. The first to be found developmentally are pairs. A pair exists when person A chooses person B and B reciprocates, choosing A. A triangle appears when A chooses B and B chooses C chooses A. Four individuals choosing each other in the same way make a square on the sociogram. More than four make a circle and a series of individuals connected by choice or rejection, whether or not these choices are reciprocated, make a chain. An over-chosen individual, with lines coming to her or him from every direction, is called a star. One can be a star of rejection as well as of choice. Those who neither choose nor are chosen are isolates, while those who make and receive far fewer than the average number of choices are called under-chosen.

The appearance of these substructures indicates the degree of differentiation or complexity of organization of a social entity. In the developmental studies that Moreno made (discussed below), pairs showed up first, followed by the more elaborate structures. One of the values of the sociogram is that it gives a picture of the whole group while keeping the position of each member of the group in sight.

Sociometric Networks

In the age of the Internet and the World Wide Web with websites like Facebook, Twitter, LinkedIn, and the like, social networks are a familiar concept. For decades, new college graduates and others looking for employment have been advised that networking is the most effective way to succeed. The invention of computers and especially the Internet has established a medium by which we can communicate with almost any number of others, and do so practically instantaneously. A new science of network theory has developed a mathematics of networks and the concept of networks is being applied in physics (as Moreno predicted), biology, sociology, social psychology, economics, and other disciplines.

Social networks and networking were not so familiar when Moreno discussed them in the first edition of *Who Shall Survive?* Psychosocial networks are larger social structures hidden in the sociograms of communities. The study of these sociometric networks at the Hudson training school was initiated by an unusual happening: 14 girls ran away from the school in 14 days. This was strange because there had been only 10 elopements in the preceding seven months. In addition, there were a number of other girls who were considered sociometrically predisposed toward running away but who did not join in with the 14 runaways. Moreno suspected that the 14 runaways were somehow connected, although they lived in four different cottages and were not all acquainted with each other. Using the sociograms, Moreno was able to identify the links, which connected the girls in a chain, a network, even though none of them knew all the others in the network.

Runaways seldom leave alone. They leave in pairs or in small groups. When a girl is contemplating eloping, finding a partner with the same thoughts reinforces the motivation of both, eventually triggering attempt. In the case of the 14 runaways, a strong current was developed through the network, with each member contributing more or less desire to run. The other students who were considered to be predisposed toward elopement but did not join the 14 were not linked to the runaway network.

Unlike some of the smaller social structures, pairs, triangles, and the like, sociometric networks are not readily apparent. At the same time, there were several phenomena that suggested that such structures existed. Rumors spread in an irregular way through the school. Students were noticed to be doing or saying similar things in different parts of the community even though they were not acquainted with each other. The search for networks in the sociograms that could explain these occurrences began. It started with one individual who had a line that went out to any member of a different cottage. A line to someone in a third group that came from this second person was found, and so forth, until the chain stopped with a person who had no connection with another cottage. This chain was considered to be the main line of communication of the network. Then the connections that each member of the main line had within her own group were added. These were the side branches of the main line. For each of these members, a search for links to other cottages was made. When these were found, they and their connections were added to the network.

Using this method, five large networks were found in the Hudson training school community. There was some overlapping with girls who belonged to two or more networks. Only a few of the individuals in a network knew each other personally. The majority was connected to one another by hidden links. Networks serve as channels of communication for the transmission of news and opinions, no matter how far apart their members may be geographically.

Rumors were continually running through the Hudson training school community. To demonstrate the dynamic effect of networks, Moreno tested the hypothesis that the spread of rumors would follow the paths of the networks that had been mapped. He started a rumor and watched how it spread through the community. The rumor was first given to a well-connected individual in one of the largest networks, identified as Group I. As predicted, it spread rapidly through Group I before it entered other groups. It was also predicted that Group V would be the last network to receive the rumor because there was no overlap between that group and Group I. That prediction was also verified.

The network research done at the Hudson training school was based on the sociograms of the proximity in living criterion. That was a strong criterion that changed slowly, providing some consistency in the identified networks. The network is related to and molded by the currents that run through it (Moreno, 1960e). If an idea or opinion reaches a person who rejects it or does not see it as important to pass along, that individual and any who are only connected through that person will not become a part of the network for that idea or opinion. News, gossip, and opinions that do not hurt the network member are passed along with little resistance, but if information concerns certain sensitive activities, sexual ones, for example, or if it concerns illegal ventures, the individuals involved are very careful. They try to keep the particulars restricted to others who will not expose them and away from the larger networks. This seldom works and few things remain secrets for very long. For that reason, a user of illegal drugs in an unknown town or city usually has little difficulty in finding a source for replenishment of his/her supply.

A community or neighborhood may be a unit physically, but it is actually broken up into parts, which extend beyond it into other units:

> The local districts are, so to speak, transversed by psychological currents which bind large groups of individuals together into units, irrespective of neighborhood, district, or borough distinctions. These networks are the kitchens of public opinion. It is through these channels that people affect, educate, or disintegrate one another. It is through these networks that suggestion is transmitted. In one part of a community a person has the reputation of honesty; in another part of dishonesty. Whatever the actual facts may be, this reputation is due to two different networks in which travel two different opinions of him. (Moreno, 1960e, p. 78)

Moreno maintained that there are many specific patternings of these networks and that different types of networks will be found to characterize different communities. He predicted that the size of networks would be found to cover a wide range; some limited to an individual locality while others extended to several communities and some will even extend across the country (Moreno, 1934). The psychosocial network theory of J. L. Moreno explains the tenacity of phenomena such as racial and ethnic prejudices, existing as currents running through and connecting individuals and groups widely scattered over the country.

THE SOCIOGENETIC LAW

Moreno's first systematic sociometric work was conducted with school-children. The first hypothesis that Moreno wanted to test was that social organization evolved from a simpler form to a more complex one over time. Although the answer seems obvious, Moreno wanted to produce evidence that could support it. To study this assumption, Moreno and Jennings conducted observational studies of infants and sociometric studies in a public elementary school.

The work with infants took place in an unidentified institution but quite likely the Plymouth Institute in Brooklyn. Groups of nine babies, within a day or two of the same age, were placed in proximity with each other on a daily basis. They were observed for several kinds of interactions, including looking at the other, crying with the other, smiling at the other, trying to grasp the other, and touching the other.

From birth on, there was no interaction until 20 to 28 weeks. Infants were isolated and self-absorbed. Moreno labeled this stage "organic isolation." From 20 to 28 weeks, the infants began to react to their neighbors, the babies closest to them. Moreno called this "horizontal differentiation." At about 40 to 42 weeks, a new phenomenon appeared. One or two of the infants received a disproportionate amount of attention from the others, creating a "vertical differentiation" in the group. What Moreno would come to call the sociodynamic effect had made its appearance. Although the study continued to the age of 18 months, no further stages of differentiation were noted (Moreno, 1934).

The studies of schoolchildren took place in Public School 181 in Brooklyn, New York. Moreno and Jennings gave sociometric tests to every class in the school from kindergarten through the eighth grade. The criterion was proximity: "You are now given the opportunity to choose the boy or girl whom you would like to have sit on either side of you. Write down whom you would like first best; then, whom you would like second best. Look around and make up your mind. Remember that next term your friend you choose now may sit beside you" (Moreno, 1934, p. 13). As far as the literature goes, this was the first systematic sociometric test and experiment ever conducted.

The results of the tests clearly show increasing complexity in the social organization of the student groups from kindergarten to the eighth grade. These are reflected in the sociometric structures that appear in the sociograms of the various groups. As noted above, the simplest structure is mutual choice or pairs. The number of pairs steadily increases with class level. Triangles, squares, circles, and chains begin to appear in the second grade and increase in number through grade eight. Other features of the experiment involved the choices between genders. The choices for a member of the opposite sex were highest in kindergarten and first grade, accounting for 35 percent and 32 percent of the total choices. In the second grade, the choices dropped precipitously to 8 percent and declined even further to zero in the sixth grade. In the seventh grade, this cleavage between sexes began to change, and choices across sexual boundaries started to reappear. They rose to more than 10 percent in the eighth grade.

These findings can be interpreted as supporting Freud's notions of a homosexual developmental stage based on his theory of the sexual instinct. Moreno, however, had a different interpretation of the phenomenon. He suggests that the complex problems of learning how to interact in accordance with the rules of the society in which one lives are simplified by eliminating the special demands of intersexual relationships. It is easier for the members of each sex to master social interaction without the added dimension of a different gender.

Unchosen students ranged from a low of about 15 percent in the sixth and seventh grades to a high of 45 percent in the first grade. The percent of unchosen in other grades hovered at just less than 30 percent. The overchosen, stars, ranged from five in kindergarten and the seventh grade but otherwise averaged about two.

Summarizing this work with children, Moreno suggests that three periods of social organization can be identified. The first is a presocialized period covering the years up to seven to nine. Groups formed during these ages tend to be unstable. There are many isolates and few mutual pairs, the basic sociometric structure for stability. Choices tend to be diffuse and do not lead to cooperative interaction to achieve a specific goal. Groups in this period require adult assistance to function effectively.

From seven to nine years on, children are able to form independent social groups that can function without adult assistance. As a matter of fact, during this period, there is a cleavage with adults, and groups in this period develop their own codes of conduct. Interrelationships are sufficiently differentiated to grasp social codes. Groups are able to organize around a specific goal and work cooperatively to achieve it. This is the first socialized period.

The third period, the second socialized period, begins at about age 13 or 14 and continues on into adulthood. This period is the organization of the adult members of a society with all its complexity and differentiation. The more technologically advanced a society is, the more differentiated and complex is the social organization.

Moreno suggested that the increasing complexity of social organization associated with age and maturity recapitulates the history social organization in humankind. In other words, he hypothesized that the social organization of humankind has evolved with history. Moreno called this theory the sociogenetic law. He saw it as analogous to the biogenetic law, the notion that higher, more complex organisms have evolved from simpler ones.

The public school studies fell far short of Moreno's goal of a sociometric study of a community. The school was at best a very partial community. The members of it, the students, spent only a few hours a day in it. To extend his research into the larger community in which the school was embedded meant including the families and neighborhoods from which the students came. This was obviously too overwhelming a project to contemplate. Moreno looked for a smaller contained community, one more like Mitterndorf, in which to carry out his dream of a scientific, sociometric analysis and restructuring of an entire community. He soon found it in the New York State Training School for Girls at Hudson.

THE SOCIODYNAMIC EFFECT

One might expect that sociometric choices would be randomly distributed within a group, that they would fall along a normal probability curve like the distribution of so many psychological measurements, such as intelligence test scores, or physical measurements, such as height and weight. This does not happen. The results of every sociometric test ever conducted show a distinctive feature. A few members of the group are far more highly chosen than others, while a slightly larger number receive no choices or far less than average. Studies have empirically demonstrated that the differences, compared with a random distribution of choices, are statistically decidedly significant (Moreno & Jennings, 1938). Bronfenbrenner (1943), using sophisticated mathematical methods, has provided further evidence that sociometric choice deviates significantly from chance expectancy. Distributions of sociometric test scores regularly form a J-shaped curve rather than the familiar bell-shaped probability curve. Furthermore, the frequency with which mutuality of choice (A chooses B and B chooses A) appears is many times that which could be expected by simple chance. Moreno considered these clear indications that some factor or agent is influencing the distribution of the positive and negative choices made in the context of a sociometric exploration.

Moreno labeled the phenomenon of overchoice of a few the psychodynamic effect and sometimes called it the psychodynamic law. It appears to be found in all populations and groupings. It can vary in degree but seems to be universally present. The effect may be greater in groups with great diversity along racial, economic, and cultural dimensions.

In the training school study, within seven cottages of 26 students each, 2 percent of the population received 8 percent of the choices; 8 percent received 23 percent of the choices; 25 percent received 58 percent; 35 percent shared 5 percent; and 20 percent were not chosen by anyone.

SOCIOMETRIC THEORY OF LEADERSHIP

Individuals who are over-chosen in a community have exceptional influence over a community's activities, values, and attitudes. Sociometric stars of attraction, therefore, are considered leaders in their groups. This notion accounts for the title for Helen Jennings's book, *Leadership and Isolation* (1943), in which she made comparisons of those girls of the Hudson training school who were over-chosen with those who were under-chosen or not chosen at all.

Moreno identified three types of leadership in *Who Shall Survive?* (1953c) and later in an article (1950). The three types are (1) the popular leader; (2) the powerful leader; and (3) the isolated leader. Moreno used sociograms to demonstrate the different types and those are reproduced here.

These social atoms display only positive choices. Figure 9.1 is the social atom for individual BL and shows that she receives many choices from the girls who live in the same cottage with her. BL in turn gives her choices to cottage mates. The only two girls from other cottages who chose her are themselves rejected and isolated in the community. Moreno identifies this as the social atom of a popular leader who has great influence within her group although not in the community at large.

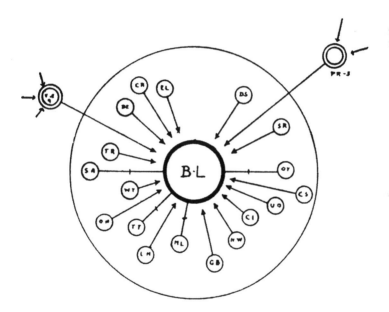

A POPULAR SOCIOMETRIC LEADER

BL is the center of attraction from twenty individuals. Eighteen of these twenty live with her in the same home group, the total population of which is 25 members at this time. The population of this cottage has fluctuated between 25 and 31 individuals. BL is attracted to four individuals (SA, TT, ML and OY) of her own home group. Thus she would be classified as a popular leader. But the two attractions coming to her from outside her group are from two isolated and rejected individuals, VE of C9 and PR of C3 and the attractions from inside her group come from individuals who are singly almost cut off from the chief currents of the community. Therefore, notwithstanding the fact that BL commands quantitatively a great direct influence, this influence is limited to the area of her own cottage, C8.

Figure 9.1   Social atom of a popular leader.
Source: *Who Shall Survive?* with permission.

Figure 9.2 is centered on individual LP. LP is chosen by four members of the community, two of them from her own cottage. LP chooses all four of those who chose her; they are all mutual choices. When we look at the social atoms of those who choose LP, we find that these individuals are themselves highly chosen, receiving even more attractions than does LP. LP's four choices receive attractions from well-chosen individuals in other cottages. Through her mutual connections with highly chosen members of the community, LP exerts influence throughout the community, even though she receives only four choices directly. This, Moreno says, is the sociogram of a powerful leader.

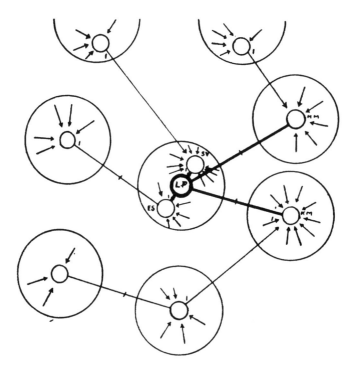

A POWERFUL SOCIOMETRIC LEADER

LP of C6 is the center of attraction from four individuals: SV and ES both of her own cottage, MM of C1 and KM of C7. She is the first choice of these individuals as is indicated by the numeral 1 on the side of the line extending from each of them to her. She makes use of four of her five choices and appears attracted in return to SV, ES, MM and KM with each of whom she forms a pair. Quantitatively she would be classified as an individual of average direct influence, but through SV, ES, MM and KM, she commands by indirection nearly one hundred individuals, of whom fifty-eight are indicated in the chart. She actually has a powerful position in the community.

Figure 9.2   Social atom of a powerful leader.

Source: *Who Shall Survive?* with permission.

Figure 9.3 shows the structure of an isolated sociometric leader. A and B are mutual choices. Not only that, they are the exclusive choices of each other. Neither makes use of the other choices, five, at their disposal. B is the choice of four other individuals, all of whom have received many choices. Through indirect linkage, B is an individual who has great influence in the community. However, A, being the only choice of B, has great influence with B and, indirectly then, upon the community. Moreno coined the term *aristotele* to describe this structure: "A single tele relationship which produces, through indirect links, a large network of influence is called 'aristotele'" (1953c, p. 324). This leader may be thought of as "the power behind the throne."

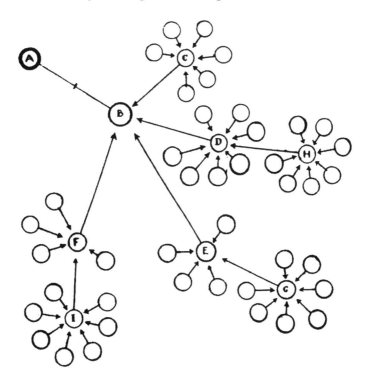

STRUCTURE OF AN ISOLATED SOCIOMETRIC LEADER
A single tele relationship which produces, through indirect links, a large network of influence is called "Aristo-tele."
Individual A is the first and exclusive attraction of B and B is the first and exclusive attraction of A. (Both individuals, A and B, make use of one choice only from the five at their disposal.) Except for the one tele from B, A is *isolated* in the community. But B is also the first choice of C, D, E and F, who in turn, are the centers of attraction of 6, 8, 5 and 5 other individuals respectively. Among these latter 24 individuals are three persons, G, H and I, who are the center of 7 attractions each. The effect of the one tele from B to A is to connect A, like an invisible ruler with a main psychological current, and to enable him to reach 50 persons potentially predisposed towards him.

Figure 9.3   Social atom of an isolated leader.
Source: *Who Shall Survive?* with permission.

TELE

Tele is one of the more enigmatic if not esoteric of the Morenean concepts. It was introduced by Moreno to account for the fact that the distribution of choices during sociometric testing, and especially the occurrences of mutual choice, deviated so far from a normal distribution. Moreno discussed tele in many passages. Cukier (2007) lists more than 50 items concerning tele in her list of Morenean quotations, and yet, like spontaneity, it is a difficult notion to fully comprehend.

In his attempt to explain the phenomenon that he would call tele, Moreno recalled events from his experiences with the *Stegreiftheater* in Vienna. In *The Theater of Spontaneity*, he wrote that at times some of the spontaneity players appear to be joined by an unseen connection of feelings. They "have a sort of heightened sensitivity for their mutual inner processes. One gesture is sufficient and often they do not have to look at one another, they are telepathic for one another. They communicate through a new sense, as if by a 'medial' understanding" (1947e, p. 68). It appears as if they are communicating with each other without words or gestures. The capability seems to grow with experience.

The social atom is relatively easy to describe and is readily apparent in the sociogram. It is much more difficult, Moreno (1937b) says, to describe the process that attracts individuals to one another or that repels them, that flow of feelings of which the social atom and the networks are apparently composed. Those feelings are associated with our perceptions of other people. Underlying this flow of feelings are real processes in people's life situations that make them sensitive to real processes in other people's life situation. These interpersonal sensitivities result in feelings that are positive or negative and of varying degrees of intensity. Tele is an experience of some real factor in the other person. It is an interpersonal phenomenon, not the emotional response of a single person. It is the feeling basis of intuition and insight (Moreno, 1946a). As suggested in the thought experiment in the previous chapter, tele is operating between group members at the first meeting (Moreno, 1972a).

Moreno called upon two other concepts to help delineate the concept of tele: transference and empathy. Transference was a major concept in Freud's system and was considered of great importance in understanding the relationship between the analysand and analyst. Transference is, of course, a fantasy. The analysand is portrayed as projecting characteristics of someone else, usually a parent, and the accompanying feelings upon the analyst. Moreno agreed that this was a real phenomenon. He argued, however, that in addition to this unreal aspect of the relationship, another process takes place. The analysand sizes up the analyst and assesses what kind of person the analyst is. "These feelings into the actuality of this man, physical, mental or otherwise are 'tele' relations" (1959b, p. 6).

When two people meet for the first time, their perceptions of each other are in all probability a combination of tele and transference. Each perceives accurately some but not all aspects of the other accurately. Tele, Moreno says, doesn't really change, but we don't see everything in the other person at first. It is through continuing contact that our awareness grows and develops. Transference, on the other hand, is irrational and changes in transference are not related to present perceptions of the other.

Transference and tele, Moreno concludes, are linked together. Transference is a distortion of tele. It is a one-way process, while tele, Moreno insists, is an interpersonal process, "like a telephone, it has two ends" (1953c, p. 53). Over time, people in a relationship see each other more and more authentically as tele replaces transference. This affects the dynamics of the relationship, either deepening it or resulting in a cooling off of the relationship (1954b).

Empathy is the other concept that is often used in explaining interpersonal relationships. Introduced in the study of aesthetics by psychologist Theodore Lipps, empathy was first described as feeling oneself into a work of art. Now it also means experiencing the feelings of another person. Moreno agreed that empathy is a veridical process. But, like transference, empathy is a one-way process. As such it cannot account for the mutuality that occurs in sociometric experiments (1953b, 1955d, 1959b, 1960c).

> Telic reciprocity proposes that A and B are an interactional, cooperational unit, that they are two parts of the same process although occasionally at different points in space and time. Telic sensitivity is, therefore, a two-way process, sensitivity of the parts "for one another": it is by experience mutual and reciprocal, what benefits one benefits the other. It is productive because it is both ways and continuous. It can be compared with telephonic communication. Empathy is a telic fragment which emerges in the course of individuation and self-integration. It proposes that A and B are separate individuals, they are acting side by side. It is a one-way process, sensitivity which one has for the other. . . .
>
> It is an uncanny sensitivity for each other which welds individuals into unity. In genuine love relations the partners share each other's cleverness as well as each other's limitations. Love is a telic relationship. In life itself we are expected to be sensitive for the feelings of the person with whom we are interacting at the time. Watching the behavior of partners and putting ourselves into their situations, mentally reversing roles with them, we are continuously getting clues how they expect us to act. In turn, we are giving them clues how we expect them to act. (Moreno, 1955d, p. 276)

Tele is a function of spontaneity. For this reason, it is important that the participants in sociometric testing be carefully warmed up fully to the task of expressing their choices. Just as individuals can be trained to be more spontaneous, their capacity for tuning in to telic communication can be increased. Moreno developed a sociometric perception test that serves as a training exercise. It is presented in six steps in *Who Shall Survive?* (1953c, p. 325). In the first step, the individual identifies all the others in the situation under consideration. Next, he establishes how he feels about each of these other people, just as if he were taking a sociometric test. The third step is to guess how these others would choose him if this were a sociometric test. The fourth step involves guessing how the others who are part of the situation would choose each other. The next action is to have oneself rated by someone else who is familiar with the situation, and the sixth and last step is to check the validity of this work by conducting a sociometric test of the individuals involved. Moreno hypothesizes that it might be possible through the "training of many generations in the conation and cognition of tele, in role enactment and role perception, [that] we will be able to penetrate the social universe . . . and communicate with individuals at a distance without meeting them physically, attaining the effects of extrasensory perception without an extrasensory function" (1953c, pp. 327–328).

There are a number of events that are attributed to telic processes, several of which occur frequently in psychodrama groups. Zerka Moreno (2000a) discusses one that is quite common but can still generate a feeling of the uncanny. Many psychodrama groups are truly synthetic groups in Moreno's terms, composed of people who have not previously met. In a psychodrama, the protagonist is asked to select a member of the group to serve as an auxiliary ego, that is, to represent an absent person from the protagonist's social atom, perhaps a family member. At the end of the drama and in sharing with the protagonist, the auxiliary says something like, "I don't know why you picked me for that role, but I have had the same kind of experience that person had." It is also common that members of the group anticipate being selected to become an auxiliary. A frequent statement heard during sharing is: "I knew you were going to pick me to be your mother (father, sister, brother, uncle, etc.)."

During the years that I was a student at the Moreno Institute and eventually the Director of Training, a phenomenon occurred that was difficult to explain other than by tele. The training program after about 1968 consisted of three sessions a day, most of which involved a classical psychodrama with a student as protagonist and another student or staff member directing. It was not unusual for the group members to return to the residence to find a message that there had been a call for one of the group during the psychodrama session. The call was often for the group member who had been the protagonist and usually it was from the person with whom the protagonist had been exploring his/her relationship. I have a deep regret that I missed a great research opportunity by not keeping track of calls received during group sessions and noting what percentage of them were for protagonists.

The concept of tele can account for events not related to the psychodrama theater. Many of us have had the experience of thinking about or being concerned for someone and, as we are warming up to calling him/her, we receive a call from him/her. Nowadays it may be an email instead of a phone call. Another phenomenon, not so common, that can be attributed to tele is the experience that some people have of suddenly knowing that someone close to them has passed away. It is often very dramatic, like waking up in the middle of the night with a powerful sense of the death of a significant other.

At the very least, tele phenomena tell us that we know more about people than we allow ourselves to believe. The skepticism of science has entered society at large and we get trained not to accept our intuitions about others. Social conserves such as "don't judge a book by its cover" steer us away from trusting our spontaneous sizing up of the other person. Tele is not a concept that is easy to understand or accept because it has the quality of nonlocality. Although tele is somewhat mysterious and conventional psychology cannot account for it, it can be understood from the perspective of David Bohm's vision of the universe. In this theory, all the subatomic particles of the universe, including those of which we and everybody else are composed, share information about the whole universe. Tele, then, is a matter of tuning in to information that is already in us.

ROLE THEORY

Role theory in the Morenean system accomplishes a number of goals. It characterizes the relationship of interacting individuals, identifying the types of actions that can be expected. Role theory provides a theory of personality. It describes the dynamic interaction of the individual with society through which individuals together create society, while society, in turn, shapes the behavior of the individuals. Roles and role relationships form what we know as the culture of a society.

Moreno liked to point out that the concept of role originated in drama and that the discipline of sociology adopted it long after its use in the theater. In the conventional theater, a role is the finished product of the playwright's creativity. It describes in great detail how the actor who takes the role will look and act. The role identifies the character's social status and determines every interaction with every other character in the drama. Attitude and every speech to be made, every action to be taken are determined by the role. It allows for the minimum of creativity and calls for a minimum of spontaneity on the part of the actor. Taking a role in conventional drama is one extreme of a continuum of role behavior, the other extreme being role creating (Moreno, 1960c, 1972a). Society, more specifically culture, serves a function akin to that of a script with respect to the roles we take in life. Social roles provide templates for the actions that are considered appropriate for people in a role relationship (Moreno, 1953b).

Moreno, whose greatest interest was creative activity, was most interested role creating, how roles are created. The *Stegreiftheater* (theater of spontaneity) that he devised in Vienna required the players to create their roles in the moment of presentation. There was no script to guide them, no rehearsals in which to prepare, only a theme or a situation from which they had to create the drama. His observations of the spontaneity players as they created their roles became the first step in developing his role theory.

The Genesis of Roles

Moreno distinguishes three kinds of roles: psychosomatic roles, psychodramatic roles, and social roles. Psychosomatic roles deal with physiological functions; the eater, the eliminator, and the sleeper are some of the first that emerge. Developing later are the roles of the crawler, the walker, and so forth. All skills have a psychosomatic role component. According to Moreno's developmental theory, the newborn human infant does not initially distinguish between self and the universe. The sense of self grows out of repeated experiences of physiological functions, such as eating. The sensations from sucking, milk in the mouth, esophagus, and stomach establish the connections between them, forming the role of the eater. The other psychosomatic roles, such as the eliminator, evolve in the same manner. Finally, the experiential associations between the psychosomatic roles establish the sense of a physical self.

Psychodramatic roles are wished for roles and when an individual is unable to take or enact such a role, act hunger ensues. Psychodramatic roles are stimulated by observation of the acts of others, parents, older children, actors on TV shows, and stories heard or read. They may be realistic, capable of playing or taking, or they may be fantastic, such as the roles of fairies and ghosts, Batman and other heroes, and hallucinations or delusions. Psychodramatic roles are the stuff of children's free creative play and children possess many such roles and much act hunger. Young boys in their play drive trucks, win great battles, and perform heroic feats. Young girls become mothers, create homes, and engage in other play activities according to that which the culture designates. Psychodramatic roles are in no way limited to children, however. Psychodramatic roles may be responsible for the major changes in lifestyle and occupation that are termed midlife crises. Just as psychosomatic roles give rise to a physical self, the psychodramatic roles establish a psychological self.

The roles that are enacted and recognized in the culture of a group are social roles. They comprise the entire professional, occupational, family, recreational, ethic, or nationality roles in a culture. Many individuals in a culture represent a social role, such as the father role. Each father is both alike and different from every other father. Every father creates the father role in a unique and individual way. It is the common elements of all the fathers that comprise the social role of *the* father. As taken by the individual, it is the role of *a* father.

The social role has a strong influence on all the individuals who take that role. Social roles are conserves, which exert a coercive pressure on the members of a culture, offering norms for taking the role and sometimes demanding or restricting certain actions. For example, in many cultures, a father is required to provide financial support for his children and is prohibited from abusing them. Behavior in some roles is highly regulated by law. People in professional roles, lawyers, doctors, judges, and policemen, for example, may be required to have a prescribed education or training and to be licensed before they can practice. Roles that carry certain power over other people, such as policemen or judges, also have restrictions defining when and how that power can be used. Social norms, values, and ethics may also be associated with other roles, such as teachers, religious leaders, and government officials.

Role Theory Concepts

Moreno employs a number of terms in his discussion of role. These include role-playing, role taking, and role creating. Moreno is not totally consistent in his use of these expressions, and they are neither tightly defined nor totally distinct from one another.

For Moreno, role taking is an actional process. It is the enactment of an established role, a conserved role. The prime example is that of an actor taking a role in a play. The playwright has created all the roles. The actors' actions, words, and interactions with the other characters in the play are prescribed. There is minimal room for the actor to alter the performance. Role taking, in Moreno's view, consists of engaging with one or more others in a role that has already been created, and opportunity for spontaneity and creativity is at a minimum. At times Moreno seems to limit role taking to the conventional drama, although in other passages it is obvious that role taking is what we do in real life: "Real action in a role may be called role taking or 'being' in a role in life itself" (Moreno & Zelany, 1961, p. 643). Here culture rather than a script provides norms and constraint upon one's actions. Social roles, though they may be prescriptive, are not as structured or restricting as are roles in the theater.

Role-playing, on the other hand, is an experimental procedure, the acting out of a role in a simulated situation, such as in children's creative play or in psychodrama or role training. Rehearsing for an upcoming situation, such as an interview for a job, is an example. Role-playing is a method of learning to enact a role more successfully and is the basis of psychodramatic role training. Since its introduction by Moreno, role-playing has found its way into training in numerous vocational activities.

Role creating is exactly what it sounds like: the creation of a role from scratch. The spontaneity players of the *Stegreiftheater* were routinely required to create the roles that were assigned to them. This illustrates the maximum degree of role creating, while role taking in the conventional theater represents the minimum degree. It is easy to see that role-playing may be the means of role creating, and that role taking may include a degree of role creating. Moreno promoted the idea of greater role creating in the sense of entering into every interaction with recognition that it was unique and offered an opportunity for a creative originality.

Moreno also uses the concept of role perception, the perceiving of another person taking a role. Role perception is almost always a preliminary step to taking a role. For example, we perceive our parents in father and mother roles before we, ourselves, take those roles in life. Moreno also indicates that there is some degree of role-playing, even if it is only fragmentary as a mental rehearsal, prior to role taking. Role-playing can serve to increase one's adequacy in specific roles that one takes in life. It also is a way of promoting understanding of others in roles that we do not take. A male, for example, can achieve some degree of comprehension of the world as experienced by a woman, and vice versa.

Role terminology became complicated by the fact that there are alternative role theories from sociology and social psychology and some identical words have different definitions (Coutu, 1951). This problem began to develop at about the time that Moreno introduced his role theory in the first edition of *Who Shall Survive?* In the same year, 1934, students of George Herbert Mead, who had died in 1931, published *Mind, Self and Society*, a book compiled from student notes taken during Mead's lectures with Mead listed as the author.

Mead was a philosopher and social theorist, a close friend and colleague of John Dewey, and a leading figure in the school of pragmatism. Mead developed a theory of roles that had much in common with Moreno's ideas. He rejected determinism and was convinced that autonomy and creativity existed. He considered that human interactions occurred in role relationships. His work inspired the school of symbolic interactionism, which has many similarities to Moreno's role theory, as well as a spate of role theory and experiments in sociology.

The process Mead describes and calls role taking is an internal, psychological process in which the participant of an interaction with another imaginatively puts him/herself in the role of the other, using the information thus obtained as a guide for his/her own actions. Mead seems to be saying that in social interactions, each participant has an awareness of the patterns of action, which the participants can be expected to produce. One accesses this information by doing what a psychodramatist might consider a mental role reversal. Role taking, for Mead, requires what Moreno called role perception of those with whom one is interacting.

Role Theory of Personality

A role is the tangible and functioning form that the self takes in a specific situation in relation to another person (Moreno, 1961b). "Role playing is prior to the emergence of the self. Roles do not emerge from the self but the self may emerge from roles" (Moreno, 1946b, p. 157). Moreno suggests that concepts such as self, ego, or personality are essentially the collective of roles that one takes or has taken in life. This is not to be construed as meaning that a role should be viewed as a part of the self. It is a pattern of behavior, skills, a way of perceiving, and the attitudes one takes to accomplish something that satisfies a need or desire. When we are successfully creating or taking a role, we embody it. Our entire self, body, mind, and emotions, our whole person, is engaged in the enactment:

> The role is not considered separate from a person's essence, as the clothes he puts on or takes off, but an existential part of his being, the part that makes up his ego with other roles. The personality may emerge from the roles. . . . The psyche is an open system with the roles in various stages of development. It is not a container into which the roles fit, like pick-up sticks in a tube. (Moreno, 2000b, 235)

Lewis Yablonsky (1953), student, colleague, and friend of Moreno, offering an operational theory of roles, discussed the dynamics of the interpersonal role relationship. The first step is the warming up of the actors to each other and to the situation in which they encounter each other. Each actor sizes up the situation and other participant (or participants), deciding whether or not to engage in interaction. This warming up process may be almost instantaneous in an emergency situation or when two people are well acquainted and have developed a bond of trust or, in Morenean terms, are each other's mutual positive choice. The warming up process may be relatively slow and cautious if the actors are unknown to each other, have mistrust of each other, or if the proposed interaction is perceived to have important and long lasting effects on the actor's life. The warming up may also vary from superficial, as in the warm-up to buying stamps at the post office, to profound, as in the warm-up to a life-changing act such as proposing marriage.

Once the actors have warmed up to each other and are satisfied that a rewarding interaction is possible, they act out their respective roles to the best of their abilities. Each act is unique, no matter how many others in similar roles have engaged in similar acts. Each moment is unique. Each actor brings a unique set of experiences to the act. The actors affect each other in unique ways. All of this novelty requires spontaneity. Even the reenactment of a familiar and highly defined role, even a role in the theater, requires a minimal degree of spontaneity. Life roles are not so explicitly defined. Every situation is at least a little bit different, and spontaneity is what makes it possible for us to adjust our behavior to the novelty of each situation. Spontaneity, as Yablonsky notes, is a necessary concept in order to comprehend role behavior in action.

CREATING SOCIETY

There are psychological theories that consider behavior from the standpoint of the individual, minimizing social influence on how we act. There are other theories that emphasize the role that society plays in how people behave, minimizing the effect of the individual. Morenean theory sees an even balance between the two extremes. The society in which we live provides a lot of ready-made roles and rules that greatly affect the development of the ego of its members. The social role of the mother, for example, influences how mothers relate to their children at all ages. However, there is a constant interplay between a society and its members. At the same time that her culture is influencing a mother's behavior, her behavior is influencing the social role of mother. Roles, therefore, provide a dynamic connection between the individual and society. Social roles make demands and put expectations on the individuals. Simultaneously, the Spontaneity-Creativity of the individuals and their sociometric attractions to each other are constantly changing and expanding the culture in which they occur. There is a reciprocal ongoing interaction between individual and society.

Members of a culture have considerable awareness of the roles in that culture. Children as young as six or seven can demonstrate a grasp of a number of common roles. Asked to "show me what a policeman does," children will act out directing traffic, chasing a criminal, and other policeman activities (Moreno & Moreno, 1945). In spontaneity testing and training, psychodrama, and sociodrama, people demonstrate a considerable capacity to produce accurate and valid role enactments of the roles in the culture in which they live. This ability is usually far greater than the individual himself is aware and greater than could be expected from examination of one's role history.

However, Moreno states, roles really do not need to be defined. They take form spontaneously and define themselves as they emerge in our interactions with each other. New roles are constantly being created and existing ones modified. Some roles become obsolete and cease to exist in a culture; inventions and social change call for the emergence of new, previously unimaginable roles.

A CALL FOR FURTHER RESEARCH

Moreno concluded his major opus with a list of sociometric hypotheses. The list includes his basic assumptions such as "mankind is a social and organic unity" (1953c, p. 606). Many, if not all, are invitations to further research. The 21 pages of hypotheses in *Who Shall Survive?* represent a gold mine of topics and ideas for theses and dissertations in the field of sociology. They also offer an excellent synopsis and general survey of Moreno's sociometry.

10 Psychodrama and Sociodrama

> Everybody who has ever participated in a psychodrama is both fascinated and stunned by the impact of spontaneous play. This form of theatre starts out on an empty stage with no script, no professional actors and no rehearsals. There is only the protagonist with his or her story which through the unique psychodramatic techniques expands into a full play, be it tragedy, satire, or comedy. The psychodrama has a strong psychological impact on the protagonist, the co-actors, and the group present.
>
> —Z. T. Moreno, (2000b, p. 1)

Psychodrama has been utilized predominantly in the mental health field, so much so that it is widely considered a method of psychotherapy. As Zerka Moreno indicates in the above quote, psychodrama is intrinsically a dramaturgy, a method of creating dramas. Although Moreno first used spontaneity techniques to resolve a marriage problem and later developed the psychodramatic method with patients in his sanitarium, he was always mindful of the many other potential applications of psychodrama. In particular, he thought of psychodrama as a method for normal, well-functioning people to better understand themselves and their relationships with others, an activity that is sometimes referred to as personal growth and development.

Psychodrama is known for the intense emotional arousal that many protagonists experience, which can make possible the catharsis of integration, the element that Moreno asserted was the goal of psychodrama. Although describing events and experiences, as happens in many forms of psychotherapy, can stir up strong emotions feelings associated with those events, putting the whole body into reenacting such moments, as happens in psychodrama, is far more effective in affective arousal. Action techniques also allow for a much fuller expression of the feelings engendered. For Freud, acting out was *resistance* to psychotherapy. For Moreno (1955c, 1959b), the acting out of one's desires and feelings in a controlled setting *was* psychotherapy.

As Zerka Moreno points out, it is both stunning and fascinating to watch a psychodrama unfold as a protagonist seeks resolution of a troublesome worry, anger at an employer, problems in a marriage, the pain of loss of someone near and dear, feelings of despair and inadequacy, frustration with one's profession or career, or rage at oneself to the point of wanting to destroy oneself. The protagonist and the director take the stage. The protagonist identifies the situation or issue that he/she wants to explore. A drama unfolds in which the protagonist provides the content and the director provides the method and techniques by which the protagonist presents a story from his/her life. Group members assist by taking roles of the people in the protagonist's life who are not present in the session. Time and again the drama leads from the current problem to an experience earlier in the protagonist's life that was not resolved satisfactorily, leaving the protagonist with strong negative emotions that are revived by the present situation. An integrative catharsis frees the protagonist from the past, allowing him/her increased spontaneity to solve today's problems.

The story of how Moreno first used spontaneity drama to address the marital problems of one of his spontaneity players has been told in Chapter 2 of this book. Barbara, the sweet, demure young actress of the spontaneity theater, had become a splenetic, resentful hellion in her marriage. Moreno first gave her roles in the spontaneity dramas in which she could express herself in ways that were threatening her marriage. Then Moreno had her, with husband George, enact their day-to-day relationship together on the spontaneity stage. Audience members commented to Moreno that these dramas seemed to touch them more deeply than the other spontaneity dramas and the living newspaper dramas that the group presented. Moreno contended that the audience was more moved by the Barbara and George dramas because they recognized that what they were watching was real, the genuine experience of the actors, not just talented players creating dramas spontaneously.

THE BEGINNINGS

Moreno was drawn early to drama. He engaged children in Vienna in spontaneous acting out of stories. He joined the group of thespians who met at Café Museum and, with them, founded the *Stegreiftheater*. Moreno claimed that his legendary search for a new king of Austria was the first psychodrama. That production could also be considered a sociodrama since it dealt with a social problem, and also as a role test, even though none of those words had been coined at the time. These concepts all developed much later. His treatment of the relationship of *Stegreiftheater* player Barbara and her husband, George, on the stage of the *Stegreiftheater* more closely resembled the psychodramas that he conducted later at Beacon Hill Sanatorium. He used similar spontaneity theater techniques in his private medical practice in Vöslau. Moreno conducted spontaneity testing in the Impromptu theater. At the Hudson training school, he introduced spontaneity tests and spontaneity training, role tests and role training, and psychodrama therapy. These events all took place before 1934. However, it was at the Beacon Hill Sanitarium after 1936 that he systematically developed and employed psychodramatic psychotherapy, the application of psychodrama for which it has become the known worldwide.

In 1936, J. L. Moreno purchased an estate that sat high above the Hudson River in Beacon, New York. The property that included a 31-room mansion had originally been the summer home of a wealthy industrial family. More recently, it had been occupied by a boarding school for boys that had failed financially during the Depression. The estate became a psychiatric hospital licensed by New York State after Moreno acquired it. It was here that he began systematically developing the therapeutic application of psychodrama, building on what he had learned during his experiences with the *Stegreiftheater* in Vienna, the Impromptu theater in New York, and the New York State Training School for Girls at Hudson. The carriage house of his new property was converted into a psychodrama theater (for more details, see Marineau, 1989).

For a number of years, Moreno was the only person who directed psychodrama sessions. He soon established a reputation for successfully treating severely disturbed schizophrenic patients with his new method. As Moreno's success became known, many psychiatrists referred their psychotic patients to him. At this time, the 1930s and 1940s, the only other widely recognized psychotherapy was psychoanalysis and Sigmund Freud had repeatedly insisted that with psychotic and narcissistic individuals no transference could take place. Therefore psychoanalytic treatment could do them no good, he maintained. Lack of transference does not preclude psychodramatic treatment, Moreno said.

Moreno (1940c) wrote an article in which he discussed his approach to the psychodramatic treatment of psychosis as well as several case studies. He explained that the psychotic experiences of the patient couldn't find adequate or satisfactory expression in the real world. They remain locked in a vague and confused subjectivity. Through the imaginary reality offered by psychodrama, the psychotic productions of these patients can be experienced on the psychodrama stage. Many such patients welcome an opportunity for expression in a setting that relaxes the bonds of the reality principle that have so restricted them heretofore. Auxiliary egos help patients to realize roles that they have not previously been capable of realizing.

> The psychodrama actually functions as a milieu that will reflect the patient's psychosis in such a way and on such a level that he can see his psychotic experiences objectified. As the treatment progresses, this objectification begins to interest the patient and continues to do so, more and more. For him the world of reality and of socialized action has become so unstable—so "unreal"—that a new and imaginary world is a necessity as an anchor for him if his experiences are not to be permanently reduced to the level of false signals and symbols. (1940c, pp. 116–117)

The creation of this imaginary reality tailored to the individual's inner world and in which all his hallucinations, delusions, thoughts, feelings, and roles are valid provides a satisfaction that could not be achieved in the world of reality. This is the first step in treatment and takes place on the psychodramatic stage. The patient, Moreno maintained, does not need to live continuously in the imaginary reality that psychodrama creates. Periodic psychodrama sessions are all that is ordinarily necessary to satisfy the fantasy world, and the rest of the time the patient can live in the ordinary reality of sanitarium life. Moreno describes how carefully timed immersions in the imaginary reality are used to assist the patient to function in that everyday reality.

Moreno presented two fascinating descriptions of the psychodramatic treatment of delusional patients. One, reported in three separate articles, relates the treatment of a woman in search of an imaginary lover (1944, 1959c, 1969a). Relatives of a young woman, identified as Mary, sought treatment for her at Moreno's sanitarium. Mary became a problem when she began searching for a man, John, whom she claimed was her lover. She sometimes entered private houses convinced that he might be within.

Moreno uses the treatment of Mary to illustrate his rationale of psychodrama in the treatment of delusional patients. The first step was to give her, on the psychodrama stage with the help of auxiliary egos, the imaginary world she had constructed in her mind. Through a maneuver that he called therapeutic deceit, he convinced Mary that John had been inducted into the army. An auxiliary was chosen by Mary to represent John in psychodrama sessions. It became apparent that Mary was much better connected to her imaginary world than to the world of real people around her. The auxiliaries allowed her to experience this imaginary world in a concrete way but one in which she discovered that it was not as perfect in psychodramatic reality as in her fantasy. As her acceptance of the auxiliary egos in the roles that she had created increased, Moreno gradually directed her into accepting them as they were in the reality of the real world. Eventually, John's death was announced. She experienced a long period of grief supported by those who had originally taken auxiliary roles. The final step, clarification, meant informing her of the therapeutic deceit that had been required to secure her initial compliance with treatment.

Moreno (1957b, 1959c) tells the intriguing story of Karl, a butcher from Yorkville, a German area of New York City, who was convinced that he was Adolf Hitler and had somehow been replaced by "that imposter in Berlin." Again Moreno lets this Adolf Hitler act out his story on the psychodrama stage with auxiliaries taking the roles of his henchman, Goering, Goebbels, Hess, Ribbentrop, and others. In psychodramatic reality, he returns to Germany and calls a meeting of his war cabinet to plan the future of Germany.

> For many weeks we had sessions with Hitler at regular intervals. We provided him with all the characters he needed to put his plans of conquering the world into operation (technique of realization). He seemed to know everything in advance; many things he presented on the stage

came very close to what actually took place years later. He appeared to have a special sense for fitting himself into moods and decisions that were made thousands of miles apart from him. In fact, at times we speculated whether he, the patient, was not the real Hitler and the other in Germany his double. We had the strange experience of feeling the real Hitler among us, working desperately on finding a solution for himself. We saw him often with his mother or sweetheart along, bursting out in tears, fighting with astrologists for an answer when he was in doubt, praying in his solitude to God for help, knocking his head on the wall, fearing that he might become insane before he could attain the great victory at other times, he portrayed moods of great desperation, feelings that he had failed and that the Reich would be conquered by its enemies. (1959c, p. 196)

At one point his mood became very dark and he asked all his Gestapo leaders to die with him and shot himself. Moreno wrote that years later when Hitler killed himself in a Berlin bunker, he recalled how the butcher from Yorkville had predicted world history so closely.

A turning point came one day when Hitler announced that he wanted a haircut. A barber was called and cut his hair as Hitler prescribed, onstage. As the barber was preparing to leave, Hitler suddenly pointed to his mustache and demanded, "Take this off!" The barber immediately did as requested. Hitler rose from his chair, pointed at his face, and began to weep. "It's gone, it's gone, it's gone, it's over!" he moaned. "I lost it! I lost it! Why did I do it? I shouldn't have done it!" (1957b, p. 199).

Gradually a change took place and people could see changes in his body, his facial expressions, and the words that he spoke. He now asked to be called Karl instead of Adolf. He wanted his wife to be present for the psychodrama sessions. He kissed her warmly on the stage. He eventually made a good recovery, Moreno reports.

Still another case of the treatment of psychosis (Moreno, 1946a; Moreno, 2012) is the account of the case of a young man treated before the establishment of the Beacon Hill Sanitarium. In his discussions with students at the Moreno Institute, he elaborated on this case to illustrate his idea of creating an auxiliary world. The patient, identified as William, was diagnosed as schizophrenic and believed that he was Christ. His family was wealthy enough during these early days of the Depression to rent a small house for William's treatment. Moreno hired a group of other young men, mostly college students, to serve Moreno as psychiatric aids and William as disciples. With the guidance of Moreno, an imaginary world was constructed to fit the needs of the patient, allowing him to act out and experience his psychotic fantasies. The auxiliary world created to fit the subjectivity of the schizophrenic patient is "filled with roles and masks, with fictitious objects" Moreno (1946a, p. 222) says. As the patient gains satisfaction from the auxiliary world, the auxiliary egos, over time, turn into real persons with whom the patient can establish genuine relationships.

Moreno used psychodrama to address other problems beside psychosis, of course. He was a pioneer in working with the interpersonal problems of marital relationships (Compernolle, 1981). His first paper describing psychodramatic marriage therapy, "Inter-Personal Therapy and Psychopathology of Interpersonal Relations," was published in 1937. Another article on the subject, "Psychodramatic Treatment of Marriage Problems," came three years later (1940b). Moreno's thoughts about marriage relationships and the treatment of the interpersonal problems between intimate partners are as relevant today as they were groundbreaking in their time. Anyone conducting marriage therapy today would likely profit from reading Moreno's approach to marital problems. Moreno (1941c, 1948a, 1966d) also wrote on how psychodrama can be used in premarital counseling to predict a couple's chances of making a successful marriage. Zerka Moreno (Toeman, 1945) published a plan for research involving premarital couples to predict success in marriage.

Moreno's practice of psychodrama evolved over these early years. Initially, Moreno treated the patients of the sanitarium individually, taking the patient into the psychodrama theater along with one or more of the sanitarium nurses who served as auxiliaries. After the session, Moreno sometimes conducted an analysis of the session, gauged to the readiness of the patient to hear it. The analysis involved comments from the director and the auxiliaries about the protagonist's performance. Over time, the staff of the sanitarium and Moreno noticed that the patients seemed to have a heightened sensitivity for other patients. Moreno began taking them into the theater as group members in psychodramatic sessions. Later, when psychodrama training events were being held, patients were often included with non-patient trainees in psychodrama sessions.[1]

THE METHOD

Over the years, J. L. Moreno published a number of articles on psychodrama in journal articles, in his books, and in books edited by others. There are now dozens of books by many other authors on psychodrama in many languages and hundreds of journal articles that discuss all aspects of the psychodramatic method, its techniques, and the applications of psychodrama to various populations and situations. Many describe the application of psychodrama to specific kinds of problems, both in clinical and nonclinical settings.

At the annual conference of the American Psychiatric Association in 1946, Moreno read a paper on psychodrama and group psychotherapy. He later published it (1946b). In this article, he describes the five instruments of psychodrama and adds a brief discussion of catharsis and audience therapy. Reprints of this basic paper on psychodrama were given to every visitor to the psychodrama theater of the Moreno Institute and every psychodrama student learns about the five instruments of psychodrama.

The Stage

The first instrument of psychodrama is the stage. Although Moreno constructed two psychodramatic stages, one in the First Psychodrama Theater at Beacon Hill Sanitarium and the other in the New York City Moreno Institute, he maintained that any area could be designated as the stage, the space in which the drama will take place. The stage is understood to be beyond the limitations of ordinary reality. It is a space in which the world of fantasy as well as the world of reality can both be experienced. On the psychodrama stage, surplus reality reigns and the protagonist may not only speak again to a deceased mother, but also listen to her responses and experience her embrace. On the stage, the delusional patient can act out the delusion (Moreno, 1940, 1944). This is a much more satisfying process for the delusional person than the conventional ongoing argument with the psychiatrist about the unreality of the delusion. To the paranoid individual, the delusion is more real than the psychiatrist. Dreams, ghosts, and even God can be given three-dimensional, physical embodiment on the psychodrama stage, allowing the protagonist to engage, encounter, and even physically struggle with them.

The Protagonist

The protagonist is the second instrument mentioned by Moreno. The protagonist is a group member who steps out of the group and provides the subject matter, the content of the drama. There are several ways in which one may become the protagonist. The protagonist is asked to present his/her private world on the psychodrama stage, not to be an actor as in the theater but to act him/herself spontaneously and freely. He/she is urged to express all thoughts and feelings and to express them more fully than life sometimes allows. A number of techniques are utilized to assist the protagonist in warming up to the role. Self-presentation, soliloquy, role reversal, and the mirror are but a few of them. The aim, Moreno says, "is not to turn the patients into actors, but rather to stir them up to be on the stage what they *are*, more deeply and explicitly than they appear to be in life reality" (1946b, p. 251). The protagonist may act out a current problem that istroubling, a scene from the past, a desired role or a fantasy role for which reality has not provided an opportunity, or an anticipated future situation. Almost anything is possible with the magic of the psychodrama stage.

The Director

The psychodrama director is a dramaturge. The content of the drama comes from the protagonist. A psychodrama is an externalization of the internal, the memories, thoughts, and feelings of the protagonist. The director has the responsibility of coming up with the proper dramatic techniques through which the protagonist can turn those thoughts and feelings into psychodramatic action, action that accurately reflects the protagonist's subjectivity and communicates it to the group. The director also has a responsibility to the audience, to keep the members of the audience in rapport with the protagonist during the drama.

The director has the responsibility to see that the protagonist is not harmed by the psychodrama. Like any powerful instrument, psychodrama misused can be hurtful to participants. It is the director's obligation to see that this does not happen. For example, in psychodramatic therapy, a group member may be seeking to deal with the residuals of a severely traumatic experience like, for example, the death of a child. Although it may be in the protagonist's best interests to experience and express fully the terrible pain of that loss, it is in the hands of the director to make sure that in doing so the protagonist is not re-traumatized but, rather, that the experience leads toward resolution and acceptance of the tragedy that life has brought.

The most successful psychodramas occur when protagonists achieve the spontaneity state. This is an altered state of mind somewhat akin to, yet different from, a hypnotic state. The spontaneity state tends to happen when the protagonist experiences a high level of trust in the director. Then, as in hypnosis, the protagonist turns over some degree of intellectual or ego functioning to the director, allowing the fullest arousal and the most complete expression to his/her emotions. This requires great confidence in the director's expertise. Once asked what the most important personal characteristic was that one needed in order to be a director, Moreno replied without a pause, "Courage." It is courage that is needed to go with the protagonist into the deepest, darkest areas of the protagonist's private world in order to attain release from the monsters and ghosts that may be lurking there. The courage of the director may be what gives the protagonist the courage to explore this territory. Psychodrama can feel like a risky undertaking, especially for one new to it. It is trust in the director that allows one to take that risk.

Unlike the relationship between the psychoanalyst and the analysand, where analysts keep an objective distance between themselves and their analysands, the director and the protagonist enjoy a fuller relationship. It is permissible, Moreno writes, that the director may laugh and joke with the protagonist and just as permissible to confront or shock the protagonist. Moreno's position clearly underscores the fact that in psychodramatic therapy, the director is a real person and utilizes his/her own spontaneity in the directorial role. The psychodrama director's individuality and personality are expected to become integrated into his/her personal style as a director.

The director of a psychodrama session is also responsible to the group members, some of whom enter the drama as auxiliary egos. He is in charge of the sharing session. After the drama has reached dramatic resolution and the director indicates that it has come to a close, the director invites the group members to share *their* personal life experiences that connect them to the protagonist and the themes and events that the protagonist has presented. The psychodramatic protagonist has stepped out from the group as the original protagonist stepped out from the chorus in ancient Greek theater and expressed pain and concerns that are not only the protagonist's, but that are also the pains and concerns of the group. At the conclusion of the drama, as the protagonist returns from the spontaneity state to the more ordinary state of awareness, and from the psychodrama stage to the group, he/she often feels psychologically exposed, aware of having made public his/her deepest subjectivity. As group members relate their own experiences, identifying with the protagonist, the latter quickly realizes that he/she is not alone in the way he/she has experienced life. Fears of having revealed too much of oneself quickly fade, and the individual who has stepped out of the group and placed his private life upon the stage for everyone to see once again feels incorporated back into the group. The process of sharing is discussed in greater detail below.

Auxiliary Ego

Auxiliary egos make up the fourth instrument of psychodrama. In a psychodrama, a protagonist may want to examine his/her relationship with a supervisor or boss, but that person is not a part of the group. How can this interpersonal relationship be explored when one party to it is not present? The solution lies in assigning the role of the absent significant other to a member of the group, who then becomes an auxiliary ego, a helping or supporting being. The auxiliary helps both the protagonist and the director, serving as kind of a bridge or connecting link between them. The auxiliary assists the protagonist in dramatizing the protagonist's life and helps the director by expanding the role of the significant other.

Auxiliaries were particularly important in Moreno's work with psychotic patients, and he often used staff members especially trained to do this work. In addition to taking the roles needed by the protagonist, often that of hallucinatory voices or images and delusional psychodramatic roles, the auxiliary explores the relationship of the assumed role and the protagonist. The auxiliary may interpret the role and may act as a therapeutic guide and serve as a bridge to the world of reality (Moreno, 1978).

In working with groups of nonpsychotic people, auxiliary egos are group members. Most, but not all, psychodrama directors encourage protagonists to select their auxiliaries. The protagonist is asked and encouraged to select the group member that the protagonist thinks can best take the required role. The protagonist's choice may rest on physical characteristics, such as age, body size and shape, or voice, or on some psychological characteristic. The initial responsibility of the auxiliary is to enact the role as closely as possible to the manner in which it is presented by the protagonist. The ease and degree to which this is accomplished is often uncanny and the protagonist is taken aback at how quickly and how accurately the auxiliary plays the role of his wife or her husband. This catapults protagonists deeper into their feelings and enhances the spontaneity state. The drama then increases its impact upon the audience.

Auxiliaries usually understand immediately and intuitively when the protagonist has accepted them in the assigned roles. The auxiliary feels fully engaged with the protagonist and experiences the protagonist's emotion and responds to it. Once this happens, experienced directors encourage auxiliaries to trust their spontaneity and expand their portrayal of the role, exploring with the protagonist the protagonist's perception of the relationship. This sets the stage for the third function of the auxiliary, which is to interpret more fully the significant other to the protagonist. The expansion of the role by the auxiliary is tested by role reversal. When the auxiliary has added a new element to the role of the significant other, the reaction of the protagonist usually makes it clear whether the protagonist can accept the possibility that the significant other would say or do what the auxiliary has produced. Nonetheless, at some point a careful director will reverse roles and with the protagonist in the role of the significant other inquire if the thought or feeling added by the auxiliary feels authentic. The protagonist is the final arbiter.

The Audience

The fifth and final instrument that Moreno identifies is the group or audience. The audience of a psychodrama is usually established ahead of time as a group. The group represents the social world of the protagonist, hence world opinion. The protagonist steps out of the group, as the original actor in ancient Greek theater stepped out of the chorus, to proclaim the pain of society. Group members are the protagonist's cohorts, his/her companions and fellow beings. The audience also is the source for the auxiliaries that the protagonist requires to tell his/her story; they are that part of the world that learns about this story. They provide the witnesses for the protagonist's story. They are those who, through sharing, inform the protagonist that he/she is not alone with whatever pain is experienced. The audience both helps the protagonist and is helped by the protagonist. In the protagonist's exploration of his/her pain, members of the group are provided an opportunity to experience, explore, and expunge their own pain along with the protagonist. "The audience sees itself, that is, one of its collective syndromes portrayed on the stage" (Moreno, 1946b, p. 251).

THE PSYCHODRAMATIC PROCESS

There are many ways in which a psychodrama group is established. Patients in a psychiatric hospital or unit may be assigned to a psychodrama psychotherapy group. A private practice practitioner may form psychodrama groups for psychotherapy, for personal growth and development, or for other ends. A psychodrama trainer teaches others to direct psychodrama in a training group or training workshops. A practice that is no longer prevalent is the public session that Moreno initiated in 1942 at the Psychodramatic Institute, 101 Park Avenue, in New York. In order to familiarize people with psychodrama, Moreno conducted weekly demonstrations of psychodrama (Moreno, 2012). Anybody could attend, although the groups were mostly made up of students and mental health professionals. The Psychodrama Institute eventually moved to 236 W. 78th Street and, beginning in 1961, public sessions were conducted every night from "Monday to Saturday at 8:30" (*Announcement*, 1960; Hunting, 1966). Open to everyone, the attendees paid a small fee. The Morenos or a psychodramatist trained at the Institute conducted the session. The ethics of public sessions has since been questioned, and Jonathan Moreno (1994), son of J. L. and Zerka and a well-known bioethicist, has written that the practice is not ethical under today's standards. I have written on a procedure by which I think psychodrama can be ethically demonstrated in a public session (Nolte, 2008).

Regardless of how the group comes together, there are certain consistencies in the conduct of psychodramas. A psychodrama session typically consists of three different parts: warming up, the action phase, and sharing. Warming up in this context means preparing for action and begins as the group forms and ends with the selection of a protagonist. The action portion of the session is the psychodrama proper, and sharing takes place at the end of psychodramatic action when members of the group reveal how the drama has affected them.

The Warming Up Phase

The warming up process is an aspect of the Canon of Spontaneity-Creativity (Moreno, 1953; Chapter 5, this volume). Warming up with respect to a psychodrama session has been the subject of a number of articles in the psychodrama literature because the success of a psychodrama is so heavily influenced by the appropriate warming up of both protagonist and director. Moreno (1937a) noted that the first problem a therapist confronts is how to get the patient started. Paul Cornyetz (1945) analyzes the process of warming up, especially with respect to a newly forming group. Enneis (1951), Yablonsky and Enneis (1956), and Sacks (1967) discuss several ways of warming up a group to action by making use of the spontaneous interactions of group members. Other articles on the warming up process are by Weiner and Sacks (1969) and Robbins (1973). Kipper (1967) offers a theoretical discussion of spontaneity and the warming up process. Another approach to the warming up phase of a psychodrama session is the central concern model developed by James Enneis at St. Elizabeth Hospital (Buchanan, 1980). The idea behind this model is to discover the group member who best represents an issue that affects all the members of the group.

There are two different warming up processes to be considered. The first is the warming up processes of the individual group members as they approach the group meeting. This consists of the thoughts and feelings that a member experiences when anticipating the session. These may be positive feelings toward other members of the group or for the activities of the group, or they may be negative thoughts and anxiety about going to the session. The person may be ambivalent, recognizing the positive results that may be gained from the group and, at the same time, anxious about engaging in psychodrama. Whatever the thoughts and feelings of the individual members, they are deeply involved in the warming up process of the group.

The second part of the group warming up process begins with the group members gathering in the place where the group meets. It ends with the selection of a protagonist for a psychodrama. Warming a group up to involvement in the group's activities is the responsibility of the director. There are many ways to accomplish the task, and how the director proceeds can depend upon a variety of factors. If a group is new, meeting for the first time, the director will want to transform an aggregate of individuals into a group of related people (Cornyetz, 1945). It was noted in the chapter on sociometry that a number of persons meeting for the first time has an infrastructure in terms of the positive and negative feelings that the people have for each other. Moving from an aggregate to becoming a group means assisting group members to begin the process of identifying these attitudes. Identifying attitudes that group members have toward group goals is also a tactic that assists a group to move into action.

An ongoing therapy or training group provides a slightly different situation than a meeting of strangers. The group gathers with its structure more familiarly known to the members. Group participants know each other better. Telic relationships have been forming. Group members are more aware of the problems and issues that others are struggling to resolve. However, there has been a time interval since they last met and things change. Warming up in these groups is catching up with what has happened since the group last met.

In training workshops consisting of a number of sessions in a short period of time with the same group of participants, the most important warming up phase is to the workshop itself, usually the first session. Although there are different formats for training, the trainer will usually want to know what each of the attendees is seeking from the workshop. Some possible agendas are personal work as protagonist, directing with supervision, and theoretical understanding. When all the members of a training group are aware of what each wants from the experience, there is an increased possibility of maximizing everybody's desires.

The use of games, fantasies, and other structured exercises has been used to facilitate the warming up of groups, especially brand-new groups (Weiner & Sacks, 1969; Robbins, 1973). These activities, called "warmups," serve as icebreakers and are intended to reduce the anxiety that the newcomer often brings to the first session of psychodrama. This practice has become *de rigueur* for some trainers and practitioners who begin every psychodrama session with some sort of group exercise. The most effective warm-up, however, is created on the spot by the director to meet the specific needs of the group. It will take into account characteristics of the participants, the purpose of the group, the situation in which the group meets, and other factors. The warm-up may be simply a statement of observations that the director has made of the group as it assembles, a reflection upon a current event that, the director can assume, has affected everybody, or an impression of the group's mood. Use of an exercise pulled at random from the director's collection of warm-ups can actually interfere with the spontaneous warming up process of the group, warming the group up and away from issues with which it needs to deal.

In therapy groups, the psychodramatic director-therapist may have reasons to select the protagonist. Warming up the group and getting all members as involved as possible in the session is still required. In addition, the director will need to warm the selected group member up to the role of protagonist, and, at the same time, warm the other group members up to that person. The success of the group session will depend in large part upon the director's expertise in accomplishing both goals.

In training groups and personal growth and development groups, consisting of highly functioning individuals, a practice based on sociometry that has become widely applied allows group members to choose a protagonist for each session that the group meets. Typically, the members of the group are invited to indicate a desire to be a protagonist. If two or more present themselves, each prospective protagonist is asked to indicate the issue that he/she wishes to explore. Group members are then asked to make known their first choice for the current session. The rationale for this method is based on the notion that the psychodrama is a group creation. From sociometric theory, one can assume that the telic relationships of the group play a significant dynamic in warming up individual group members to the role of protagonist. In addition, the aim of the psychodrama is not only to benefit the protagonist, but also to benefit the group itself. "The audience sees itself, that is, one of its collective syndromes portrayed on the stage" (Moreno, 1946b, p. 251). The issue and protagonist chosen by the group enhance the probability that the session will be meaningful to all involved.

The Action Phase

The protagonist and the director take the stage. In Moreno's terms, they are the co-producers of the psychodrama. A drama is a story and this story comes from the protagonist's life experiences, frequently experiences that have disturbed the protagonist's equilibrium. As a story, a psychodrama should have a beginning, development, and resolution or denouement. The therapeutic and esthetic values of a psychodrama are not unrelated. The first problem of the director is how to help the protagonist begin, another warming up process.

There are an infinite number of ways to begin a drama. The protagonist may have a scene that he/she wishes to present. If the protagonist has described the issue with sufficient detail, the director may suggest a beginning scene. When the issue is not clear, a frequently used technique is to ask the protagonist to soliloquize about it, perhaps while walking about the stage. From the new information revealed, a starting point may become obvious. More often than not, the first scene of the psychodrama will be an experience in the protagonist's current life.

The next step is setting the scene. Here the director encourages, aids, and abets the protagonist in creating a specific place and time on the stage. Again the image of children playing house comes to mind. "This will be the kitchen, and here's the living room, and that's the children's bedroom back there," a little girl says. Her companion takes over, "You be the daddy, I'll be the mommy, and Betsy can be our little girl. You're just coming home from work." Using a few simple props, chairs, a table, perhaps pillows and boxes, the protagonist identifies and creates the room or locality in which the action will take place. Setting the scene has several functions. It warms up the protagonist to the spontaneity state preparing him/her for the action to ensue. At the same time, the audience is "warmed up" to the protagonist, pulled into the protagonist's life story and into the spontaneity state.

The spontaneity state is an altered state of mind, akin to, but distinguishable from, a hypnotic state. It is the state that children often attain when totally involved in play. Entirely in the moment, there is a distorted sense of time. When they look at the clock at the finish of a psychodrama, both protagonist and audience are often surprised at how long or how short the drama was in terms of hours and minutes. It is when spontaneity is at the highest that the protagonist can play him/herself the most naturally, when it is easiest to accept the auxiliary egos as the individuals for whom they are stand-ins. It is also then when the auxiliaries seem to automatically and naturally fall into their assigned roles. The psychodrama stage becomes an extension of life space into which audience members can step as protagonist and auxiliaries, very different from the conventional theater, where the proscenium arch separates the space, the stage upon which the rehearsed and prepared actors perform, from the audience in the auditorium.

After the scene is set, the auxiliary egos are introduced through the fundamental technique of psychodrama, the role reversal. When a significant other is introduced into the drama, the director commonly asks the protagonist to reverse roles, become this other person and show rather than tell the auxiliary and the audience who this person is and how this person looks, walks, talks, and thinks. This is a very economical way to present the significant other and instruct the auxiliary ego on how to relate to the protagonist.

When these preparations are complete, the director says to the protagonist, "Show us what happens," and the action begins. The protagonist, with the help of auxiliary egos, shows the director and the group a recent event in his/her life that has left the protagonist puzzled, anxious, angry, sad, frightened, or otherwise troubled. The director keeps the drama in the present even when an event from the past is reenacted. The psychodramatic reenactment is happening in the here and now.

Depending upon the matter in question, the psychodrama may remain in the present with the protagonist exploring his/her relationships with the members of his/her social atom. The drama may explore the future when the protagonist is anxious about events yet to come. In this case the director helps the protagonist externalize and reenact events in a future projection. And quite often, the psychodrama leads into an exploration of past experiences.

It often happens that the protagonist's emotional reaction in the initial scene of the psychodrama strikes the director as excessive. The protagonist seems to be overreacting to the events portrayed. The director then asks, "When in your life have you had these feelings before?" If the director has been perceptive, the protagonist will recall one or more instances when he/she has experienced the feelings associated with the current situation. Emotion is a bridge that can connect the present to the past.

The past events that psychodrama activates tend to be associated with potent and sometimes overpowering emotion. They include experiences in which a child's or adolescent's spontaneity has been squelched, sometimes abusively. As children we have a tremendous amount to learn and there are many agents of education exerting their influence upon us: parents, teachers, older children, and other adults who exercise their authority over us. We are taught how to conduct ourselves, how to feel about many things, including other people, and what to think about a wide variety of issues, problems, and situations. Lessons are often subtle and we learn them as if by osmosis. At other times, especially if we have violated a rule of conduct, the consequences are accompanied with strong feelings of embarrassment, guilt, and even shame.

Far too many children are subject to a variety of abuses. There is physical abuse from parents who use it as a means of correcting a child's behavior, and sometimes to satisfy the parent's own needs. There is emotional abuse in the form of harsh words, accusations, denunciations, and threats of punishment or loss of love and support. There is sexual abuse from parents, older siblings, and strangers. There is neglect from alcoholic or emotionally disturbed parents. Even the best of parents under stress from work, an interpersonal relationship, or other provocation can treat a child unfairly. Abuse of children mostly takes place out of sight of the world and there is more of it than we imagine. Is there anybody who has not experienced some degree of unfair treatment during childhood? Not only do these occurrences generate intense emotion in the child, feelings of rage, fear, and emotional pain; under the circumstances, the child is usually unable to give expression to these emotions. The child's weakness compared to the adult's strength results in suppression and, under certain conditions, repression of these intense emotions.

These experiences can have a great emotional impact that lasts into adulthood. Eric Berne (1971), the originator of Transactional Analysis, suggests that they lead to "existential decisions" in which one comes to conclusions about one's place in the world vis-à-vis other people. Abuse experiences lead us to decide that we are not worthy, not as good as others. Such decisions, even if they are succeeded by more positive opinions, can be reactivated even into adulthood. The events that lead to negative feelings about oneself appear with great regularity in psychodramas, accompanied by the expression of long-suppressed emotion.

A problem with untoward events of this nature is that they undermine a child's natural spontaneity. Moreno's engagement with children in the gardens of Vienna, as described in his writings (1946a, 1989a) and in Chapter 1 of this book, was an early and largely intuitive attempt on his part to repair the damage done. He writes:

> It was . . . a crusade of children for themselves, for a society of their own age and their own rights. Children took sides—against adults, grown ups, social stereotypes and robots—and for spontaneity and creativity. . . . I permitted them to play God if they wanted to. When they missed, just as I was treated when my arm was broken, I began to treat children's problems by letting them act extemporaneously, a sort of psychotherapy for fallen gods. (1946a, p. 3)

And later he began treating adults, as well, using a more systematic method of letting them act extemporaneously: the psychodrama. Experiencing an event the second time, Moreno taught, allows us to let go of it. Childhood is not the only time that terrible things happen to people.

A psychodrama is a unique and unrepeatable occurrence. It can take an infinite number of forms. There are, however, a few motifs that appear with some regularity. A common pattern begins with the protagonist reenacting a scene from current life, followed by reenactment of an early life experience called to mind by the emotion aroused, a reparative scene. The drama then returns to a repeat of the first scene, where the protagonist's new insight is allowed to enter the action.

From the first therapeutic employment of spontaneity theater techniques, the treatment of the marriage of Barbara and George, described in Chapter 2, audience members asked why these dramas touched them so much deeper than others. Members of psychodrama groups note that the psychodrama consistently induces a more intense reaction in them than does even the best-acted conventional drama. The reason, Moreno states, is that protagonists on the psychodrama stage are presenting themselves, their own problems and conflicts, not those created by another person, the playwright, and assigned to them. It is the difference, Moreno says, between a spectator watching a motion picture of a volcano erupting and a person who watches the eruption in real life. The psychodrama does for every person what the conventional drama had done for Hamlet, Macbeth, or Oedipus—it makes one a hero:

> In the therapeutic theatre an anonymous, average man becomes something approaching a work of art—not only for others but for himself. A tiny, insignificant existence is here elevated to a level of dignity and respect. Its private problems are projected on a high plane of action before a special public—a small world, perhaps, but the world of the therapeutic theatre. The world in which we all live is imperfect, unjust and amoral, but in the therapeutic theatre a little person can rise above our everyday world. Here his ego becomes an aesthetic prototype—he becomes representative of mankind. On the psychodramatic stage he is put into a state of inspiration—he is the dramatist of himself. (1940a, p. 240)

Sharing

The drama comes to a conclusion. The director and the protagonist sit down in the group, and sharing begins. In the early years of the development of psychodrama, Moreno often concluded the session with a discussion of the protagonist's performance. He might make comments on their performance or offer some interpretations, whatever he thought would have a positive result for the protagonist. Members of the group were allowed to join in the discussion. Then one day he stopped doing this, and the practice of sharing began. Zerka Moreno (2006) relates how this came about. After a session with a young woman patient, the group included psychiatrists who were offering their various interpretations with little regard for the feelings of the protagonist. Moreno noticed her confusion and distress in reaction to the professional talk about her work, effectively excluding her from her own experience. He became indignant and confronted the group members. "Do you have children?" he demanded. "What is your relationship with your daughter? Here we share our hearts, not our brains" (Z. T. Moreno, 2006a, p. 22). He forbade professional discussion and advice giving immediately following psychodramatic work. Thus personal sharing in lieu of professional analysis was instituted and has become the final part of every psychodrama session.

In sharing, the members of a psychodrama group relate to the protagonist and to the other group members the personal life experiences of which they were reminded by the protagonist's portrayal in the drama. As we participate in a psychodrama, we are touched by the emotions and themes that the protagonist explores. Both feelings and subject matter activate memories of experiences in our lives Perhaps the drama is the story of the protagonist's loss of a husband or wife through an unwanted divorce. Members of the group are reminded of and talk about the stories of their own divorces, the breakup of love relationships, the effect of the divorce of their parents, and many other similar events. Sometimes we remember experiences that don't seem to be particularly connected with the protagonist's story. Nonetheless, these are appropriate incidents to share.

Several goals are accomplished in sharing. The ostensible purpose of sharing is to give something back to the protagonist who has revealed intimate details of his/her life story with the group, enlarging their knowledge and understanding of the human condition. The protagonist, in the midst of a psychodrama, becomes fully engaged in the moment being reenacted, and the presence of the group tends to fade away. At the conclusion of the drama, he/she may feel a bit unsettled and wonder at how much of his/her life he/she has shared with the group. There can be a feeling of having been emotionally unclothed. In sharing, group members honor the protagonist by letting him/her know how the drama has touched them and how they are connected by similar themes, feelings, and events. In the vernacular of group dynamics, the protagonist, who has stepped out of the group and onto the stage, is reintegrated into the group.

Important for the protagonist, sharing also serves a beneficial purpose for group members. During a psychodrama, especially when the theme is a basic existential issue, such as isolation or death, and the protagonist has expressed intense feelings, the emotions stirred up in the audience members are also intense. The drama may have achieved a high degree of resolution for the protagonist, but it is as if a great wave of emotion has moved from the stage and inundated the audience. Sharing provides group members an opportunity to release some of the emotional tension that they experienced during the drama. It is like letting the wave die down so that the emotional waters are calmer.

Sharing has positive results for the protagonist and for individual group members. It is also good for the group as a group. During the drama, the group has learned about the protagonist. During sharing, group members learn more about each other. The group learns more about the group.

PSYCHODRAMA AS THE HERO'S JOURNEY

I have long noted a similarity between a psychodrama session and Joseph Campbell's concept of the hero's journey, found in his *Hero with a Thousand Faces* (1968) and *The Power of Myth* (Campbell & Moyers, 1988). Campbell lists 17 fundamental events in heroic tales, although it is rare that one myth contains them all. The following is a simplified sketch of the hero's journey.

The journey begins with a call to adventure that often comes when there is a threat to the well-being of one's village. Someone must right a wrong, recover a lost object, discover a secret, or find an amulet that will serve as a boon to save or preserve peace in the village. Called to adventure from within or without, the hero leaves familiar surroundings of the village and crosses a threshold into unknown and magical territory. With the aid of a guide, the hero sets out on a journey into the unknown. The first step is crossing the threshold between the familiar everyday world of the village and the unknown territory that lies beyond. It is a strange and magical world, Campbell says, something like the world of dreams that does not seem to obey the rules of the everyday world. The hero embarks upon adventures and confronts or is confronted by a variety of characters, some of whom are helpful and some of whom are dangerous. The hero is forced to undergo trials in which he/she must conquer fear and face dangers. After conquering those who would thwart him/her, the hero finds that which he/she is seeking. The hero now returns to familiar territory, the village from which he began the journey, and shares the fruits of the journey with the other members of the community.

As the hero accepts the call to adventure, a call that may come from within or from an outside source, a group member, volunteering or selected by the group, becomes the protagonist of the group's psychodrama. As the hero crosses the threshold, the protagonist leaves the group and steps upon the psychodrama stage, a place where the rules of ordinary reality do not necessarily hold. There a director who is familiar with the magical space serves as the protagonist's guide. The protagonist finds that he/she is in a strange territory where anything can happen. The protagonist can visit events from the past or in the future. Anything that the protagonist has experienced or that the protagonist can imagine takes form on the stage. Here the protagonist must confront anxieties and fears and ghosts from the past. With the help of the guide and auxiliary egos, the protagonist faces powerful figures from his/her current and past life, figures that have thwarted or frustrated him/her in the past. By confronting them on the stage and overcoming them, the protagonist takes their power and strength into him/herself. Having prevailed over the obstacles of the journey, the protagonist then returns to the "village," the group, and is welcomed back as the group members share their own stories. Psychodrama makes us the heroes of our own lives.

THE PSYCHODRAMA MOVEMENT

Psychodrama attracted a lot of attention just as sociometry had before it, and from many of the same people, social psychologists, social workers, educators, and guidance counselors. Psychologists and a few psychiatrists were added to the mix. By 1940, Moreno was offering training in psychodrama at Beacon Hill. That year's issue of *Sociometry* announced the Moreno Institute, a summer training program of three months, consisting of lectures and training in the techniques of the psychodrama applied to educational guidance, marriage counseling, mental disorders, and social maladjustments. The list of topics to be presented was ambitious and included sessions on the warming up process, the psychodramatic concept of catharsis, the auxiliary ego, psychodrama in education and in problems of delinquency. The fee for the three-month program was a modest $375, and that included room and board. In today's dollar, it would amount to approximately $4,800, or about $50 per day.

Moreno created the Sociometric Institute and Theater of Psychodrama that soon became referred to as the Psychodramatic Institute, located at 101 Park Avenue in New York in 1942. He organized the Society for Psychodrama and Group Psychotherapy the same year (renamed the American Society for Group Psychotherapy and Psychodrama a year later). Three Bulletins for the Society for Psychodrama and Group Psychotherapy were published in the journal, *Sociometry*, in 1943 and 1944 (1943a, 1943b, and 1944) for the purpose of establishing communications between workers in psychodrama and group psychotherapy. These documents listed Moreno's activities at the Psychodramatic Institute in New York City and referred to psychodrama programs in other locations. During 1943 and 1944, the Bulletins listed following events that took place at the Psychodrama Institute:

1. A demonstration of psychodrama was given for students from College of the City of New York, Hunter College, Brooklyn College, Queens College, New York Medical College, and Sarah Lawrence College.
2. A sociodrama on the topic of the Nazi–Jewish conflict was conducted at one session.
3. "The atmosphere of a small craft before, during and after combat was portrayed by actual participants" at another.
4. A psychodramatic approach to dance was conducted.
5. A psychodrama of dreams was conducted.
6. The psychodrama treatment of a religious psychosis, during which the protagonist "went to hell and up to heaven," was conducted, apparently at an open session.
7. The application of sociodrama to anthropological problems was presented.

The Bulletins listed psychodrama programs and projects in a number of communities scattered throughout the country:

1. St. Elizabeth Hospital, Washington, DC, reported by Frances Herriott and Margaret Hagan.
2. Elgin State Hospital, Elgin, Illinois. A psychodramatic clinic was directed by psychologist Dr. Theodore Sarbin.
3. The Neuropsychiatric Institute of the University of Chicago. A psychodramatic clinic was directed by Dr. Alfred P. Solomon.
4. Howard State Hospital, Howard, Rhode Island. Dr. Gerhard Schauer conducted sessions of group psychotherapy for mental patients.

5. Duke Hospital, North Carolina. Louise Anne Sullivan directed the psychodrama project there.
6. Child Guidance Clinic, Raleigh, North Carolina.
7. Public School 157, Brooklyn, New York, where Nathan Shoobs initiated a psychodrama program for treatment of delinquency problems.

Other items noted were a leadership training workshop conducted by Ronald Lippitt at the New School of Social Research and the use of psychodramatic techniques in the training of leaders for Boy Scout units, conducted by Lippitt and Alvin Zander (1943a). It is obvious, almost from the start, that the psychodrama method was being applied in other ways than as psychotherapy. Another Bulletin (1943b) also indicated that Moreno read papers at the Institute for Psychoanalysis, Chicago, Illinois, and at the Institute on Personality Development, New York, New York. He gave demonstrations of the psychodramatic approach to marital problems for the Society for Social Research at the University of Chicago. He presented a paper on his work with psychotic patients at a program on group psychotherapy at the Chicago Institute for Psychoanalysis, as well as giving lectures and a demonstration of psychodrama at Vassar College.

Reports of psychodrama research were reported in one Bulletin (1944). One researcher planned to relate autism to Moreno's concept of auto-tele. One study was designed to relate the Thematic Apperception Test with psychodrama. Another proposed to examine the field concept in comparison to the concept of the psychodramatic situation. Others include a study of the psychodramatic techniques intuitively used by great playwrights and psychodrama as a projective technique. The Bulletins clearly showed how active Moreno was in demonstrating the broad parameters of psychodrama and how much he was in demand as a presenter on his new method. Psychodrama was off to a promising start.

World War II produced a large number of psychiatric victims among the veterans who fought in their country's various services. This greatly increased the number of psychiatric admissions to Veterans Administration (now Veterans Affairs) hospitals. The need for psychotherapy was far greater than the supply of psychotherapists could meet, and as a result an urgent demand for group psychotherapy emerged. Moreno found himself increasingly called upon to present lectures and demonstrations of psychodrama at institutions all over the country. Eventually dozens of hospitals and mental health agencies offered psychodramatic group psychotherapy among their services (J. L. Moreno, 1965a).

Mental health professionals from all over the world started coming to train in the Moreno Institute for psychodrama. In 1951, Moreno, with Zerka at his side, took his first trip back to Europe. This was the trip mentioned in Chapter 7 during which he organized the International Committee of Group Psychotherapy in France in 1951. Other trips followed and psychodrama began to spread throughout European and South American countries. The Morenos were instrumental in the organization of international conferences for both group psychotherapy and psychodrama.

In "The First Psychodramatic Family" (Moreno, Moreno & Moreno, 1963), Moreno created a fable called Johnny Psychodramatist (pp. 1–3). Obviously borrowing from the legend of Johnny Appleseed, which was also based on a real person, Johnny Psychodramatist plants circular stages of several levels:

> It was a stage upon which the moon shown its friendly light. [Johnny] stepped upon it and acted the friendly neighbor, the strong courageous man, the bringer of luck. . . . All the stage needed was a world to act upon it. From now on he initiated every man who came to him to be and act what he was in his fantasy. The story of Johnny who can build a stage for everyone out of the seed in their mind spread, and stages began to blossom and grow all over. (p. 204)

The fable seemed to be becoming actuality.

ZERKA MORENO'S CONTRIBUTION TO PSYCHODRAMA

Zerka Toeman came into J. L. Moreno's life in 1941, when she brought her mentally ill sister to Beacon Hill Sanitarium for treatment. Moreno admitted the sister, Naomi, and hired Zerka. Naomi recovered and left the sanitarium. Zerka remained. She became Moreno's secretary, muse, lover, collaborator, wife, mother of his son, and primary bearer of his mission after his death. She was also his first professional auxiliary ego in the psychodrama theater. Zerka's influence upon J. L. Moreno and the development of psychodrama can hardly be exaggerated. She was simultaneously *his* auxiliary ego and copartner in their mission to promulgate and implement the methods that were intended to promote a fairer and more peaceable society. The interaction between the two was dynamic, creative, and immediate. Moreno (1970a) has written an account of their initial meeting in which it is apparent that he knew at first sight that this was the person that his life had been lacking, his muse. Zerka (2012) has written at some length not only about that first meeting, but also about the entire 34-year relationship.

Zerka has said that she did not initially consider ever becoming a director of psychodrama. Like many mental health practitioners in the early years of psychodrama, she assumed that only Moreno could direct a psychodrama. She was committed, she said, to becoming the best auxiliary ego instead. Moreno insisted that she could learn and encouraged her to do so. Zerka not only learned to direct, but she developed a style of directing of her own. Moreno's directorial style emphasized and explored the protagonist's social atom. When he directed, the drama focused on the interactions of the protagonist with the significant people currently in the protagonist's life. Zerka's style more often led to critical events in the protagonist's past. Zerka Moreno was Moreno's star student and became a psychodrama director *par excellence*. During the years when Moreno was traveling all over the country to demonstrate psychodrama at universities, state psychiatric facilities, and VA hospitals, Zerka always traveled with him. Their presentation typically began with a talk by Moreno about his theories and philosophy followed by a demonstration psychodrama session. By 1950, the demonstration was often conducted by Zerka.

Both Morenos produced papers on psychodrama method, theory, and technique. J. L. Moreno wrote at least 50 articles on psychodrama and the three volumes entitled *Psychodrama*. Zerka was given credit in the last two in the form: "In collaboration with Zerka T. Moreno."

Probably two dozen of Zerka's approximately 50 publications are on psychodrama, method, and techniques. Her discussions of psychodramatic techniques especially are arguably more helpful to the student of psychodrama than are those of Moreno. Moreno discussed the techniques of psychodrama in several articles but preferred teaching them by demonstration (1951b, 1952, 1954c, 1958a). His writings on psychodrama dealt more with the rationale, theory, philosophy, and dynamics of psychodrama, and justifying the use of action methods over the verbal techniques of other methods. Zerka Moreno's articles are practical descriptions of techniques. One reason why Zerka's articles may be more helpful than J. L. Moreno's is that although Moreno invented the method and most of the techniques of psychodrama, he was always the director, never the protagonist or auxiliary ego. Zerka's extended experience in action on the psychodrama stage gave her experiences that Moreno did not have. Her analysis based on her experience was quite helpful in understanding and learning to take auxiliary roles.

While still Zerka Toeman, she wrote about her experiences of being an auxiliary for the psychotic patients that Moreno was treating in the early years of her presence at Beacon Hill Sanitarium (Toeman, 1946). Another paper on the double appeared in the first issue of *Sociatry* (Toeman, 1948a). Her additional articles on method and technique include: "Psychodrama in a Well-Baby Clinic" (1952); "Psychodrama in the Crib" (1954); "The Reluctant Therapist and the Reluctant Audience Technique in Psychodrama" (1958b); "A Survey of Psychodramatic Techniques" (1959); "Practical Aspects of Psychodrama" (1969b); "The Function of the Auxiliary Ego in Psychodrama with Special Reference to Psychotic Patients" (1978); and "Time, Space, Reality and the Family: Psychodrama with a Blended (Reconstituted) Family" (1991). Perhaps her most important article on the practice of psychodrama is "Psychodramatic Rules, Techniques and Adjunctive Methods" (1965). This paper represents the first attempt to provide a written account of the basic guidelines for the practice of psychodramatic psychotherapy. Many of the 15 rules apply equally well to nonclinical applications of the method and are as relevant today as they were 50 years ago.

Zerka also wrote on the history of sociometry (Toeman,1949) and group psychotherapy (1966a), as well as theoretical articles on spontaneous learning (1958a), on theory (1971, 1986, 1987, 2000a), and on ethics (1972, 1986). Moreno had often contributed chapters to edited tomes on group psychotherapy. After his death, Zerka became the spokesman for psychodrama, and contributed chapters to *Comprehensive Group Psychotherapy*, edited by Kaplin and Sadock (Z. T. Moreno, 1983); *The Evolution of Psychotherapy*, edited by Zeig (Z. T. Moreno, 1987); and *The Evolution of Psychotherapy: A Meeting of Minds*, also edited by Zeig (Z. T. Moreno, 2000a).

As Zerka's skill grew, Moreno began turning more and more teaching responsibilities over to her, appointing her Director of Training for the Moreno Institute. For a number of years, Zerka conducted the active training sessions. Moreno came to the theater periodically, sometimes directing a psychodrama, always leading discussions of the method or theory. The evening session was held in the Moreno house instead of the theater, and the day's work was discussed. By the late 1960s, he no longer attended sessions in the theater, but he held private sessions with each student in his living room. Instead of the didactic session in the evening, the group would have another action session in the theater.

After J. L. Moreno's death in 1974, Zerka Moreno kept the Moreno Institute training program in operation. Moreno's inactivity for some years before his death meant that the transition was barely noticeable. Students had been coming for a long time to train under Zerka and continued to come for that purpose. They came from everywhere, from all over the United States, from Europe and South America. Training groups were quite cosmopolitan.

Zerka was now able to accept invitations to travel to other countries to conduct workshops and spread the Morenean methods abroad. In her autobiography, Zerka lists 24 countries that she visited repeatedly, and I suspect that there may have been even more. There are now multiple Zerka Moreno Institutes teaching psychodrama all over the world.

Moreno gave much credit to Zerka during his lifetime. He called her his muse and by that term meant more than is easily apparent. His description of their meeting and Zerka's discussion of their relationship in her autobiography make it clear that Moreno's tremendous creativity owed a lot to their interactions. Zerka triggered Moreno's spontaneity and vice versa. A simple example, Zerka writes that from time to time she would make a casual remark that she assumed was of no particular significance. Moreno would stop what he was doing and ask her to repeat her remark. He would reply, "'That's very important. Come on, let's get to work.' Totally unexpected, out would come a significant piece of writing" (Moreno, 2012, p. 254). The resulting creativity was enormous and manifested in many facets. His personality, which was anything but shy, the fact that he was the originator of the methods, and the fact that he could absorb abundant amounts of acclaim meant that Zerka's contributions tended to get overshadowed. It was only after his death that the fullness of her part in the development and dissemination of psychodrama and group psychotherapy were recognized.

PSYCHODRAMA TODAY

J. L. Moreno kept tight control over psychodrama training for many years, and training at the Moreno Institute was the only way of receiving a certificate attesting to one's competence in using the method. For a long time, there was no fixed course of training. A student attended workshops at the Institute until Moreno decided that an adequate level of competence had been reached. This was usually after the student believed him/herself to have reached that level. In 1963, Moreno responded to student requests for a more predictable schedule of training and set 16 weeks of attendance as the criterion for receiving a certificate as Director of Psychodrama. Three other certificates were also awarded. After four weeks of training, one received a certificate as Auxiliary Ego; after eight weeks, Assistant Director of Psychodrama; and after 12 weeks, Associate Director.

He also called for the Council of Fellows of the American Society for Group Psychotherapy and Psychodrama to develop a certification process. This was not accomplished until after his death. In the meantime, Moreno began accepting training credit from several training programs conducted by outstanding former students. These included the psychodrama training program of St. Elizabeth Hospital, directed by Jim Enneis; the psychodrama training program at the St. Louis State Hospital, under the direction of Leon Fine; and a training center in California with Martin Haskell and Lew Yablonsky as directors. Prospective candidates for certification could complete half their training at one of these agencies, the rest at the Moreno Institute. More training centers were added later.

A committee on certification, appointed by the Council of the American Society for Group Psychotherapy and Psychodrama, announced the establishment of the American Board of Examiners in Psychodrama, Sociometry and Group Psychotherapy in 1975. The board has established two levels of certification: Certified Practitioner and Trainer, Educator, Practitioner. There is also a status known as Practitioner Applicant for Trainer for Certified Practitioners who have declared their intent on becoming certified as a Trainer, Educator, Practitioner. Certification is based on a written examination and a demonstration of skill. At this writing, there are a little more than 400 individuals in the United States who are certified at one or the other levels. There are many more practitioners of psychodrama than are reflected in that figure. From this writer's perspective, only a small percentage of those people who attend training workshops choose to become certified.

The mental health professions have not been particularly welcoming to the psychodrama method in the United States and the method's nonclinical potentials have barely been exploited. Psychodrama has been far more warmly embraced in other countries, especially in South America, Europe, Australia, and New Zealand. There are thousands of psychodramatists practicing in dozens of countries. Psychodrama has long been known in Japan and in the past 10 years there has been an escalating interest in other Asian countries. It can now be said that psychodrama is known and practiced worldwide.

SOCIODRAMA

Moreno created a third form of spontaneity drama in addition to the spontaneity theater and psychodrama. He introduced the idea of sociodrama in a series of presentations given in Chicago at the University of Chicago and the Illinois Conference on Family Relationships, in Detroit at Wayne University, and at the Sociometric Institute, New York, in 1943. Moreno also published an article on sociodrama in *Sociometry* (1943a).

The difference between psychodrama and sociodrama is closely related to Moreno's role theory and the distinction between social, or collective, roles and individual roles. Social roles, *the* role of *the* husband, *the* wife, *the* teacher, *the* store clerk, are identifiable roles that are taken by numerous individuals in a culture. They are culture specific; each culture has a certain set of such roles. A social role, say, of the wife, will vary in some degree from one culture to another. The social roles have a strong influence upon those who take them.

The psychodrama addresses private problems, the problems of the protagonist and the members of the psychodrama group. The sociodrama is intended to address social problems, often the misunderstandings that arise between different cultures. To achieve this goal, sociodrama works with representative types within a given culture and not private individuals. It constitutes a nonclinical application of the same spontaneity techniques of psychodrama. It is a method of sociotherapy. Moreno's search for the king of Austria, the event that he calls the first psychodrama, was more of a sociodrama because it was an attempt to deal with the social problems of leadership in postwar Austria.

Sociodramas take many forms. Moreno considered the living newspaper performances of the *Stegreiftheater* in Vienna, which he later produced in the United States, to be sociodramatic. They are sociodramatic because news events serve as a mirror in which a culture sees itself in action. Dramatization of news articles in the theater brings them to life in three dimensions in a way that the newspaper, limited to words, cannot. In the theater, the roles and the setting were portrayed in the manner characteristic for the particular subculture in which the event occurred. Moreno also conducted living newspaper sessions at Carnegie Hall in 1931, this time with the members of the group playing the roles. More often than not members of the group played the roles being explored in a sociodrama, rather than having those roles played by spontaneity trained actors as it happened in the *Stegreiftheater*.

Like psychodrama, sociodrama has three phases: the warming up process, the action phase, and sharing and discussion. Sociodramas can be structured in any number of ways. Whatever the structure, the issues being explored typically come from the group and represent social problems or conflicts that are contemporary and topical.

Sociodrama is frequently applied as an educational or training method, and one of the earliest collections of articles on sociodrama was entitled *Psychodrama and Sociodrama in American Education* (Haas, 1949). The papers covered the use of role-playing techniques at the elementary, junior high school, high school, and college levels. Many of the selections demonstrate a modest understanding of psychodrama and sociometry and a poor grasp of the distinction between these methods. They repeatedly establish, however, that students at all levels readily take to learning by action and that role-playing is a universal talent.

Sternberg and Garcia (1989) have an extensive list of applications of sociodrama in their more recent book entitled *Sociodrama*. They identify several ways in which sociodrama can be used with respect to conventional theater. Pointing out that playwrights from the time of ancient Greek theater have consistently dealt with social problems, they explain how sociodrama can be used to explore the dynamics of a theme that a writer has chosen for a play. Sociodrama can be used in the training of actors (see also Garcia, 1981) as well as in rehearsal to allow actors to expand the role beyond the limits of the script in order to gain a better understanding of the character that they are portraying. Sternberg and Garcia describe the use of sociodrama in teaching history and social studies, foreign languages, and the study of other cultures. They also refer to sociodrama in the teaching of literature and professional skills.[2]

Moreno (Moreno & Borgatta, 1951) describes a session of sociodrama with a group of personnel managers, consultants, public relations men, industrial psychologists, working in various branches of industry. These individuals had a special interest in dealing with industrial problems. The purpose of the session was to demonstrate the type of work that can be done with sociometric techniques.

The sociodrama literature contains a number of articles on the use of sociodrama in the exploration and learning of professional skills. Examples are: on training teachers, Lima-Rodriguez (2011); on training middle management, Synnot (1992); on training staff who work with older people, Wiener and Traynor (1987–1988); and on teaching medical personnel transition to palliative care, Baile and Walters (2013).

Sociodrama provides a powerful means of exploring moral and ethical issues. Moreno took special interest in racial conflict. After rioting occurred in Harlem in the summer of 1943, he conducted one or more

sociodramas in which perceptions of white and black people were produced, according to a paper published in *Sociometry*. Both white and
black New Yorkers attended:

> The procedure was so designed that some of the actual rioters and
> victims of the riots should be brought to the theatre as if it would be a
> psychodramatic session, but the method was to leave it entirely open
> whether they will be put on the stage to portray their individual experi-
> ences. The idea was rather to have a number of individuals on the spot
> who could serve as informants of what they have gone through. The
> plan was that if they would not act in person, they could transfer their
> experience to some of our auxiliary egos who, in turn, would translate
> them into role-creating action. (Moreno, 1943a, p. 443)

The sociodrama was not intended to explore the individual situations of
the participants. It was focused on exploring the conflict between the two
cultures with representatives of both cultures present and taking part. The
scene was an employment office that dealt with both black and white appli-
cants. A common situation developed in which two black girls were denied
jobs because of their race.

> [A] collective complaint which every Negro has against the white peo-
> ple as a group. The sociodrama began to develop from then on almost
> upon its own momentum. The girls returned home and told their par-
> ents that they had failed to get the jobs. A brother who was in the army
> and just home on furlough, got into a frenzy over what he heard from
> his sister. Then tension began to mount in the audience. One spectator
> after another tried to act out his own variation of the conflict, the col-
> ored problem in the army followed the colored unemployment problem
> and a spontaneous mood began to spread all over the audience and
> up to the stage, similar to the one which must have existed in Harlem
> before and on the day of the riots. (p. 444)

Moreno does not tell us more about this session. We can assume that the
white members of the group, whatever they knew intellectually about life in
Harlem, had a much deeper appreciation for the problems that confronted
the black population. From Moreno's brief description of the session, we
don't know if whites dramatized the problems with which they were confronted in their interactions with blacks.

Knepler (1970) describes using sociodrama with the members of a conference on mental health in Connecticut. The conference's objective was
to deal with resistance to the establishment of a regional mental health
center. "The sociodrama emerged as a 'warm, humorous, and spontaneous' presentation of the conference's chief concern and was evaluated by the
sponsors of the conference as 'an extraordinarily effective catalytic tool' in

loosening up the conference participants and helping them to focus more frankly upon central issues" (p. 130).In the same article, Knepler writes about the use of sociodrama in dealing with other community problems. One such application was with an organization dealing with housing for the poor. Another was attacking conflicts between police and citizens.

Moreno conducted a number of sociodramas in which there was a reenactment centered on a world-renowned person. These included "The Sociodrama of Mohandas Gandhi" (1948b); the trial of Adolf Eichmann (1961a); and the assassination of President Kennedy. The latter was presented as a joint trial of Oswald and Ruby in 1964. These sessions were held on the Sunday before the annual conferences of the American Psychiatric Association. They were always well attended by the psychiatrists who were in town for their profession's annual meeting, and the presentations always drew much publicity. According to Zerka Moreno (2012) the trial of Oswald and Ruby was reported in *Time* magazine.

Sociodrama has experienced a resurgence of interest in recent years, not only in America, but also in South American and European countries, and in Australia and New Zealand as well. This is the result of practitioners trained in psychodrama focusing their attention on social problems and finding new, nonclinical applications of spontaneity techniques. There is a growing literature on sociodrama as shown in the online bibliography of psychodrama: www.pdbib.org. Books by Sternberg and Garcia, mentioned above, and by Rosalie Minkin (2001) have been published. A special feature of the Sternberg and Garcia book is a chapter in which a dozen sociodramatists from several countries discuss their sociodramatic activities. A Fourth International Conference on Sociodrama was held in Iseo, Italy, in September 2013, and a fifth is scheduled for 2015.

NOTES

1. My first two-week training session at the Moreno Institute coincided with admission of a woman who was convinced that she had been divorced from one husband and married to another man through radio waves. Her first psychodramas were integrated into the training event.
2. I recall taking part in a presentation at an annual conference of the ASGPP on the use of sociodrama in exploring poetry. This was probably in 1964 or 1965, and I have forgotten who the presenter was but I remember moments in the session quite vividly.

11 Psychodramatic Theory

"Psychodrama seems to be known more for its applications than for its theories," writes Peter Kellermann (1992, p. 33) in a book that has been highly regarded in psychodrama circles. Kellermann suggests that psychodrama should be considered a "collection of unsystematic treatment interventions." Kellermann is wrong; there is an extensive body of theory associated with psychodrama and psychodrama is a method based on "a system of thought, a view, a philosophy of the world, a synthesis of methods that hang together and whose breakup produces confusion instead of enlightenment, invites disaster instead of producing cohesion" (Z. T. Moreno, 1969, p. 4.) Kellermann perpetuates a belief, common today, that psychodrama requires additional non-Morenean theoretical support. Many current psychodramatists combine psychodramatic techniques with one of the non-psychodramatic theories of psychotherapy. Books and papers have been published recounting these combinations of psychodrama with other methods. Some examples are: psychodrama combined with various theories of family therapy (Guildner, 1983, 1990; Hollander, 1981; Dodson, 1983; Williams, 1989; Perott, 1986; Remer, 1986); with psychoanalysis (Aronson, 1990; Kellerman, (1995); Lebovici, 1956a, 1956b); with Adlerian therapy (Dushman & Bressler, 1991; Starr & Weisz, 1989); with object relations theory (Powell, 1989; Holmes, 1992); and with Transaction Analysis (Holtby, 1975; Jacobs, 1975). These combinations raise the question of whether practitioners are conducting psychodrama or practicing another kind of psychotherapy utilizing psychodramatic techniques. Moreno addressed this issue when he complained that his methods had been widely adopted but the philosophy upon which they were constructed had been left behind "on library shelves." His entire life and his life's works had been dedicated to changing society, of creating "a superdynamic community" based on the principles of Spontaneity-Creativity and faith in the good intentions of our fellowmen. He perceived associating his techniques with other methods as potentially maintaining the status quo, the very thing he had set out to alter.

Contrary to the notion that psychodrama lacks theory is the existence of a number of theories linked to the psychodramatic method. They include the theory of Spontaneity-Creativity (J. L. Moreno, 1953c); the concept of the moment (J. L. Moreno, 1941c); action theory (J. L. Moreno, 1953c); tele (J. L.

Moreno, 1937a, 1941a; Z. T. Moreno, 2000a); role theory (J. L. Moreno, 1944); surplus reality (J. L. Moreno, 1953c, 1965b; Z. T. Moreno, 2000b); and, most important of all, Moreno's (1940b) concept of catharsis. These theoretical ideas as well as Moreno's view of psychopathology are the subjects of this chapter.

AN EXISTENTIAL, PHENOMENOLOGICAL METHOD

Nowhere is Moreno's existential, phenomenological philosophy more apparent than in psychodrama (J. D. Moreno, 1974, 1977; J. L. Moreno, 1954a, 1956a, 1969a). Psychodrama regards human behavior from a very different perspective than does conventional psychology and psychotherapeutic methods that are based on a logical-positivist philosophy. An example is the Morenean definition of psychodrama: "Psychodrama can . . . be defined as the science which explores the 'truth' by dramatic methods" (Moreno, 1946a, p. 249). Truth, as Moreno used the word in this definition, has caused some confusion and even consternation among psychodramatists. Moreno put the term in quotation marks. This indicates that he is using the concept as understood by the father of Existentialism, Søren Kierkegaard. That is, it is subjective truth as perceived and understood by an individual, as contrasted with historical fact. We all have experiences that we can recall with varying degrees of clarity and vividness. We are absolutely certain that certain things happened, that this person said this and did that to me or someone else, and then the other person responded in this way or that way. This is our truth. It is what we "know" happened. It is the truth that we swear to tell as a witness in court.

Two participants in an event may experience it very differently. Each has his/her truth of what happened. Cognitive dissonance can be considered as the collision of two contradictory truths.

THE MOMENT

One's truth is one's truth in the moment. Memory is remarkably susceptible to modification. How we recall an event in the present is how that event can affect our actions. This is so important in psychodrama, where the protagonist is encouraged to produce his/her subjective truth in dramatic action upon the psychodramatic stage. Making an experience concrete and tangible allows us to extract a new truth from an old event (Z. T. Moreno, 1994).

The moment (the present, the here and now) is critically important to understanding the psychodramatic method (J. L. Moreno, 1941c). The psychodrama, whether it involves the protagonist's experiences from the past or in the future or is the dramatization of a fantasy or dream, takes place in the present. The protagonist is encouraged to stay in the present by using present tense and by acting out behavior here and now rather than describing a recollection of an event. The reason for this is very logical. Though an event may have taken place in the historical past, the reenactment of it is the reenactment of the protagonist's present memory of it. How we understand an event as it unfolds is substantially influenced by many subjective elements. Two individuals involved in the same experience will have two different perceptions and interpretations of what happened. They will have different memories of the event. We also know that memories are seldom fixed. They are subject to change over time. Aspects of what is remembered of an experience change or disappear with time. Therefore, relying on the memory of the protagonist, we can only dramatize the protagonist's *present recollection* of a past event. The same principle is true for future events. In this case we are dramatizing protagonist's here and now anticipations of what *might* happen in the future.

THE SITUATION

The human being is looked at as an organism-in-an-environment from the perspective of conventional psychology. In existential psychodrama, on the other hand, the human being is perceived as an individual-in-a-situation. The situation includes not only a physical environment, but a social one, as well. The individual is not only a human being, but also a particular human being in this moment. The individual carries into every situation a history of all the prior situations that one has experienced, and all the learning that one has accumulated prior to this situation. Since every individual has a unique history of experiences, every individual-in-a-situation is a unique event. The psychodrama itself is a unique event and it can only take place in the moment.

Observing a psychodrama of an event from the protagonist's past from the perspective of conventional psychology, one may wonder how accurately the psychodrama portrays the original event. That might be considered a legitimate question from an historical point of view. This point of view would raise the question of validity: How valid is a psychodrama? From the existential position it is a meaningless question. Validity is existential validity and depends only on how faithfully the drama expresses the protagonist's memory of the event (Moreno, 1956a). It is the meaning of an event in the present moment that influences the protagonist's emotions and actions.

PSYCHOPATHOLOGY AND PSYCHODRAMA

In his discussions with the students of the Moreno Institute, J. L. Moreno often said that there weren't many people who were psychotic. There really weren't many people who were neurotic, he would add. "But," he continued, "Everyone is normotic." Moreno's position diverged from Freud's dictum that neurosis was the price we paid for the benefits of civilization. Freud believed that everyone was neurotic until they had been successfully psychoanalyzed. By normotic, Moreno meant that we respond poorly to surprise and the unexpected in life:

> A change may take place at any time in the life-situation of an individual. A person may leave or a new person may enter his social atom, or he may be compelled to leave all members of his social atom behind and develop new relationships because he has migrated to a new country. A change may take place in his life-situation because of certain developments in his cultural atom. He may, for instance, aspire to a new role. . . . Or he is taken by surprise by new roles in his son or his wife which did not seem to exist in them before. . . . Influences might threaten him from the economic, psychological and social networks around him. (Moreno, 1940a, p. 223)

When one's spontaneity is adequate to deal with the change in events, one can retain one's equilibrium:

> As long, however, as he is unable to summon the spontaneity necessary to meet the change, a disequilibrium will manifest itself which will find its greatest expression in his interpersonal and inter-role relationships . . . It is a peculiarity of these disequilibria that they have their reciprocal effects. They throw out of equilibrium other persons at the same time. The wider the range of disequilibrium, the greater becomes the need for catharsis. (p. 224)

There is almost no limit to the sources of disequilibrium, Moreno wrote. The relationship of the body to the mind or the mind to the body can result in inadequacy of performance. The thoughts and actions we have in relation to others, and the thoughts and actions others have toward us can push us off-balance. Life may be too complicated for one person and too simple and boring for another. Almost anything can throw one off-balance:

> Practically speaking, there is no sphere of the universe imaginable, whether physical, mental, social or cultural, from which there may not emerge, at one time or another, some cause of disequilibrium in a person's life. It is almost a miracle that an individual can achieve and maintain any degree of balance, and man has continually been in search of devices which will enable to attain or increase his equilibrium. (p. 228)

The vast majority of problems that people bring to psychotherapists are existential problems, problems of dealing with life and with the repercussions of the unexpected events for which we were not able to summon sufficient spontaneity to successfully meet. This formulation fits Moreno's basic notion that humankind as a whole has paid too much attention to conserves, the end products of creativity, and insufficient consideration to spontaneity and its role in the creative process. It is not civilization itself that is the problem, as Freud proclaimed. It is society's emphasis upon the conserve and society's failure to emphasize the importance of spontaneity in meeting life's challenges that has resulted in the current state of affairs.

It is no surprise that Sigmund Freud introduced the medical model into psychiatry at the same time that he decided that the nature of hysteria and other neuroses were psychological in origin instead of being neurological illnesses. He was trained as a doctor, and in medicine the notion that symptoms are an indication of an underlying malfunctioning physiology that calls for specific treatments to correct has been a powerful and successful model. How successful it is for understanding and dealing with psychological functioning is still a question (Wampole, 2001).

For Moreno, psychotherapy involved learning to be more spontaneous rather than treatment for an illness or disorder. The need for psychotherapy resulted from the learning of social conserves that failed in moments of surprise and that led to misinterpretations of the situation and inadequate actions. Psychodrama provided a means of reinterpreting the learned meaning of previous experience as well as increasing one's spontaneity.

Morenean theory is normative rather than pathologizing. Most theories of mental illness and psychotherapy are originated by mental health practitioners and based on observations of and attempts to explain behavior that is considered psychopathological. Moreno's theories emerged from his work with and observations of essentially normal, functioning people, the children in the gardens of Vienna, the prostitutes of Vienna, the villagers of Mitterndorf, and the actors of the *Stegreiftheater*. The normative feature of psychodrama makes it especially suitable for applications that go far beyond psychotherapy.

ACTION THEORY

"However important verbal behavior is, *the act is prior to the word* and 'includes' it" (Moreno, 1955c, p. 17, italics and quotation marks in the original). The human being is an actor, Moreno asserted, and an inter-actor. He believed that action was the *raison d'être* of humankind. Freud believed that it was possible to delve into and discover the hidden secrets of the unconscious through the free associations of his patients. Moreno put his protagonists on their feet and into action on a psychodrama stage. He engaged the entire person, mind, and body in the psychotherapeutic endeavor.

It is easy to see the difference between describing an event verbally and reenacting it. No matter how carefully a therapist (or other interviewer) probes and questions the narrator, a reenactment with a skilled psycho-dramatic director will produce a much fuller picture. The actions of moving in space, setting the scene of the event, reversing roles with significant others who took part in the event, and then with the help of auxiliary egos actually reenacting what happened unfolds far more from the protagonist's memory than can be obtained by verbal recollection. Much of what would otherwise remain outside awareness emerges in the reenactment, assisted perhaps by soliloquy. "The more the [protagonist] becomes involved, the less conscious he is of his actions; it is like seeing the acting out of the unconscious itself" (Moreno, 1955c, p. 14).

In an article on acting out in psychotherapy Moreno pointed out several problems that are encountered in psychoanalysis that are resolved by psychodrama. Transference, for example, to the therapist is minimized by the use of auxiliary egos. Transference is directed toward the individuals taking the roles of significant others, and at least partially resolved through role reversal, which gives the protagonist an opportunity to understand the other more fully, to replace transference with tele.

Acting out in psychoanalysis is considered an unacceptable alternative to rational understanding of unconscious impulses, achieved through free association and the interpretations of the analyst. It is deemed resistance to getting better psychologically. The controlled acting out of the psychodrama method affords the therapist an opportunity to observe the protagonist's deepest thoughts and motivations. It also allows protagonists to observe themselves.

The act hunger that we experience is always looking for opportunities to be expressed. This includes destructive and self-destructive desires. Acting out one's urges in psychodrama under the direction of a skilled therapist-director can reduce the need to express them in real life.

A director of conventional theater, Martin Esslin (1976), gives us an analysis of drama that both emphasizes drama as communication and calls attention to the interaction between actors and audience. Drama, he points out, communicates more fully and in a simpler, more direct, and quicker way than literary narrative. The author of a story may be able to convey the attitude of a character as well as his speech but must use many words in doing so. The author has also to depend upon the reader to grasp the intended meaning. The actor (or the protagonist in a psychodrama) conveys in an instant through body language, facial expression, words, and tone what the author may need paragraphs to communicate.

Half of the dramatic experience is the interaction between the audience and the actors, Esslin points out. It is the audience that determines the success of a play, finding it either acceptable or unacceptable. Acceptable means that the performance carries conviction. The audience must feel that the situation being presented feels right for it to be acceptable. As I have noted elsewhere, psychodramas tend to carry the conviction that a theater company hopes its dramas achieve. That is why the audience members of the *Stegreiftheater* found the Barbara and George dramas more moving than the other offerings of the spontaneity theater. They carried conviction because they were the real experiences of real people. The occasional psychodrama that fails in this respect is, for the most part, the result of individuals who have been so seriously hurt by their life experiences that they have lost touch with the inner core of themselves.

Esslin also identifies what Moreno called the co-conscious that an audience sometimes develops:

> Moreover—and this is one of the most attractive and mysterious characteristics of the drama—some sort of collective reaction, a consensus, will often develop in an audience, and will in a stage performance tend to become manifest both to the actors and to the audience itself. Anyone who has ever acted on a stage will confirm that the collective reaction to a play is palpably real. The audience, in some senses, ceases to be an assemblage of isolated individuals; it becomes a collective consciousness. (1976, p. 24)

Having shared a common experience, the audience has become a group. Esslin notes that this phenomenon will often develop in the conventional drama. It is an almost universal effect with psychodrama. Watching the struggles of a fellow human being, the protagonist, we respond emotionally as if the dramatized experience were happening to us. When it is clear that the protagonist has been unethically treated by a parent or other authority figure but does not express the anger that is appropriate to the situation, we develop an act hunger. We feel the anger and want the protagonist to give expression to it. At times a great tension builds up in the group as we wait for the protagonist to act.

The psychodrama director, of course, is especially concerned with the impact upon the protagonist. In relating an experience from one's past as one may do in a conventional psychotherapy session, one may very well reexperience the feelings associated with it. However, as anyone who has been a protagonist can affirm, that is a very weak reexperiencing compared with what happens during the psychodramatization of that event. It is the intensity of reenacting the past that makes catharsis of integration possible.

SPONTANEITY

The theory of Spontaneity-Creativity is the cornerstone for all Moreno's contributions, and psychodrama is certainly no exception. Moreno believed that participation in any of the action methods—a sociometric experiment, role training, psychodrama, and sociodrama—increased the spontaneity of both groups and individuals. Psychodrama was most specifically designed to assist participants live their lives more spontaneously. It is modeled after life but does not have the finality of life. On the psychodrama stage, the protagonist is free to experiment, to respond to situations, past or present, in many ways, to create new responses to old situations, and to create adequate responses to new situations.

Moreno's early systematic use of psychodrama included the spontaneity testing and spontaneity training that he conducted at the Hudson training school not only to promote better relationships within the institution, but to help the students deal more effectively with life problems when they reentered society outside the school.

In Chapter 8, I suggested that Moreno's concept of spontaneity could be associated with physicist David Bohm's concept of the implicate order, identified as a subtle order of energy. To the extent that this comparison is valid, spontaneity involves access to an energy in which every part contains information of the whole. Spontaneity, then, connects us with the whole universe.

ROLE THEORY

Role theory is an important feature in the practice of psychodrama. Moreno maintained that everybody has a capacity to take far more roles than life provides the opportunity and that we long to take far more than is possible. We have our official roles, but we also have many psychodramatic roles, roles in which we would like to act but for many reasons cannot. The more socially isolated and under-chosen one is, the fewer are the roles that become available. One result is antisocial behavior.

When life blocks us in giving expression to important roles, act hunger results. This not only is disruptive to our interpersonal relationships, but, Moreno (1953b) believed, is a major source of anxiety. Moreno assisted psychotic patients by allowing them to experience their fantastic worlds first to satisfy this act hunger. Then he led them to reconnecting to the world of consensual reality through the auxiliary egos who had peopled their delusional worlds. He understood problems in marriage to arise from the situation in which the psychodramatic roles of one partner had no counter-role in the other. A majority of psychodramas feature interpersonal role conflicts in which one or both partners of a relationship expect actions from the other that are not forthcoming. Many also portray inner role conflicts, such as social pressures to take unwanted roles.

Many psychodramas, especially when centered on problematic relationships that are ongoing, involve some degree of role training. An unsuccessful interaction between the protagonist and a significant other is enacted. After a role reversal or two and maybe other interventions, the director comes back to the opening scene and lets the protagonist try other ways of playing out the original interaction. Role training is also utilized to prepare the protagonist for future events that are a source of anxiety to the protagonist.

TELE

Some of the phenomena in psychodrama that are attributed to tele were mentioned in the discussion of the concept of tele in Chapter 8. There is more. As a group assembles for a psychodrama session, a lot of communication is occurring. Some is direct and observable, verbal as people speak to each other and nonverbal in facial expressions and body movements. Tele is a major aspect of this communication and there are varying degrees of awareness among individual of the currents of thoughts and feelings that are streaming through the group. Group members are, nonetheless, responding to them. Everyone has had the experience of being in groups that make them feel secure and confident, and everyone has had the experience of being in groups that make them feel anxious and vulnerable. In the vernacular we talk about the "vibes" of a group, good vibes and bad ones.

The emotional currents swirling around in a group have a significant impact on the groups' actions. One of the more subtle effects is the role that these currents play in warming up group members to the role of protagonist. It has become a customary practice by many psychodrama directors to make use of these emotions by having group members select the protagonist. This is done by having those individuals who wish or are willing to take the protagonist role make a brief statement about an issue that the psychodrama would explore if they were the protagonist. Group members make their choice in action by placing a hand on the protagonist whose issue most interests them.

It is customary to think of a psychodrama as the protagonist's drama and refer to it as Betty's drama or Tom's drama. However, it is really the group's psychodrama, not only because the members of the group are involved either as auxiliary egos or simply as observers, but also because the telic communications in the group have influenced the themes portrayed.

SURPLUS REALITY

"It can well be said that psychodrama provides the subject with a new and more extensive experience of reality, a *surplus reality*, a gain which in part justifies the sacrifice he made by working through a psychodramatic production" (J. L. Moreno, 1953c, p. 85). In the Morenean scheme we can find three different realities: consensual reality, social reality, and surplus reality. Each of us lives in a unique world composed of a combination of these realities, a universe that is unlike, in its entirety, the world of any other individual who lives or who has ever lived. Luckily, there is a significant part of all these individual universes that overlaps.

Consensual reality has mostly to do with the physical reality of the world in which we live. Science is the great human endeavor through which this reality has been explored and, to a large extent, mastered. There is widespread agreement about the validity of the laws and discoveries of classical science. This reality is the primary domain where individual universes overlap. It provides sufficient commonality for people to cooperate and collaborate with each other in the search for the security and sustenance necessary for survival.

Social reality is the reality of sociometry. This is the reality of interpersonal interaction. It is the world of encounter, of attraction and rejection, of tele, of social and cultural atoms, sociometric networks, and eventually all humankind. Our perceptions of this world are far more diverse than those of the physical world. There is enough commonality for societies and cultures to come into being. There is not sufficient understanding of the laws that apply to social functioning for societies to foster the well-being of all their members. Moreno hoped to establish methods that would uncover the laws of society and increase opportunities for everyone.

And then there is the third reality, surplus reality, the world of dreams and daydreams, fantasies, delusions, hallucinations, and illusions brought into concrete and tangible form on the psychodrama stage (J. L. Moreno, 1965b). According to Zerka Moreno (2000b), there is the visible objective reality of everyday life that I like to call consensual reality. But there is another invisible reality, surplus reality, in subjective thought and fantasy. It may be unseen but it is very real and often the reality with which the psychodramatist is dealing. (Z. T. Moreno, Blomkvist, & Rutzel, 2000).

Life, J. L. Moreno (1939) points out, is too narrow and constraining for most of us to create all the roles that we crave to experience. There are certain invisible dimensions in the reality of living, not fully experienced or expressed, and that is why surplus operations and surplus instruments to bring them out are needed. The protagonist can experience the roles denied by life on the psychodrama stage with psychodramatic techniques and the assistance of auxiliary egos. One can also explore how one's life would change with a different childhood or a different profession. On the psychodrama stage, one can live one's life the way one wants. Anything is possible with the surplus reality that psychodrama makes available.

Psychodrama gives dreams a three-dimensional existence. For Freud, dreams were the royal road to the unconscious, and he interpreted them. The purpose of dream psychodrama, on the other hand, is not to analyze or interpret dreams but to give the protagonist control of the dream process (1951a, 1959b). Nonetheless, the psychodramatization of dreams usually brings a lot of clarity to the symbols and elements in the dream. Psychodramatization of recurring nightmares is especially helpful to a protagonist. This procedure, properly carried out, almost always results in cessation of these unwanted and disturbing events. As Moreno told Sigmund Freud, his purpose was not to analyze dreams but to help people to dream again.

Psychodramatists often refer to scenes that are not based on the protagonist's actual experience as "going into surplus reality." In actuality, psychodrama itself is surplus reality in which the protagonist can reverse roles and become her husband or his wife, something that the other realities don't allow.

In psychodrama, a man can play the role of a woman; an adult can play the role of a child or of a person who has died. An empty chair can serve as an auxiliary ego and the protagonist can reverse roles with a picture on the wall or a sofa in the living room. Psychodrama is surplus reality.

The inner reality that is the source of surplus reality is indeed very real and essential in understanding creativity, human behavior, and psychodrama. It is the inner world of imagination and fantasy where great ideas, great inventions, and great deeds germinate. There is no reason to think that artist Marc Chagall was acquainted with J. L. Moreno and his idea of surplus reality. However, he would have understood it. In a speech delivered at Chicago University, Chagall said, "Our whole inner world is reality, perhaps even more real than the apparent world. To call everything that seems to be illogical a fantasy or fairy tale is to admit that one does not understand nature" (McMullen, 1968, p. 198). That certainly applies to the nature of human existence.

CATHARSIS

The concept of emotional catharsis as a therapeutic factor in psychotherapy has, over the years, stirred considerable controversy. Some theorists have regarded catharsis as a major therapeutic vehicle, while others have rejected it as of little or no value in accomplishing therapeutic goals. Empirical studies aimed at evaluating its therapeutic efficacy, surveyed by Nichols and Zax (1977), have produced mixed results. The possibility that catharsis can be counterproductive has been supported by research evidence (Bandura & Walters, 1963). A number of phenomena, all involving intense emotional expression, have been labeled catharsis (Scheff, 1979). Catharsis has been described in so many ways that Kellermann (1992) wonders if different authors are referring to the same phenomenon.

Catharsis is a concept of special interest to psychodramatists because J. L. Moreno (1940a) ascribed the salubrious effects of psychodrama to catharsis. He also expanded the notion of catharsis as it is used by contemporary psychotherapies as well as from its original Aristotelian description. In this way, Moreno created continuity between the aesthetic and therapeutic catharsis. Catharsis has received considerable attention in the psychodrama literature since J. L. Moreno's (1940a) first article on the issue. Karp (1968), Z. T. Moreno (1971), Ginn (1973), Kellermann (1984), Blatner (1985), and Bemak and Young (1998) are among those who have dealt with the topic. Their articles serve as resources for the current treatment of catharsis.

Catharsis as Discharge of Affect

Sigmund Freud first introduced the term *cathartic method* into psychiatry to describe Josef Breuer's discovery that when one of his patients, in hypnotic trance, recalled the event in which one of her myriad hysterical symptoms had initially occurred, the symptom disappeared. Freud was favorably impressed when Breuer, his erstwhile friend, colleague, and collaborator, related this cure to him. At the time, Freud was still intent on a university career in physiological research and had not begun the neurological consulting practice that was to lead to his eventual fame. Hence it was some six or seven years later, after he had begun his private practice, that he adopted Breuer's technique of investigation under hypnosis. Freud met with such initial success that he persuaded Breuer to publish their *Studies on Hysteria* (1895/1957) in which they claimed they had discovered a cure for hysteria. Freud called the intense expression of emotion that the method entailed abreaction.

At this time, Freud considered affect to be the residual of unexpressed instinctual excitation. When it was blocked from expression, strangulated, he said, it could become toxic, creating hysterical symptoms. By discharging the strangulated affect, abreaction relieved the symptoms.

His faith in abreaction faded as he discovered that the cures that he was effecting tended to be temporary. Most of his patients relapsed. The original symptoms returned within a year or so after treatment ended. He was greatly disappointed and gave up hypnosis in favor of free association.

Although Freud abandoned the cathartic method and abreaction as a therapeutic process, not all his psychoanalytic colleagues did. Among the theorists who were at one time associated with Freud, perhaps Wilhelm Reich was the one who was most impressed with the importance of unexpressed affect and the therapeutic importance of expressing it. Reich's ideas are found today in organismic therapy, bioenergetics, and radix. These current neo-Reichian modalities retain emphasis upon expression of emotion, utilizing techniques designed to elicit catharsis. Other therapeutic modalities stressing catharsis, most of which developed in the 1960s or early 1970s, include Primal Therapy (Janov, 1970), New Identity Process, sometimes referred to as "Casriel's scream therapy" (Casriel, 1972), and Gestalt therapy (Perls, 1969). Many long-established psychotherapy methods have followed Freud in rejecting the therapeutic efficacy of catharsis, although some careful researchers have reported positive results from abreactive catharsis (e.g., Nichols & Efran, 1985; Greenberg & Safran, 1987).

Many of the therapies that highlight catharsis emphasize expression of, release, or discharge of emotion. Although Freud's original hydraulic conceptualization of emotion (Fritz Perls called it Freud's excretory theory of emotion) has been discarded, many therapists still seem to regard emotion as something that, if expression of it is blocked, is stored up somewhere inside the body. It can have pathological consequences until it is released or discharged. The error is in regarding emotion as though it is a substance or something that can be stored. Nichols and Efran (1985) point out that emotions express relationships and do not express possessions.

Emotion can be thought of as the initial reaction to the situation in which we find ourselves or to a significant change in the situation (which actually makes it a new situation). The word itself is derived from the Latin *emovere*. "The term, which literally means 'to move out,' was initially used in the sense of moving a crowd out of the forum . . . that is, in the sense of an authoritative force moving a resisting mass" (de Rivera, 1977, p. 11). An important characteristic of emotion is that under the influence of a strong emotion we feel ourselves being moved—and often say so. "When we are moved by emotion we feel the desire to hit, hug, or whatever, even though our judgment may check this action. We are passively being moved rather than acting and yet this movement seems to be coming from *within* us" (p. 12). Emotions then can be regarded as instructions on how to behave in the situation in which we find ourselves. There may be factors that stand in the way of carrying out those instructions. For example, a situation may stimulate both anger and fear of expressing that anger. Example: A parent refuses a child's desire to do or have something that generates a reaction of anger at the parent as well as fear of the consequences of expressing it. The memory of the event years later can bring back the emotions that belong to it.

Aristotle and Spectator Catharsis

It is not surprising that Moreno should begin his discussion of catharsis with Aristotle, who explained why people liked to attend the tragedies of ancient Greek drama, why they liked to watch events they would not want to happen to them. In his *Poetica*, Aristotle (1951) explained that spectators of the tragedy experienced a *Katharsis*, a purging of fear and pity. Although scholars believe that there may be a lost volume of Aristotle's writings in which he may have expanded on his ideas of *Katharsis*, all we know is that he perceived tragedy as purging the spectator of fear and pity. Moreno considered his spontaneity theater, from which he created psychodrama, to be a return to the original Greek drama that evolved from spontaneous songs sung in praise to Dionysus.

Moreno accepted Aristotle's analysis of catharsis as valid but noted that Aristotle had not considered the role that spontaneity plays in the catharsis: "The spectator is witnessing and experiencing this human tragedy for the first time; these emotions, these roles, these conflicts and this outcome are in this constellation a novelty for him" (1940a, p. 224). The cathartic effect relies on novelty and surprise, the fact that the spectator does not know what to expect. The spectator experiences the most powerful catharsis with the first viewing. Even though a spectator may want to see the play again, even several times, catharsis is diminished by each performance as the drama loses novelty for the spectator. The play has become a conserve. It is no longer surprises. Eventually the spectator will no longer be interested in seeing it again.

The novelty of the first performance is one factor that helps determine the magnitude of catharsis that the spectator experiences. A second element is the extent to which a spectator identifies with the symbolic characters portrayed by those of the hero or other actors.

The greater a spectator's social and psychodramatic roles correspond to the symbolic roles portrayed on the stage, the greater is the catharsis produced by the drama. The degree to which the spectator can enter into the life upon the stage, adjusting his own feelings to what is portrayed there, is the measure of the catharsis he is able to obtain on this occasion. (Moreno, 1940a, p. 226)

The Actors' Catharsis

The spectator's catharsis described by Aristotle is a passive catharsis. Moreno's attention was centered on the impact of drama upon the actors. Because the actor embodies the role rather than merely observing it, Moreno thought that the cathartic impact of drama is more powerful for an actor than for a spectator. This is especially true when the actor's part is one that touches upon the actor's personal experience (Z. T. Moreno, 1971). Moreno called this active catharsis and said that it is inspired by the religions of the East and Near East that held that "in order to become a savior . . . [one] had to make an effort; he had, first, to save himself" (1940a, p. 227).

The psychodramatic concept of catharsis includes both active and passive catharsis, catharsis of the actor and catharsis of the spectator. In conventional theater, actors must take their respective roles many times in rehearsals and in performances. Their problem becomes accessing sufficient spontaneity to keep their performances fresh and new. The situation in psychodrama is quite different. Here, instead of an actor in a symbolic role on the conventional stage, we have private individuals with their private tragedies on the psychodrama stage. There is no script and no rehearsal. Everything happens for the first time. Protagonists must, with their own spontaneity, create both roles and action. The drama is created and produced simultaneously. There is only one performance of a psychodrama.

Moreno has now extended the concept of catharsis considerably beyond Aristotle's conception of something taking place in the spectator of the tragedy. Catharsis is something that occurs in the actors, as well, even more potently than in the spectator. And it occurs in life outside the theater. More than by seeing roles enacted and emotions expressed by others, it is by acting out roles that touch one deeply, roles that involve feelings to which one relates most meaningfully, that one masters those feelings and those roles.

Moreno's preoccupation with the actor's catharsis became the foundation of psychodrama. Because the drama in psychodrama comes from the protagonist's own life, the protagonist is always ensured of having a special affinity for his part, actually his parts for he has a special interest in all the roles in his psychodrama. Of historical interest is the fact that in the initial period of the development of psychodrama, Moreno tended to conduct psychodramas with only a single patient and a staff of auxiliary egos, reflecting the overvaluation of the actor's catharsis as compared with spectator catharsis. It was by happenstance that he became aware that patients benefited significantly from observing and taking part in their fellow patients' psychodramas, reconfirming the validity of the concept of spectator catharsis and its therapeutic effectiveness.

Abreaction

Abreaction from psychodramatic perspective is essentially catharsis as it is conventionally conceived in mental health circles. It is the same process that Freud described, the expression of affect associated with an old and often repressed event. The occasion for abreaction comes about as the result of a universal human experience, that it is sometimes necessary or advisable for us not to give expression to our feelings. From time to time, we find ourselves in situations in which intense emotions are aroused but, for any of a number of reasons, are not expressed. This is especially frequent in childhood, in which, for instance, a child may be afraid to express anger toward a parent. For many families, there are emotions whose expression is strongly discouraged. In one family, it may be anger. In another, fear in males may be interpreted as cowardliness or weakness, and the young boy who expresses it may be humiliated. Even in adolescence and adulthood, most of us find ourselves in relationships with family members, teachers, colleagues, supervisors, and others in which discretion often dictates that we not be completely spontaneous with our emotional responses. In other words, we learn to suppress if not repress, deny, or otherwise withhold rather than express what we feel in many situations. Although therapeutic amelioration is certainly not required for every instance of this sort, any event in which emotion is not expressed can become the potential for abreaction.

Abreaction is relatively common in psychodrama, much more so than in non-actional psychotherapies. This is because the entire self, physical and mental, is put into action in psychodrama. Abreaction is a function of memory and psychodramatists learn quickly that memory is a neuromuscular activity, not simply a neurological one. Protagonists routinely report that many details of an experience come to mind through the act of reconstructing a scene from their past.

Abreactions usually occur spontaneously. The skilled psychodrama director seldom seeks to precipitate abreaction. It happens unexpectedly and is often startling to the protagonist who typically tries to block expression of the emotion. Abreactions give psychodrama a dramatic impact. Zerka Moreno (2006c) expressed concern that this has led psychodrama to be viewed as a method of relief from emotional tension. The intense outburst of emotion of abreaction is not the therapeutic mechanism of psychodrama. Abreaction happens and plays a significant role in psychodramatic psychotherapy, but the catharsis of integration is the ultimate goal.

The psychodrama director must learn to be comfortable with intense displays of emotion, a characteristic that often may be absent in practitioners of non-actional methods. The experienced director will be careful to facilitate a complete expression of the emotion that has overwhelmed the protagonist and does nothing that might interfere. Psychodramatic action may touch upon a profound grief that may seem to both protagonist and group members to have no bottom and that it will go on forever. The director knows, however, that any emotion, when it has been sufficiently expressed, will diminish and then another one will take its place. Sound psychodramatic practice usually calls for the psychodramatist to continue the drama after abreaction has occurred.

Other therapies that emphasize abreaction as a healing event often deal with emotions in a nonspecific way. Clients who present anger as a problem may be instructed to "get it out" by various means, such as screaming and yelling or beating a pillow or a mattress with a tennis racket. Clients may even be given instructions to express the anger this way at home in private. The practitioner of psychodrama is not willing to deal with emotions in this abstract manner. If a protagonist says, "I want to deal with my anger," the psychodrama director will ask, "Who or what are you angry with?" The director will establish a scene, complete with auxiliaries, in which the client's anger has meaning. The protagonist will then be encouraged and facilitated in expressing the anger, perhaps to discover a more important feeling that the anger may be masking.

Catharsis of Integration

Here is Moreno's description of what happens in psychodrama:

As the [protagonist] takes part in the production and warms up to the figures and figureheads of his own private world he attains tremendous satisfactions which take him far beyond anything he has ever experienced; he has invested so much of his own limited energy in the images of his perceptions of father, mother, wife, children, as well as in certain images which live a foreign existence within him, delusions and hallucinations of all sort, that he has lost a great deal of spontaneity, productivity and power for himself. They have taken his riches away and he has become poor, weak and sick. The psychodrama gives back to him all the investments he had made in the extraneous adventures of his mind. He takes his father, mother, sweethearts, delusions and hallucinations unto himself and the energies which he has invested in them, they return by actually living through the role of his father or his employer, his friends or his enemies; by reversing the roles with them he is already learning many things about them which life does not provide him. When he can be the persons he hallucinates, not only do they lose their power and magic spell over him but he gains their power for himself. His own self has an opportunity to find and reorganize itself, to put the elements together which may have been kept apart by insidious forces, to integrate them and to attain a sense of power and of relief, a "catharsis of integration" (in difference from a catharsis of abreaction). It can well be said that the psychodrama provides the subject with a new and more extensive experience of reality, a *"surplus" reality*, a gain which at least in part justifies the sacrifice he made by working through a psychodramatic production. (1953b, p. 85)

This statement is full of meaning, at least for the seasoned psychodramatist, but it is not necessarily a passage that would clarify the meaning of the catharsis of integration to practitioners of other methods. The integrative catharsis is the ultimate goal of psychodrama. It involves confronting and making peace with factors from both within and outside oneself, factors and experiences that, when they occurred, threw the individual off-balance and out of harmony with self and/or world. As integration is achieved, bit by bit, equilibrium is restored, and the protagonist feels newly empowered and experiences a sense of harmony. Freed of ghosts from the past, the protagonist is more at peace. Old psychological wounds and hurts may be healed, and the individual may be ready to forgive adversaries who once seemed to make life difficult.

Integration entails a change in perception. That change may include perceiving a significant other in a new way. It may result in a change in the interpretation of an event or experience. It may give rise to a change in the protagonist's self-perception or in the protagonist's sense of relationship to the world at large. The new perception, to be truly integrative, is experienced in a deep and convincing way. The protagonist is convinced that the new perception is more accurate than the old. The group members feel the same way. In Esslin's (1976) concept, the psychodrama is acceptable.

All the basic psychodrama techniques, role reversal, soliloquy, the double, the mirror, and future projection, generate the information that can lead to the protagonist's new understanding of self, others, and events. In role reversal, we look at situations from the perspective of the significant others who share the experience with us. Soliloquy gives us time to explore our own thoughts and feelings more thoroughly than life often provides. The double helps us articulate feelings that remain preverbal for us. In the mirror, we can observe ourselves from a distance. Future projections allow us to test out different reactions to assess the consequences of them.

A simple psychodrama will help illustrate how integration can occur. The protagonist, we will call her Beth, is a psychology student who has had a negative experience with a practicum supervisor who put her in a situation in which she was scared for her physical safety. She would like to confront him with his negligent behavior but has not been able to do so. The psychodrama begins with a reenactment of the experience in which the supervisor leaves her in a small interview room in a prison, alone with a male prisoner who has been convicted of rape. He had given her no instructions nor did he say when he would return. The scene easily brings back the fear that she had felt in the situation.

Beth is next given a chance to confront the supervisor, whose role is taken by a group member. Facing him, she finds it impossible to remind him of his mistreatment of her, let alone express the anger she had been feeling toward him. Concretization of bodily feelings that she feels while facing him brings to mind an experience with her father when she was a young child. The scene is reenacted. She is four or five years old and in the family living room, singing and dancing to commercials on the TV when her father comes home from work. He scolds her for making so much noise and tells her to turn off the TV and quit. She feels like she has been a bad child and is crushed by his scolding.

Beth is reversed into the father's role and interviewed by the director, who asks "him" why he treated his young daughter so harshly. Beth-as-father replies that things were not going very well at work and that when he came home he wanted some peace and quiet. "You have really hurt her feelings," the director points out. "She feels terrible."

"I didn't mean to do that," the protagonist-in-role-of-father says. "Now I feel bad."

"If you could do it over," the director asks, "would you do something different?"

Beth-as-father thinks for a minute, then replies, "Yes. I think I would ask her to teach me how to sing and dance to commercials on TV."

The protagonist has produced a perfect reparative scene. She is reversed back into her four-year-old self and teaches the auxiliary father how to sing and dance to TV commercials, the music provided by the group members.

During the process of the drama, the director had learned that the father was not living at the time of the drama. Beth is given a chance to have a talk with him before letting him go back into the cosmos. Both express love and regrets for missed opportunities during his lifetime.

Now the protagonist is ready to confront the supervisor. Beth and the auxiliary stand face-to-face for a few moments. "Are you ready to tell this guy off?" asks the director. "No," she replies. "I would like to tell him how scared he made me and ask him to please not do this to other supervisees. I would like to make sure that he doesn't so something like that to someone else."

"Go ahead," the director says, impressed with her mature approach to the situation.

She tells the auxiliary supervisor how terrified she had been when he left her in a small room with a rapist. In a strong and assertive voice she demands, "Please don't do something like that to anybody else."

The director calls for a role reversal. The auxiliary-as-Beth repeats her words. The Beth-as-supervisor is silent. "What do you feel?" the director asks. The protagonist looks puzzled. "I don't feel a thing," she replies. "I could care less what this woman thinks. She is nothing to me."

The director reverses Beth back into her own role. Now she is angry and she tells the supervisor what a poor excuse for a practicum supervisor he is and that he probably has no more concern for his patients than he has shown for her. He should be kicked out of the profession, she thinks. The director suggests that she doesn't need him in her life anymore and suggests that she push him out of her psychodrama. This she does with relish.

There were several moments of integrative catharsis in this psychodrama. The first was occasioned by the role reversal with the father in the scene from the past. In his role, the protagonist could experience her father coming home from a busy or frustrating day, seeking peace and quiet and a chance to relax, being easily irritated by the noise of a young child singing and dancing to the TV set. Informed that his actions had hurt his young daughter, in his role she felt his regret at the outburst at the young child. The solution that she came up with in his role was inspired. It put her, as a little girl, in the dominant role of teacher to her father as a student. It is quite possible that it also fulfilled a common desire of children to have more time with a parent, particularly a parent who spends much of the day earning a living.

Questions about psychodrama are always raised in the minds of those of us who have been trained in the ways of conventional science. Questions that many people have are: How do we know that the dramatization of an event from childhood by an adult is faithful to what actually happened? And how trusty is the role reversal in a situation like this? These are questions of validity, critically important to psychologists and sociologists, and raised by them with respect to sociometry and psychodrama. The answer to both questions is: It doesn't really matter.

Memories like this protagonist produced are enfolded in the body like information is enfolded into a holographic plate or the explicate order is enfolded into the implicate order. They can and do have an effect on our behavior in subtle ways outside our awareness. Recalling an event brings with it the emotion associated with the experience. Emotion, after all, is about relationship and memories always involve relationships. Emotion is a primary trigger for recall of past events, so much so that we can say that emotion is the bridge to the past.

Memories are also very susceptible to alteration. In training groups, we have found it almost impossible to reproduce in the afternoon an event that happened in the morning. Memories should not be considered historical accounts of the past. Machines such as video and movie cameras can capture an event faithfully; the human body cannot.

In psychodrama this is not a critical matter. If a memory of an old event is having an effect upon a person, it is not the historical event but the here-and-now memory of that event that is having an influence—and that is precisely what is produced in psychodrama.

Questions about the validity of the role reversal are answered in a similar way. How accurate is Beth's portrayal of her father? If he were present, would he say and do that which Beth does in the role reversal? The fact is that the father in Beth's psychodrama is not the real-life father but rather Beth's perception of her father. The psychodramatist understands that and has no trouble accepting the psychodramatic father as the protagonist presents him. Moreno (1946b) defined psychodrama as the science that explores the truth by dramatic methods. Truth in this context is the subjective truth of the protagonist.

It is easy to suggest that the father's regret at having hurt his daughter's feelings and his suggestion for doing something differently are wish fulfillment fantasies of the protagonist, projected upon the father. That is certainly possible and it would be difficult if not impossible to prove or disprove. When we know a person well and have had a relationship over an extended period of time, we can anticipate how that individual will act. Reversing roles and putting ourselves in the place of the significant other provide a different way of organizing what we know about the other. We experience what we know in a subjective way rather than as observations and perceptions of the significant other. When we watch a protagonist in an encounter in which there will be a number of role reversals, we can observe distinct changes in the protagonist as they move from one role to the other, changes in posture, facial expression, tone of voice, and so on. People who have experience in role reversal report differences in subjective feelings in the role reversal. Accepting that one can never put oneself in another's place with 100 percent accuracy, we can also believe that one can reverse roles with considerable veracity. It is a psychodramatic truism that we have knowledge that we can only access in role reversal.

This has been a long discussion of one of three integrative moments in Beth's drama. The second one was the encounter in the present with the deceased father. In the scene re-creating Beth's memory of an old event, Beth interacted with the live father of a four-year-old. But there are two fathers and two Beths. There is an adult Beth and a deceased father. Knowing how often one feels unfinished business with a parent who is deceased, the director chose to let Beth have a here-and-now interaction with her father. This gave Beth a chance to express her perception of a relationship that was positive but probably with less intimacy than she could have wished for.

The third integration came out of the final encounter with the errant supervisor. Given a chance to express anger toward him, she chose a more constructive course of action: to inform him of his mistreatment of her in hopes of preventing further transgressions of the same nature to others. Now it became clear why the experience with the supervisor was continuing to plague her. She felt a need to prevent him from putting other supervisees into untenable positions. The fact that she could feel no concern or compassion in the role reversal supports the idea that role reversal is more than wish fulfillment. Beth expressed surprise that in the role of the supervisor she felt only annoyance at being confronted. She had expected to feel some regret, or at least chagrin. This served as information that her mission was futile. She could now relinquish it. The director helped her put this into the symbolic action of pushing the supervisor out of her life.

Spontaneous Improvisation

Moreno often used a strategy based on role theory to restore equilibrium. In many of the psychodramas that he describes in his publications, catharsis of integration is achieved by allowing the protagonist to take roles that life has denied. He used this routinely in his treatment of delusional patients (1940a, 1946a). Examples include his accounts of the psychodrama of Adolf Hitler (1957b, 1959c), and of the phantom lover (1944). Role assignment was not limited to the treatment of psychosis, however. The reports of the treatment of Barbara and George, and of Robert and Mary, illustrate what Moreno called the technique of spontaneous improvisation. Barbara was given prostitute and fishwife roles to counterbalance the ingénue, sweet-young-thing roles that she enacted in the spontaneity theater and in life. This reduced her need to act the hellion in the privacy of her marriage. Robert was a patient whose wife, Mary, was incorporated into the psychodramatic therapy. The couple was assigned roles such as detective and shoplifter, and welfare official and applicant (Moreno, 1946a).

Helen C. Jennings gives an engaging description of spontaneous improvisation in her treatment of a 21-year-old woman, identified as Miss K. The client had been repeatedly fired by various employers because of her indecision, lack of initiative, inability to discuss errors in her work, anxiety, and stammering, especially when talking with men. She was assigned roles in which she "played the part of the superior person who is free of anxieties and troubles which the other players may have, and parts in which she was superior to one or more of the other players" (Jennings, 1931, p. 13). The treatment, Jennings reports, was successful and Miss K developed confidence in herself, no longer stammered, and was no longer paralyzed by anxiety. Presumably she was now able to keep a job.

Reparative Scenes

Catharsis of integration is frequently attained through reparative scenes. In many psychodramas, there is a scene of what the protagonist remembers happening followed by a scene of what the protagonist wishes or thinks should have happened. The latter are called reparative scenes. In the psychodrama briefly sketched above, the scene in which the father and the protagonist sang and danced to TV commercials is one of them. Many reparative scenes are far more elaborate, as protagonists receive nurturing, encouragement, or confirmation that they were denied as children. Protagonists report that psychodramatic experiences of this nature had profound effects on them.

How and why brief psychodramatic scenes have such an impact is a phenomenon that has never been adequately explored. There are two clues. One is Moreno's discussion of the psychodramatic treatment of psychosis in which he says that brief periods of dramatizing the private world of the delusional individual are sufficient to provide the relief that they can find in the world of reality. Treatment does not require that the patient live completely in the delusional world. Carefully timed sessions in the psychodrama theater allow the individual to function in the reality of the sanitarium, and eventually outside it, as well. Another clue comes from neuroscience which tells us that fantasies are processed by the same areas of the brain that process life experience. While the reality of life cannot be erased, reparative scenes in the surplus reality of psychodrama ameliorate the effects of painful life experiences.

The Relationship between Abreaction and Integration

Abreaction and integration are rather disparate processes. Abreaction involves the expression of previously suppressed emotion while integration involves a change in one's perception. Despite these differences, the two are related and both play their part in the practice of psychodrama.

Anger, fear, and painful feelings (sadness, guilt, shame) are the most common emotions that result in abreaction. These are often called negative emotions because we designate discomfort in the relationship with those toward whom we feel them. We may avoid, suppress, or repress these feelings, which is why abreaction is possible. Abreaction of pain and fear predominately happens spontaneously and without much warning. The psychodrama director has the responsibility of facilitating a full expression of the feeling and being supportive of the protagonist who may feel overwhelmed by the emotion.

Anger is a special case. Although we may not like others to see us break down into sobs or to observe us when we are afraid, there is little social opprobrium associated with the expression of these emotions. Anger, perceived as leading to destruction and violence, on the other hand, is subject to social proscription. De Rivera's (1977) phenomenological research designates anger as the response to an obstruction that prevents one from attaining a goal. It instructs the individual to get the obstacle out of the way. Anger is energizing and it is possible that destruction and violence can result from expression of that energy. That does not mean that anger is destruction and violence.

J. L. Moreno spoke of ethical anger and Zerka Moreno wrote an article discussing the concept. Ethical anger is our response to situations in which we perceive injustice, either to others or ourselves, or when we see our sense of morality being violated:

> There are moments in life when we are justified to be angry and . . . not all anger is pathological or in need of treatment. Such moments are those in which things occur that our conscience cannot allow and in which we act upon its prompting. At such times we are, in fact, role models for others to think about and possibly to emulate in some fashion. (Z. T. Moreno, 1986, p. 147)

Parents and other authorities such as teachers have trained the average person in Western society that the expression of anger is wrong. Many of us are actually afraid of our own angry impulses. Many of us have suppressed anger on numerous occasions. As a result, anger is less apt to break through its restraints. Expression of anger in psychodrama may therefore require more assistance from the director than for other emotions.

Many psychodramas follow a pattern like this. The psychodrama begins with the protagonist confronting a significant other in the protagonist's current life with a charge of unfair or offensive behavior. It seems to the director that the protagonist is angrier than the situation calls for and he asks when the protagonist has felt this way before. The protagonist recalls a scene, often from childhood when he/she experienced a similar kind of behavior from a person in a position of authority over the protagonist, perhaps a parent or a teacher. This earlier scene is dramatized and the protagonist reexperiences the anger that could not be expressed at the time of the real-life situation. The director allows and encourages the protagonist in expressing the emotion in the psychodrama. This is abreaction, the expression of a suppressed emotion belonging to a past experience.

The abreaction is helpful in several ways. It is a completion of a hitherto incomplete transaction with a significant other. This in itself provides some sense of relief to the protagonist. It is also necessary to the esthetic of the drama. A tension builds up when the protagonist suppresses a strong, ethical anger. The group members feel this tension until the expression of the anger provides a release. The abreaction clears the way for a more profound, more valid role reversal with the significant other. When the protagonist experiences a strong emotion toward a significant other in the psychodrama, it is difficult to execute a valid role reversal. There is a temptation on the part of the protagonist to distort and caricature the significant other. The abreactive catharsis promotes the protagonist's search for the truth.

After the protagonist has fully expressed the anger, fear, or pain, the director calls for a role reversal. The auxiliary ego who has been in the role of significant other is now instructed to replay the protagonist's emotions while the protagonist observes from the role of the significant other. After this has been accomplished, the director asks the protagonist in the role of the significant other how it feels to see and hear the protagonist's feelings as the auxiliary has expressed them. The responses vary and each one is unique in some way. However, it is common for the protagonist to experience and express from the role of the significant other a sense of regret, guilt, or shame, a request for forgiveness, an explanation, or a wish to have done things differently. It is less common but it does happen that in the role reversal, the protagonist feels only defensiveness or that the significant other is not the least bit concerned about his/her treatment of the protagonist or the consequences of it. The psychodrama presented above was selected because the protagonist experienced both ends of the spectrum, regret in the role of the father and a total lack of concern in the role of the supervisor.

12 Appraising J. L. Moreno

At age 14, during an event that he labeled a mystical experience, J. L. Moreno identified himself with the universe (Marineau, 1989). That meant to him relating himself to all beings in the world, not just his family, accepting responsibility for the welfare of society. As a young man in Vienna in the aftermath of World War I, he found himself in a world of turbulence and chaos, and he sought a way to improve matters. He came to the conclusion that the fundamental source of Western society's problems was materialism. A materialistic science and technology had produced many products that were a boon to humankind—but had created others that could destroy all life. The materialistic psychologies—Freud's psychoanalysis and (much later) Skinner's behaviorism—promised to understand human behavior but reduced humanness to mechanical principles. The materialistic Communism of Marx made the position of the individual a pawn in the economic struggles of society. Religion, once a bulwark to materialism, was losing its dominance as a source of understanding. From the perspective of science, religion was an obstacle to a rational exploration of nature. Freud and Marx were both atheistic and rejected religion as superstition and the "opiate of the masses," meanwhile seeking to reduce the human being to the lowest possible denominator.

Moreno refuted such ideas. He proclaimed that the human being was more than a psychological, biological, or social organism. "Reducing man's responsibility to the psychological, social or biological department of living makes him an outcast" (1949, p. 235). Obsessed with the notion of God from early childhood, Moreno decided that a theory of God must come first:

> [A theory of God] must be attained first and is indispensable in order to make the life of any particle of the universe significant, whether it is a man, or a protozoon. Science and experimental method, if it be worthy of its claim, must be applicable to the theory of God or whatever the name which we give to a theory of the supreme value. (p. 236)

Briefly stated, Moreno's theory of God is that God is Spontaneity-Creativity and that Spontaneity-Creativity is distributed throughout the universe.

All individuals are capable of accessing spontaneity and hence potentially creative in all that they do.

> My God-universe pattern became the blueprint, the ontological guide after which I modeled sociometry, the idea of a society in which our deepest selves are realized. It is from my theological analysis and experiments that I drew the inspiration and the certainty to forge ahead in to realms which are entirely secular, materialistic and down to earth. (p. 236)

MORENO'S CONFLICT WITH FREUD

Moreno was likely unaware of the hegemony that psychoanalysis had established in American psychiatry before he came to this country. Both Marineau (1989) and J. D. Moreno (1989) suggest as much. In Austria and most of continental Europe, outside his small group of loyal followers and patients, Sigmund Freud and psychoanalysis were disdained, if not held in contempt, both by the medical establishment and by the population at large. Because of his emphasis upon sexuality, his name, if mentioned at all, was met by snickers or a knowing smile. The Viennese were likely to subscribe to Karl Kraus's definition of psychoanalysis as "psychoanalysis is that mental illness for which it regards itself as therapy" or his comment that "so-called psychoanalysis is the occupation of lustful rationalists who trace everything in the world to sexual causes—with the exception of their occupation" (Kraus, 1976, pp. 77–78). In America, on the other hand, in the early 1930s, Moreno found psychoanalysis rapidly spreading, not only in psychiatry, but also in anthropology, literature, and other fields.

Moreno often used psychoanalysis as the antithesis of psychodrama, pointing out that Freud placed his patients lying down on a couch while Moreno put them on their feet. Freud considered acting out to be resistance to analysis, while Moreno conducted therapy through controlled acting out; Freud wanted to be a blank screen to his patients, while Moreno saw the interpersonal interaction between psychoanalyst and patient as the agent of psychotherapy.

The conventional explanation for Moreno's unremitting attacks on Sigmund Freud's psychoanalysis is Moreno's jealousy of Freud's fame and the widespread acceptance of psychoanalysis. That is too simple an explanation. There are more salient reasons for his criticism of psychoanalysis. Moreno's disapproval of Freudian theory stems from the depths of the differences in the worldview between two creative thinkers.

There are some remarkable similarities in the lives of these two men who were such original contributors to human psychology. Thirty-three years apart in age, neither was born in Vienna, the city in which both spent their formative years. Born in outlying provinces of the Austro-Hungarian Empire, both were the sons of Jewish merchants, neither of whom was outstandingly successful. The families of each moved to Vienna when the sons were about four or five years old. Both Freud and Moreno were precocious young students who eventually earned medical degrees from the University of Vienna. Neither man lived out his life in Vienna; Moreno came to America at age 36, and Freud to England at age 82.

Despite these similarities, there were great differences in the ways in which Freud and Moreno encountered the world around them. Freud set his career goals early, selected a path, and moved single-mindedly down it until he was forced to accept a detour. Then he turned adversity to his advantage, finding the fame that he so determinedly sought. Freud lived a regulated life. His contacts with others were limited to a circle of close friends, his patients, and his analytic colleagues. While it would certainly be unfair to call Freud a recluse, compared with Moreno's invitation to encounter everybody in the world, Freud can be considered restrained in his life habits.

Moreno, on the other hand, seems to have ridden off in all directions simultaneously: a university student, staff member of the Psychiatric Clinic of the University of Vienna, founder of a religion, organizer of prostitutes, founder of a literary magazine, and originator of a theater. He invited everybody in the world to meet him. His lifestyle, if not Bohemian, was certainly an unconventional one. Although one can look back upon his many activities from the perspective of his later life and see the common threads, Moreno himself could hardly have anticipated how the rivulets of all his many interests and activities would eventually come together in a single major stream of thought.

A highly respected psychoanalyst and philosopher, Eric Fromm, wrote a balanced critique of Sigmund Freud's contributions. Fromm identified two features of Freud's thinking that he considers major limitations in the psychoanalytic system. They are Freud's strict adherence to the scientific materialism of his time and Freud's bourgeois authoritarian-patriarchal attitude. Psychoanalytic thinking is imbued with both of these characteristics (Fromm, 1980).

Freud acquired his investment in scientific materialism quite honestly. The logical positivism of the Vienna Circle, which had a great influence on 20th-century philosophy, emerged while Freud was still living and working in Vienna. Faith in the capacity of empirical science to fathom all the secrets of the universe was the position of his teachers, who included Ernst Brücke, one of the founders of modern physiology, and other giants of medical science, Theodore Meynert, chief of the psychiatric clinic of the university, and Hermann Nothnagel, professor of internal medicine. Freud entered medicine without a clear-cut perspective of what he would do with his life, other than that he wanted to be a scholar. It was his contact with these outstanding medical scientists that provided him with models of the role he wanted to take. It is hardly surprising that he absorbed their philosophical outlook and chose to become a medical research scientist.

Freud's commitment to the doctrines of scientific materialism underlie one aspect of psychoanalysis that brought the initial severe criticism of the medical community down upon him and earned negative public opinion, as well. To conform to positivist and reductionist demands, Freud believed he had to tie the entirety of emotional life to a biological basis. The one phenomenon in which the connection of the physiological and the psychological was well known was sexuality. By considering sexuality to be the basis of all drives, the physiological roots of psychic forces were established.

Freud's belief in determinism is reflected in his claim that every mental process, including dreams, dream symbols, slips of the tongue, and so on, was absolutely determined. He even used the term *over determined*, and maintained that through free association the determinants of even the most irrational thought or act, the meanings of dreams and of psychiatric symptoms, could be uncovered. Freud believed that he had brought psychology within the realm of science as it was understood and idealized in the 19th and early 20th century.

Freud's closed system model of psychic energy also reflects the influence of scientific materialism upon his thinking. He considered libido not only sexual in nature, but the motivating force behind all human accomplishment. To his way of thinking, each individual had a given amount of libido. It could be given direct sexual expression, converted into other passions, or sublimated, diverted into creative activity. Civilization, Freud thought, was built upon sublimated libido and the price that man paid for the advantages of civilization was to give up free and direct expression of his instincts. Neurotic symptoms appeared when one's instincts were being unsuccessfully restrained or sublimated.

In Freud's conceptualization of human beings, the major problem that a person faces is control. On the one hand, there is the id, man's animal nature expressed in raw instinct constantly striving for satisfaction. On the other hand, there are the ego and the superego, struggling to restrain id impulses and simultaneously deal with physical and social reality. Civilization, Freud held, is essentially an unnatural state of affairs, devised by humans because banding together with others of their kind offers them protection from the dangers of nature and enables them to accomplish far beyond that which is possible by an individual alone. However, there is a price to pay for the benefits of civilization. That price is neurosis. The instincts must be kept under control for if they are not restrained, one reverts to precivilized, animal behavior. It is the responsibility of the superego, derived from the control of the parents over the infant and young child, and subsequently the ego, to keep the instincts repressed and under control. When this repressive control is inadequate, neurotic symptoms erupt.

Fromm suggests that this conceptualization of the psyche was a direct reflection of the social reality of the Austro-Hungarian Empire of the turn of the century:

> Just as socially the majority is controlled by a ruling minority, the psyche is supposed to be controlled by the authority of the ego and the superego. The danger of the breakthrough of the unconscious carries with it the danger of a social revolution. Repression is a repressive authoritarian method of protecting the inner and outer status quo. (1980, p. 7)

It is certainly true that the Habsburg government was authoritarian, repressive, and reactively conservative. It had been so for generations. Threat of rebellion was frequent as nationalistic constituencies pushed for relief from arbitrary rules that were obstacles to their respective interests. It was natural then that Freud would conclude that the individual is in continual internal conflict with the id threatening to rebel against the controlling and civilizing ego and superego, just as the people are continually in conflict with the government, which must repress their rebelliousness if society is not to be destroyed.

Patriarchal-authoritarianism is also reflected in Freud's "grotesque picture of women . . . as essentially narcissistic, unable to love and sexually cool," says Fromm, and is "male propaganda" (1980, pp. 7, 8). Freud's concept of love is distorted by his bourgeois values, as well. To him loving means longing and deprivation; it lowers the self-esteem of the lover. Freud's idea of what is positive in loving is being loved in return and possessing the loved object. Basically, his model for love is the love of the little boy for his mother and is based on gratitude for satisfying vital needs, such as for food, being taken care of, and, of course, sexual needs. Not being able to possess the mother sexually out of fear of the father's revenge, Freud thought, these feelings are transferred to a more suitable sex object, that is, to an available woman. This describes love from the male's side. Women, on the other hand, he thought, are not capable of this kind of attachment to another being. They are capable only of narcissistic love, of loving themselves as they see themselves reflected in the man who chooses to love them.

Moreno encountered essentially the same scientific attitudes that Freud so readily adopted, only 30 years later. Perhaps because of the advances that had been wrought by scientific endeavor, faith in the scientific method was even stronger and more widespread than ever. Moreno's reaction was, however, quite different than Freud's. He wrote:

> The Vienna of 1910 was one of the display grounds of the three forms of materialism which has become since the undisputed world master of our age, the economic materialism of Marx, the psychological materialism of Freud, and the technological materialism of the steamboat, the

airplane and the atomic bomb. All three forms of materialism, however contrary to each other, had tacitly one common denominator, a deep fear and disrespect, almost a hatred against the spontaneous, creative self. (1947e, p. 5)

Rather than embracing scientific materialism, as Freud did (Sulloway, 1979), Moreno rebelled against it.

Nineteenth-century scientists saw the scientific endeavor replacing what was perceived as the superstition of religion with the facts and universal laws of nature and natural phenomena. It was a common attitude to see religion as the opponent of science, and the reaction of the church to both Copernicus's and Darwin's theories seemed to substantiate that position. It is well known that Freud not only considered himself an atheist, but that he considered religion to be a collective neurosis. In this respect Freud was in agreement with Marx, who described religion as the opiate of the people.

Moreno opposed the position of both. He argued that the fact that Christianity, Buddhism, Judaism, and other religions of the past have had limited success did not prove that the concept of religion itself had failed. He proposed a new sort of religion, a religion informed by the insights of science and not excluding some of the insights of psychoanalysis and Marxism.

Freud's view of humankind and his world outlook was pessimistic. He emphasized man's animal nature and focused upon the weaknesses of humankind. He saw himself as a destroyer of the pretentious illusions that man holds about himself. He attacked the illusion that man is the "rational animal" and the illusion of free will by emphasizing the extent to which every individual is under the influence of unconscious mental activity. He destroyed the illusion of the innocence of youth by proposing infant sexuality. He proclaimed all religion to be an illusion, a collective neurosis. He attacked genius by declaring creativity to be the result of redirected sexual impulses. This dark outlook upon human nature may have been justified by a world that did not treat him very kindly. In fairness to Freud, it must be stated that he and his work were often vilified and rejected without justification or a reasonable hearing. Freud felt his ostracism sharply and mentions it in his letters to Wilhelm Fliess. His negative vision may have been a position into which his identification as a scientist led him, in which his debunking of sentimentalist notions of humankind appeared to be scientific enlightenment. In any event, he saw more negative than positive in humankind, and seemed to hold out little hope for a vastly improved society. He held a Hobbesian point of view: Civilization is a thin veneer covering the basically animal nature of man, a violent and selfish nature. Control is the ultimate problem.

Brücke and Meynert were role models for Freud, and he aspired to the role of the research scientist. Moreno's role models were "Jesus, the improvising saint, and Socrates, in a curious sort of way the closest to being a pioneer of the psychodramatic format" (Moreno, 1953a, p. xxii). Moreno aspired to the role of the healer.

Moreno's explorations into the mysteries of Spontaneity-Creativity were an attempt to systematically study the phenomena of the genius, the saint, the hero, individuals who, in times of great crisis, have given new direction to humanity and averted apparent disaster. For Moreno, it was the saint or the hero that society badly needed in order to survive. He had little faith in the ability of the conventional scientist to keep humanity from continuing down its apparent path of self-destruction.

Moreno called for a functional, operational determinism in place of absolute determinism. This position acknowledges orderliness, lawfulness, and consistency in human behavior. At the same time, it is not a rigid, inflexible kind of order and law. According to Moreno's theory (1946b, p. 103), there can be truly original and creative moments, untraceable to the past. Determinism is still an issue of debate in the social sciences. Is this sense we have of freedom of will an illusion, as Freud held, or can we indeed make a difference in the chain of events that we experience as existence? Freud used his position to relieve patients of feelings of guilt. Moreno used his position to encourage responsibility and the idea that one's freedom is gained through conscious exercise of one's capacity to make choices.

Moreno's view of humankind was positive. Rather than the animal nature of humankind, what impressed him was the potential for creativity, the capacity for genius that humankind had demonstrated. He did not overlook that fact that this genius included the potential for destruction; his resolve was that if humankind can be so creative as to invent the means for its own self-destruction, salvation lies in being creative enough to escape that destruction.

Moreno's position doesn't deny that we are of the animal kingdom as Darwin demonstrated, or that much of human behavior is far from rational and motivated by impulses beyond awareness as Freud pointed out. The aspect of humanness that fascinated Moreno was not the unconscious, irrational motivation, but the apparent ability to transcend, at least momentarily, one's limitations. Spontaneity and creativity are what distinguish humankind, Moreno declared.

Freud's position on creativity bothered Moreno more than any other aspect of Freudian doctrine. Moreno accused psychoanalysis of waging "a war from the rear against all genius in order to reproach, him with his complexes" (1953a, p. xxxiv). He calls this war the vengeance of mediocrity and charges it with devaluing human nature, society, and spirit. Moreno professed to respect Freud and defended him, saying that Freud was a better scientist than many of his detractors. He also considered Freud to be a great clinician. On the issue of creativity, however, he had little but disdain and wrote:

Freud looked at man from below; he saw man "upside down" and from the position from which he looked at man he saw first his sexual organs and his rear. He was profoundly impressed, perhaps oversensitive, and he never turned his attention away from them. But one can evaluate man more advantageously by looking at him from above. Then one sees him erect, standing on his feet, eyes and head first. (1953a, p. liii)

Moreno perceived unrealized potential in humankind. It appeared to him that humankind had neglected to examine its own creative process and had focused all its attention instead upon the results of creativity. He thought that by the study of the creative process itself, he could discover the means to maximize human creativity. He dreamed of a society based upon the principles of Spontaneity-Creativity.

While Freud focused on libido as the source of psychic energy, Moreno, unencumbered by a doctrine of absolute determinism and reductionism, saw spontaneity as the energy, an unconservable energy, underlying all behavior and the key to creativity. He first became aware of spontaneity as he engaged with the children in the gardens of Vienna. Later he would study its manifestations systematically in *Das Stegreiftheater* as his players learned to create roles and dramas in the moment. From his observations, he became convinced that people could become more spontaneous and live a more creative life. He was convinced that if a whole society were based upon maximizing its individual and collective spontaneity, it could reach levels of cooperation and coordination that could maximize the extent to which it could provide benefits for all its members.

Where Freud saw neurosis as the price man paid for the benefits of civilization, Moreno saw society as a testimonial to the creativity of humankind. He saw humans as social animals, born into groups and living in groups throughout their lives. It is not surprising, then, that he originated the treatment of people in groups. Moreno's initial energies were focused upon increasing man's creativity rather than upon treating his pathology. At the same time, he was intrigued by the unique creativity in those considered psychotic and was able to bring many of them back into conventional ways of functioning. Freud saw the goal of psychoanalysis as assisting people to adjust to society. Rather than helping people adjust to a society that was causing them distress, Moreno sought to create a fairer and more just social order. "Why should we ask people to adjust to a sick society?" he asked.

A THERAPEUTIC METHOD FOR THE WHOLE OF MANKIND

Humankind had become too enamored of conserves, of the results of creative thinking, of the products of technology, and the theories and philosophies of great thinkers. Giving too much attention to the *results* of creativity, humankind had neglected to foster the creative process itself.

The key to revolution against a materialistic society lay in rediscovering spontaneity, the catalyst of and key to creativity, and living more creatively. Moreno envisioned a spontaneous-creative social order in which the well-being of everyone would be heightened. He made one attempt after another to achieve his vision.

Moreno's first endeavor at introducing spontaneity was his search for the king of Austria, an exploit that earned him some notoriety but little in the way of positive results. It was, however, the first psychodrama-sociodrama-role test, even though it was not very successful in finding a national leader. Next came the *Stegreiftheater*, the theater of spontaneity. This was more successful, according to both Marineau and Moreno. People came and the theater developed a following. However, it did not succeed in replacing the conventional theater, the goal that Moreno apparently set, according to the introduction to the third edition of *Psychodrama, first volume (3ʳᵈ Ed.) (1964)* and Fox (2006). More importantly, spontaneity drama was not having the impact upon society that Moreno and his actors sought. First of all, audiences had difficulty in accepting that the dramas were indeed spontaneous. In addition, the message was spreading way too slowly for Moreno. More disturbing to Moreno was that his actors kept turning away from spontaneity work to become actors on the legitimate stage and in the movies. When he brought spontaneity theater to America as Impromptu, he attained the same results. Although he again found appreciation for the concept, he could not see that he was generating a widespread desire for a spontaneous-creative lifestyle.

Moreno's experiences in organizing the prostitutes of Vienna in therapeutic groups led him to make a proposal for doing something similar with the inmates of the country's prisons. The Viennese groups were not conducted by a group therapist. The women became the therapists of each other. His idea was to form groups of prisoners who could do the same. He coined the terms *group therapy* and *group psychotherapy*. In 1931, the year that Moreno conducted Impromptu sessions in Carnegie Hall, he was also engaged in Sing Sing Prison classification project. The project did not turn out as Moreno had planned and hoped. He knew the reason immediately. Of all the factors that they had taken into account, the most important one, personal preference, had been left out.

Moreno and his loyal associate, Helen Jennings, set out to explore the interpersonal dimension of group life. After a sociometric testing of school-children that provided evidence for the sociogenetic law, the two addressed the sociometric study of a community. Dr. Fanny French Morse and the New York State Training School for Girls at Hudson provided the setting. Moreno and Jennings conducted the most thorough sociometric exploration and reorganization of a total community that has ever been attempted. There is no question that many of the hypotheses that Moreno had formed during his involvement with the villagers of Mitterndorf received some degree of confirmation at the school. Dozens of more limited sociometric experiments and even quasi-sociometric studies have further corroborated Moreno's findings. However, as extensive as it was, the Hudson training school study was just a first step.

Other large scale sociometric experiments, however, never happened, especially those that would have involved the sociometric organization of an open community. There were some practical reasons. The concept of sociometry has to be very carefully introduced, even to a small group. The idea of exposing one's attractions and repulsions with respect to the people with whom one lives in proximity is an unnerving if not terrifying prospect. Enlisting the goodwill collaboration of all the members of even a small community in such an endeavor is a monumental task. Moreno recognized the problems and thought that sociometry in smaller groups would have to proceed its application to larger ones.

Moreno introduced the concept of sociometric consciousness, an awareness of the beneficial effects of sociometric understanding of a group. Those who have experienced sociometric exploration realize that sociometry simply makes transparent the interpersonal dynamics that are influencing group behavior and that remain hidden until revealed by sociometry. Once these dynamics are revealed, the group has common knowledge that promotes more effective functioning. Another problem with sociometry is that it is a labor-intensive process. As the size of the group gets larger, handling the data becomes burdensome. This means that there are limitations to the kinds of groups and the kinds of criteria for which it is practical. Nonetheless, an increased sociometric consciousness is profitable in all group activities, especially if one is in a leadership role.

Although sociologists, social psychologists, educators, and others were quite excited about Moreno's methods when they were first published in the 1934 edition of *Who Shall Survive?* few really understood what sociometry was really about. The most prevalent error was in thinking that sociometry was about friendship rather than about choosing the companion with whom you wish to engage in a specific activity. They often used the non-criterion, "Who is your best friend?" a practice that Moreno consistently condemned and attempted to rectify.

Another big problem for the academic sociologist was that Moreno intended sociometry to effect changes in the group. The experiment was not complete until the criterion activity was completed, taking into account the choices and rejections that the group members had made. The sociologists were leery of their activities actually having some effect upon the groups they were studying. Their stance was reminiscent of the Prime Directive of the television show *Star Trek*. The Prime Directive forbade the personnel of a spacecraft visiting other planets to interfere with the normal and healthy development of alien life and culture. Sociologists expressed the idea that science and the application of scientific principles should be kept separate. Moreno's position, on the other hand, was that if a sociometric procedure wasn't tested, and if it didn't make a difference, you could not know that it was valid.

The sociologists, modeling the role of the social scientist after that of the physical and biological scientist, were even more reluctant to adopt Moreno's new formulation for sociological experimentation. Moreno had insisted that the subjects of a social experiment should be given researcher status. Since the experiment was a study of them, they should have a say in deciding which criteria were selected. This was the best way to ensure that the participants would be fully engaged in the experiment.

Moreno gave a number of reasons for giving the journal *Sociometry* to the American Sociological Society. I have long suspected that there was another reason that he chose not to state. I think Moreno may have come to the conclusion that sociology, and perhaps society at large, was not yet ready for sociometry. He had created the sociometric methods and techniques in order to make a positive difference in human society. He had put them into the world. Sociologists had welcomed these new techniques with enthusiasm—and then co-opted them, using the new instruments in traditional research designs instead of the purposes for which they were created. By the time that he decided to give the journal to the sociologists, psychodrama and group psychotherapy had both gained a lot of attention in the mental health disciplines. I think it is possible that Moreno decided to direct his energies in this direction, withdrawing his attention from sociometry proper.

Moreno justified his claim to be the originator of group psychotherapy over other putative founders. Other contenders for credit as founders of the method had not observed the consequences of interpersonal interactions upon the group participants as the agent of therapy. Several had merely held classes for patients to educate them on mental health topics. By virtue of his initiative in organizing with internationally recognized leaders in the field of group psychotherapy, Moreno was able to exert some degree of influence in the early days of its development.

In an open letter to group psychotherapists, Moreno (1966c) emphasized the difference between individual and group psychotherapy. In the former, the individual is the patient and the psychotherapist must understand psychodynamics; in the latter, the group is the patient and the group psychotherapist must know the structure of groups and sociodynamics that develop as the consequence of the relationships between the members. He warns that the concepts of psychological dynamics cannot be applied to group activity. Today there are so many different practices that Yalom (1985) suggests that we should speak not of group therapy but of group *therapies*. They range from methods that follow Moreno's lead in conceptualizing the group as the patient to methods that really consist of practicing individual psychotherapy in a group setting. Lecture and class methods are also called group psychotherapy in some hospitals and mental health clinics.

Some group therapists perceive the interactions of group members as providing the benefits of group therapy. Many more see themselves and their skills as the source of therapeutic effect. In psychodrama groups, Moreno's concept of each individual as the therapist of each other individual is systematized through the use of auxiliary egos and in the sharing session. Regardless of the group leader's orientation, the relationships among group members are likely responsible for the positive results that group members obtain.

Psychodrama has proved to be the most viable of all Moreno's contributions. He was probably correct when he wrote that turning from the theater of spontaneity to the therapeutic theater saved his work from oblivion. However, psychodrama has not survived without controversy or conflict. Freudian psychoanalysis had taken strong root not only in psychiatry in America when Moreno arrived, but in literature and to some degree in social science. It had set a model for psychotherapy, a 50-minute session in deepest privacy, an objective, serious psychotherapist with a penetrating eye, who limited interaction between himself and patient to verbal communication, largely on the part of the client. Moreno's practice of putting people on a stage and urging them to act out their troublesome relationships in a group setting must have seemed to be anti-therapeutic if not harmful. He violated most of the rules and conventions of conventional psychotherapy. It is not surprising that psychodrama met with resistance at first.

Psychodrama survived. Although psychodramatists represent a small proportion of psychotherapists in the United States, it has become quite popular in South American countries and in both Western and Eastern Europe, where psychodrama and sociodrama flourish. The method has attracted a lot of attention in Asian countries in the past 15 years.

The practice of psychodrama has been predominantly linked to the psychotherapy and counseling professions. There are some notable exceptions. The literature contains many examples of psychodrama and sociodrama in the field of education. Role training has been widely adopted in business and industry. Psychodrama techniques have been applied to conflict resolution, to training threat assessment investigators, and violence prevention, as well as executive coaching and teaching communication skills (see http://www.strategicinteractions.com/). Many ways of using psychodrama have been utilized by the graduates of Gerry Spence's Trial Lawyers College, in which I have had a hand (Leach, Nolte & Larimer, 1999; Garcia-Colson, Sison & Peckham, 2010).

A PARADIGM CHANGE

J. L. Moreno never attained the recognition that Sigmund Freud attained, even though Moreno's methods covered a far broader spectrum than did psychoanalysis and were more scientifically solid. Moreno claimed that there was no controversy about his ideas and that they were universally accepted. "I am the controversy," he proclaimed (1953a, p. cxiv). Many, including me, disagree with Moreno on this issue. While many of his innovations have indeed entered the mainstream of psychotherapeutic practice, some of his most important ideas have been overlooked or ignored. Zerka Moreno (1969a) addressed this when she wrote that Moreno did not originate his methods and techniques for their own sake. "They are based on a theory of life, without the comprehension of which [Moreno's methods] are meaningless, even harmful" (p. 2).

Blatner (2000) gives 10 "Hindrances to Psychodrama's Acceptance," reasons why psychodrama has been a sort of stepchild in the field of psychotherapy. He notes the competition with psychoanalysis, the fear of psychotherapists of action and elicitation of strong emotion, and the difficulties of obtaining adequate training. In addition, "The mixture of the staid professionof psychotherapy and drama seemed implausible. . . .It was hard for people to imagine such a superficial endeavor [as drama] could be turned into something healing " (p. 42), and inadequately trained psychodramatists hurt psychodrama's acceptance, Blatner wrote. He observes that psychodrama is a complex method, difficult to master. As Moreno himself did, Blatner lays many of the difficulties at Moreno's feet. According to Blatner, Moreno was a difficult person to get along with, egocentric, tactless, and extravagant in his manner. His writing style was problematic, redundant, diffuse, and turgid. Self-publishing meant distribution of his work was limited. Moreno's open sessions were shocking to the profession as was his willingness to train anybody in the psychodrama method. Finally, Blatner points out Moreno's references in his work to God, especially his concept of the I-God, the basis for some claims that Moreno was psychotic. All of the above have some validity and are the source of complaints that various people have made about Moreno, his theories, and methods.

In an article published a year after Moreno's death, three men close to Moreno each discussed his work and its impact (Borgatta, Boguslaw & Haskell, 1975). Haskell notes that both Moreno and his work were the subject of controversy because he challenged so many established concepts in psychiatry, psychology, and sociology. He adds:

> It was not at all unusual for people who adopted or even plagiarized some portions of his work to reject strongly Moreno the man and various aspects of his work. That this phenomenon occurred as frequently as it did greatly disturbed Moreno. He resented the fact that many of the sociologists and psychologists who accepted and employed the quantifying techniques of sociometry either ignored or attacked the underlying philosophy. His contributions to group psychotherapy, psychodrama, and group dynamics received similar treatment at the hands of some clinical psychologists and psychiatrists, particularly those with a psychoanalytic orientation. (p. 156)

Boguslaw commented in a similar vein:

He lived to see many of his most cherished inventions converted into lifeless rituals and intellectual toys, while spontaneity and creativity were shunted off into the back-waters of the cultural "underground" only to emerge now and again in the marketable form of "encounter groups" and related fads of group experimentation.

But in a sense, Moreno's most profound contributions were always destined for marginality in a society whose central ethos revolves about industrial production and its concomitant rationalization of everyday life. (p. 156)

In such societies, Boguslaw notes, creative individuals can only derive their inspiration from marginal situations. On the one hand, society asks them to be creative; on the other hand, it subjects them to societal norms, trying to integrate their works into established conventions.

I believe that there is another way to understand the resistance that Moreno, his methods, and theories met when he introduced them. In part, it was because of Moreno's existentialist orientation. During the period of the Religion of Encounter, he was a "heroic existentialist." That is to say, he did not write philosophical analysis of existential philosophy; he *lived* existentially. That experience infused all his later work and accounted for much of his creativity. He continued to live in the moment as much as anybody can and still survive in a materialistic society that treasures the past and looks forward to the future.

It is my opinion that J. L. Moreno introduced a paradigm change in social and psychological science. This transformation in perspective is consistent with the emergence of the notion of wholeness, that is, that everything is connected with everything else, in a number of other scientific disciplines, replacing the prevailing conceptualization of a mechanical, cause and effect universe. Briggs and Peat (1984, 1989) discuss this development in the works of David Bohm and his theory of the implicate order; Ilya Prigogene and his concept of dissipative structures; Rupert Sheldrake and his idea of morphogenesis; and Karl Pribram and his notion of the holographic brain.

"Man is more than a psychological, social or biological being," Moreno wrote (1949, p. 235), and must be understood from a cosmic point of view. "Mankind is a social and organic unity" (1953c, p. 3) and everyone is connected with everyone else. Meaningful social research incorporates the subjects as co-researchers. The therapeutic effect comes from group members, not from the therapist. These ideas stand in opposition to prevailing notions and, as such, are met with resistance.

A paradigm change, according to Kuhn (1962), seldom wins easy acceptance. The establishment, invested heavily in the status quo, fights vigorously against the new vision. Zerka Moreno touches on this in an introduction that she wrote for *J. L. Moreno* (Z. T. Moreno, 1996). Speaking of sociometry, she wrote, "For a while social scientists listened to his voice, then he was absorbed and submerged by the culture" (p. vii). Much the same can be said of all his methods. Thus group psychotherapists have, by and large, conceptualized group psychotherapy as the treatment of individuals in a group rather than as the treatment of the group itself. The sociologists who experimented with sociometry fought against social reorganization, the ultimate goal of sociometry. They also rejected Moreno's modification of the scientific method to include the subjects as co-.researchers. Many psychodramatists have imported theories of personality, psychopathology, and psychotherapy into their practice of psychodrama. This is another example of the separation of the method from the philosophy that perturbed Moreno so much.

Moreno himself acknowledged that he had failed to accomplish his goal of establishing a worldwide social order, a society in which all individuals would be granted the opportunity to achieve their highest potential, a culture in which human resources would be maximized and not wasted. He was aware that such a goal could ultimately be achieved only with the goodwill and efforts of everybody. He provided both a vision of a more satisfying social order and some tools to assist bringing that vision into being. That is no small achievement.

I believe that Moreno was far ahead of his time in both his understanding of human society and of human behavior. He demonstrated that while we create the society in which we live, that society, at the same time, shapes who we are. It is possible that the society envisioned by Moreno, one in which all individuals have the opportunity to maximize their potentials, cannot be achieved. It is nonetheless worth striving for and maybe someday in the future we will catch up to J. L. Moreno.

References

Ackerman, N. W. (1949). Psychoanalysis and group psychotherapy. *Group Psychotherapy*, 3, 204–215.

Announcements. (1960). *Group Psychotherapy*, 13, 246–247.

Aristotle (1951). *Poetics* (S. H. Butcher, Trans.). Mineola, NY: Dover Publications.

Aronson, M. L. (1990). Integrating Moreno's psychodrama and psychoanalytic group therapy. *Journal of Group Psychotherapy, Psychodrama & Sociometry*, 42, 199–203.

Aulicino, J. (1954). Critique of Moreno's spontaneity theory. *Group Psychotherapy*, 7, 148–158.

Baile, W. F. & Walters, R. (2013). Applying sociodramatic methods in teaching transition to palliative care. *Journal of Pain and Symptom Management*, 45, 606–619.

Bandura, A. & Walters, R. H. (1963). *Social learning and personality development*. New York: Holt, Rinehart & Winston.

Bemak, F. & Young, M. E. (1998). Role of catharsis in group psychotherapy. *International Journal of Action Methods: Psychodrama, Skill Training & Role Playing*, 50, 166–184.

Berne, E. (1971). *Transactional analysis in psychotherapy*. New York: Grove.

Binswanger, L. (1956). Existential analysis and psychotherapy. In F. Fromm-Reichman & J. L. Moreno (Eds.), *Progress in psychotherapy*. New York: Grune & Stratton.

Blatner, A. (1985). The dynamics of catharsis. *Journal of Group Psychotherapy, Psychodrama & Sociometry*, 37, 157–166.

Blatner, A. (2000). *Foundations of psychodrama* (4th Ed.). New York: Springer Publishing Co.

Bohm, D. (1951). *Quantum theory*. Englewood Cliffs, NJ: Prentice Hall.

Bohm, D. (1952). A suggested interpretation of the quantum theory in terms of "hidden variables" I. *Physical Review*, 85, 166–179.

Bohm, D. (1980). *Wholeness and the implicate order*. New York: Routledge.

Bohm, D. (1985). *Unfolding meaning*. New York: Routledge & Kegan Paul.

Bohm, D. (1990). A new theory of the relationship of mind and matter. *Philosophical Psychology*, 3, 271–286.

Bohm, D. (1994). *Thought as a system*. New York: Routledge.

Bohm, D. (1998). *On creativity*. New York: Routledge.

Bohm, D. & Hiley, B. J. (1993). *The undivided universe*. New York: Routledge.

Bohm, D. & Peat, F. D. (2000). *Science, order, and creativity* (2nd Ed). New York: Routledge.

Borgatta, E. F., Boguslaw, R. & Haskell, M. R. (1975). On the work of Jacob L. Moreno. *Sociometry*, 38, 14–161.

Bratescu, G. (1975). The date and birthplace of J. L. Moreno. *Group Psychotherapy and Psychodrama*, 28, 2–4.

Briggs, J. P. & Peat, F. D. (1984). *Looking glass universe: The emerging science of wholeness*. New York: Cornerstone Library.

Briggs, J. P. & Peat, F. D. (1989). *Turbulent mirror*. New York: Harper & Row.

Breuer, J. & Freud, S. (1895/1957). *Studies on hysteria*. New York: Basic Books.

Bronfenbrenner, U. (1943). A constant frame of reference for sociometric research. *Sociometry*, 6, 363–397.

Buchanan, D. R. (1980). The central concern model: a framework for structuring psychodramatic production. *Group Psychotherapy, Psychodrama & Sociometry*, 33, 47–62.

Bulletin of the Society for Psychodrama and Group Psychotherapy. (1943a). *Sociometry*, 6, pp. 349–355.

Bulletin of the Society for Psychodrama and Group Psychotherapy (1943b). *Sociometry*. 6, pp. 457–459.

Bulletin of the Society for Psychodrama and Group Psychotherapy. (1944) *Sociometry*, 7, pp. 80–82.

Campbell, J. (1968). *The hero with a thousand faces* (2nd Ed.). Princeton, NJ: Princeton University Press.

Campbell, J. & Moyers, B. (1988). *The power of myth*. New York: Doubleday.

Casriel, D. (1972). *A scream away from happiness*. New York: Grosset & Dunlap.

Chagall, M. (2003). *Marc Chagall on art and culture*. Stanford, CA: Stanford University Press.

Compernolle, T. (1981). J. L. Moreno: An unrecognized pioneer of family therapy. *Family Process*, 20, 331–335.

Cornyetz, P. (1945). The warming up process of an audience. *Sociometry*, 8, 456–463.

Corsini, R. J. & Putzey, L. J. (1956). The historic background of group psychotherapy. *Group Psychotherapy*, 9, 178–249.

Coutu, W. (1951). Role-playing vs. role-taking: An appeal for clarification. *American Sociological Review*, 16, 180–187.

Cukier, R. (2007). *The words of Jacob Levy Moreno*. Retrieved June 5, 2009, from www.lulu.com.

Damasio, A. (1994). *Why Descartes was wrong*. New York: G. P. Putnam's Sons.

de Rivera, J. (1977). *A structural theory of the emotions*. New York: International Universities Press.

Dodson, L. S. (1983). Intertwining Jungian depth psychology and family therapy through use of action techniques. *Group Psychotherapy, Psychodrama & Sociometry*, 35, 155–164.

Dreikurs, R. (1955). Group psychotherapy and the third revolution in psychiatry. *International Journal of Social Psychiatry*, 1, 23–32.

Dushman, R. D. & Bressler, M. J. (1991). Psychodrama in an adolescent chemically dependent treatment program. *Journal of Adlerian Theory, Research and Practice*, 47, 515–520.

Enneis, J. M. (1951). The dynamics of group and action processes in therapy: An analysis of the warm-up in psychodrama. *Group Psychotherapy*, 4, 17–22.

Esslin, M. (1976). *An anatomy of drama*. New York: Hill and Wang.

Forsyth, E. & Katz, L. (1946). A matrix approach to the analysis of sociometric data: Preliminary report. *Sociometry*, 9, 340–347.

Fox, J. (2006). Theater of spontaneity revisited. *Group Psychotherapy, Psychodrama & Sociometry*, 59, 51–54.

Franz, J. G. (1939). Spontaneity training in public speaking classes: A preliminary report. *Sociometry*, 2, 49–53.

Franz, J. G. (1940). The place of the psychodrama in research. *Sociometry*, 3, 49–61.

Franz, J. G. (1942). The psychodrama and interviewing. *American Sociological Review*, 7, 27–33.

Freud, S. (1901/1964). *Psychopathology in everyday life.* New York: Mentor.

Freud, S. (1954). *The origins of psychoanalysis.* New York: Basic Books.

Freud, S. (1975). *The letters of Sigmund Freud.* New York: Basic Books.

Friedman, N. (1993). *Bridging science and spirit.* Saint Louis, MO: Living Lake Books.

Fromm, E. (1980). *Greatness and limitations of Freud's thought.* New York: HarperCollins.

Gallup, G. (1941). Question wording in public opinion polls. *Sociometry*, 4, 259–268.

Garcia, Antonina. (1981). *Using sociodrama for training actors in audition and interview techniques.* Ann Arbor: University of Michigan, Microfilms International.

Garcia-Colson, J., Sison, F. & Peckham, M. (2010). *Trial in action.* Portland, OR: Trial Guides.

Gendlin, E. (1981). *Focusing.* New York: Bantam Books.

Ginn, I. L. B. (1973). Catharsis: Its occurrence in Aristotle, psychodrama and psychoanalysis. *Group Psychotherapy and Psychodrama*, 26, 7–22.

Goffman, E. (1956). *The presentation of self in everyday life.* New York: Doubleday.

Greenberg, L. S. & Safran, J. D. (1987). *Emotion in psychotherapy.* New York: Guilford Press.

Guldner, C. A. (1983). Structuring and staging; a comparison of Minuchin's structural family theapy and Moreno"s psychodramati therapy. *Journal of Group Psychotherapy, Psychodrama & Sociometry*, 35, 141–154.

Guldner, C. A. (1990). Family therapy with adoleents. *Journal of Group Psychotherapy, Psychodrama & Sociometry*, 43, 142–150.

Haas, R. B. (Ed.). (1949). *Psychodrama and sociodrama in American education.* New York: Beacon House.

Hale, A. E. (1981). *Conducting clinical sociometric explorations: A manual for psychodramatists and sociometrists.* Roanoke, VA: Royal Publishing Company.

Harary, F. & Ross, I. C. (1957). A procedure for clique detection using the group matrix. *Sociometry*, 20, 205–215.

Hare, A. P. & Hare, H. R. (1996). *J. L. Moreno.* London: Sage Publications.

Hare, P. (1986). Bibliography of work of J. L. Moreno. *Group Psychotherapy, Psychodrama & Sociometry*, 39, 95–128.

Historical Committee. (1971). A brief history of the American Group Psychotherapy Association 1943–1968. *International Journal of Group Psychotherapy*, 21, 406–435.

Herink, R. (1980). *The psychotherapy handbook.* New York: The New American Library.

Holborn, H. (1950). Wilhelm Dilthey and the critique of historical reason. *Journal of the History of Ideas*, 11, 1, 93–118.

Hollander, S. L. (1981). Spontaneity, sociometry and the warming up process in family therapy. *Group Psychotherapy, Psychodrama, & Socometry*, 34, 44–53.

Holmes, P. (1992). *The inner world outside: Object relations theory and psychodrama.* New York: Routledge.

Holtby, M. E. (1975). TA and psychodrama. *Transactional Analysis Journal*, 5, 133–136.

Howard, J. (1970). *Please touch: A guided tour of the human potential movement.* New York: McGraw-Hill.

Hunting, J. R. (1966). The public session. In J. L. Moreno, A. Friedemann, R. Battegay & Z. Moreno (Eds.), *The international handbook of group psychotherapy*. New York: Philosophical Library.

Huxley, A. (1944). *The perennial philosophy*. New York: Harper & Row.

IAGP Affiliates. (2013). *About us*. Retrieved September 15, 2013, from http://www.iagp.com/affiliates/index.htm.

Jacobs, A. (1975). Transactional analysis and psychodrama. *Transactional Analysis Journal*, 5, 69.

Janik, A. & Toulmin, S. (1973). *Wittgenstein's Vienna*. New York: Simon & Schuster.

Janov, A. (1970). *The primal scream*. New York: Dell.

Jennings, H. C. (1931). Psychoanalysis and Dr. Moreno. *Impromptu*, 1, 12–14.

Jennings, H. H. (1939). Quantitative aspects of tele relationships in a community. *Sociometry*, 2, 93–100.

Jennings, H. H. (1941a). Individual differences in the social atom. *Sociometry*, 4, 269–277.

Jennings, H. H. (1941b). Sociometry and social theory. *American Sociological Review*, 6, 512–522.

Jennings, H. H. (1942). Experimental evidence on the social atom at two time points. *Sociometry*, 5, 135–145.

Jennings, H. H. (1943). *Leadership and isolation*. New York: Longman, Green and Co.

Karp, M. (1968). Directorial catharsis: Fact or fantasy. *Group Psychotherapy*, 21, 137–139.

Keepin, W. (2008). Lifework of David Bohm. Retrieved November 14, 2011, from http://www.vision.net.au/~apaterson/science/david_bohm.htm.

Keller, H., Treadwell, T. & Kumar, V.K. (2002). The personal attitude scale-II: A revised measure of spontaneity. *Journal of Group Psychotherapy, Psychodrama, & Sociometry*. 55, 35–46.

Kellermann, P. F. (1984). The place of catharsis in psychodrama. *Journal of Group Psychotherapy, Psychodrama & Sociometry*, 37, 1–13.

Kellermann, P. F. (1992). *Focus on psychodrama*. London: Jessica Kingsley Publishers.

Kellermann, P. F. (1995). Towards an integrative approach to group psychotherapy: An attempt to integrate psychodrama and psychoanalytic group psychotherapy. *International Forum of Group Psychotherapy*, 3, 6–10.

Kipper, D. A. (1967). Spontaneity and the warming up process in a new light. *Group Psychotherapy*, 20, 62–73.

Kipper, D. A. & Hundal, J. (2005). The spontaneity assessment inventory: The relationship between spontaneity and nonspontaneity. *Journal of Group Psychotherapy, Psychodrama & Sociometry*, 58, 119–129.

Knepler, A. E. (1970). Sociodrama in public affairs. *Group Psychotherapy*, 23, 127–134.

Kohl, M. & Robertson R. (2006). *A history of Austrian literature 1918–2000*. Rochester, NY: Camden House.

Kraus, K. (1976). *Half-truths & one and a half truths* (H. Zohn, Trans.). New York: Carcanet Press.

Kuhn, T. (1962). *The structure of scientific revolutions*. Chicago: University of Chicago Press.

Leach, J., Nolte, J. & Larimer, K. P. (1999). Psychodrama and trial lawyering. *Trial*, April, 40–48.

Lebovici, S. (1956a). Psychoanalytical application of psychodrama. *Journal of Social Therapy*, 2, 380.

Lebovici, S. (1956b). Psychoanalytical group psychotherapy. *Group Psychotherapy*, 9, 282–289.

Lima-Rodriguez, L. (2011). Sociodrama, teacher education and inclusion. In R. Wiener, D. Adderley & K. Kirk (Eds.), *Sociodrama in a changing world.* Retrieved from http://www.lulu.com/product/paperback/sociodrama-in-a-changing-world/15104932.

Lippitt, R. (1943). The psychodrama in leadership training. *Sociometry,* 6, 286–292.

Marineau, R. E. (1989). *Jacob Levy Moreno: 1889–1974.* London: Tavistock/Routledge.

Mathews, S. (1895). Christian sociology. *American Journal of Sociology,* 1, 2, 182–194.

McMullen, R. (1968). The world of Marc Chagall. London: Aldus Books.

Mead, G. H. (1934). *Mind, self, & society.* Chicago: University of Chicago Press.

Meyer, H. J. (1952). Review: The sociometries of Dr. Moreno. *Sociometry,* 15, 354–363.

Minkin, R. (2001). *Sociodrama for our time.* New York: Springer.

Moreno, F. B. & Moreno, J. L. (1945). Role tests and role diagrams of children. *Sociometry,* 8, 188–203.

Moreno, J. D. (1974). Psychodrama and the future of the social sciences. *Group Psychotherapy and Psychodrama,* 27, 59–70.

Moreno, J. D. (1977). Scholasticism without God: Martin Heidegger, 1889–1976. *Group Psychotherapy, Psychodrama & Sociometry,* 30, 135–137.

Moreno, J. D. (1989). Introduction. *Group Psychotherapy, Psychodrama & Sociometry,* 42, 1, 3–12.

Moreno, J. D. (1994). Psychodramatic moral philosophy and ethics. In P. Holmes, M. Karp & M. Watson (Eds.), *Psychodrama since Moreno: Innovations in theory and practice.* London: Routledge.

Moreno, J. L. (1914). *Ein Ladung zu Einer Begegnung (Invitation to an encounter).* Vienna: Anzengruber Verlag.

Moreno, J. L. (as Anonymous). (1920). *Das testament des Vaters (The words of the father).* Berlin-Potsdam: Kiepenheuer Verlag.

Moreno, J. L. (1923). *Rede über die Begegnung (A speech about encounter).* Berlin-Potsdam: Kiepenheuer Verlag.

Moreno, J. L. (1934). *Who shall survive? A new approach to the problems of human interrelations.* Washington, DC: Nervous and Mental Disease Publishing Co.

Moreno, J. L. (1937a). Inter-personal therapy and the psychopathology of inter-personal relationships. *Sociometry,* 1, 7–76.

Moreno, J. L. (1937b). Sociometry in relation to other social sciences. *Sociometry,* 1, 206–219.

Moreno, J. L. (1939). Psychodramatic shock therapy, a sociometric approach to the problem of mental disorders. *Sociometry,* 2, 1–30.

Moreno, J. L. (1940a). Mental catharsis and the psychodrama. *Sociometry,* 3, 209–244.

Moreno, J. L. (1940b). Psychodramatic treatment of marriage problems. *Sociometry,* 3, 1–23.

Moreno, J. L. (1940c). Psychodramatic treatment of psychosis. *Sociometry,* 3, 115–132.

Moreno, J. L. (1941a). Foundations of sociometry, an introduction. *Sociometry,* 4, 15–35.

Moreno, J. L. (1941b). The philosophy of the moment and the spontaneity theatre. *Sociometry,* 4, 205–226.

Moreno, J. L. (1941c). The prediction and planning of success in marriage. *Marriage and Family Living,* 3, 83–84.

Moreno, J. L. (as Anonymous). (1941d). *The words of the father* (translated from *Das testament des Vaters* by the author and expanded). Beacon, NY: Beacon House.

Moreno, J. L. (1942). Sociometry in action. *Sociometry*, 5, 298–315.

Moreno, J. L. (1943a). The concept of sociodrama: A new approach to the problem of inter-cultural relations. *Sociometry*, 6, 434–449.

Moreno, J. L. (1943b). Open letter to contributors and readers of *Sociometry*. *Sociometry*, 6, 197–198.

Moreno, J. L. (1943c). Sociometry and the cultural order. *Sociometry*, 6, 299–344.

Moreno, J. L. (1944). A case of paranoia treated through psychodrama. *Sociometry*, 7, 312–327.

Moreno, J. L. (1945a). The future of man's world. *Sociometry*, 8, 297–304.

Moreno, J. L. (Ed.) (1945b). *Group psychotherapy: A symposium.* Beacon, NY: Beacon House.

Moreno, J. L. (1946a). Psychodrama and group psychotherapy. *Sociometry*, 9, 249–253.

Moreno, J. L. (1946b). *Psychodrama, first volume.* Beacon, NY: Beacon House.

Moreno, J. L. (1946c). Situation test. *Sociometry*, 9, 166–167.

Moreno, J. L. (1946d). Sociogram and sociomatrix. *Sociometry*, 9, 348–349.

Moreno, J. L. (1947a). Contributions of sociometry to research methodology in sociology. *American Sociological Review*, 12, 287–292.

Moreno, J. L. (1947b). Organization of the social atom. *Sociometry*, 10, 287–293.

Moreno, J. L. (1947c). Progress and pitfalls in sociometric theory. *Sociometry*, 10, 268–272.

Moreno, J. L. (1947d). The social atom and death. *Sociometry*, 10, 80–84.

Moreno, J. L. (1947e). *The theater of spontaneity* (translated and revised from *Das Stegreiftheater*, 1923). Beacon, NY: Beacon House.

Moreno, J. L. (1948a). Psychodrama of a pre-marital couple. *Sociatry*, 2, 103–120.

Moreno, J. L. (1948b). The sociodrama of Mohandas Gandhi. *Sociatry*, 1, 357–358.

Moreno, J. L. (1949). Origins and foundations of interpersonal theory, sociometry and microsociology. *Sociometry*, 12, 235–254.

Moreno, J. L. (1950). Sociometric leadership and isolation in *Who shall survive? Sociometry*, 13, 382–383.

Moreno, J. L. (1951a). Fragments from the psychodrama of a dream. *Group Psychotherapy*, 3, 344–365.

Moreno, J. L. (1951b). *Sociometry, experimental method and the science of society.* Beacon, NY: Beacon House.

Moreno, J. L. (1952). Psychodramatic production techniques. *Group Psychotherapy*, 5, 243–273.

Moreno, J. L. (1953a). Preludes of the sociometric movement. In J. L. Moreno, *Who shall survive?* Beacon, NY: Beacon House.

Moreno, J. L. (1953b). Some comments to the trichotomy, tele-transference-empathy. *Group Psychotherapy*, 5, 85–90.

Moreno, J. L. (1953c). *Who shall survive? Foundations of sociometry, group psychotherapy and psychodrama.* Beacon, NY: Beacon House.

Moreno, J. L. (1954a). Clarification and summary. *Group Psychotherapy*, 7, 327–333.

Moreno, J. L. (1954b). Interpersonal therapy, group psychotherapy and the function of the unconscious. *Group Psychotherapy*, 7, 191–204.

Moreno, J. L. (1954c). Psychodramatic frustration test. *Group Psychotherapy*, 6, 137–167.

Moreno, J. L. (1954d). Transference, countertransference and tele: Their relation to group research and group psychotherapy. *Group Psychotherapy*, 7, 107–117.

Moreno, J. L. (1955a). The birth of a new era for sociometry. *Sociometry*, 18, 261–268.

Moreno, J. L. (1955b). Canon of creativity. *Sociometry*, 18, 359–362.

Moreno, J. L. (1955c). The significance of the therapeutic format and the place of acting out in psychotherapy. *Group Psychotherapy*, 8, 7–19.

Moreno, J. L. (1955d). The sociometric school and the science of man. *Sociometry*, 18, 271–291.

Moreno, J. L. (1955e). System of spontaneity–creativity–conserve: A reply to P. Sorokin. *Sociometry*, 18, 382–392.

Moreno, J. L. (1955f). Theory of spontaneity and creativity. *Sociometry*, 18, 361–374.

Moreno, J. L. (1956a). The dilemma of existentialism, Daseinanalyse and the psychodrama, with special emphasis upon "existential validation." *International Journal of Sociometry and Sociatry*, 1, 55–63.

Moreno, J. L. (1956b). Philosophy of the third psychiatric revolution, with special emphasis upon group psychotherapy and psychodrama. In F. Fromm-Reichmann & J. L. Moreno (Eds.), *Progress in psychotherapy, 1956*. New York: Grune & Stratton.

Moreno, J. L. (1956c). System of spontaneity–creativity–conserve: A reply to P. Sorokin. In J. L. Moreno (Ed.), *Sociometry and the science of man* pp. 126–136. Beacon, NY: Beacon House.

Moreno, J. L. (1957a). *The first book on group psychotherapy, 1932* (3rd Ed.). Beacon, NY: Beacon House.

Moreno, J. L. (1957b). Psychodrama of Adolf Hitler. *International Journal of Sociometry and Sociatry*, 1, 71–80.

Moreno, J. L. (1958a). Fundamental rules and techniques of psychodrama. In J. H. Masserman & J. L. Moreno (Eds.), *Progress in psychotherapy (Vol. 3)*. New York: Grune & Stratton.

Moreno, J. L. (1958b). Research note on transference and tele. *Group Psychotherapy*, 11, 362.

Moreno, J. L. (1959a). Discussion and replies. In J. L. Moreno (in collaboration with Z. T. Moreno), *Psychodrama second volume, foundations of psychotherapy*. Beacon, NY: Beacon House.

Moreno, J. L. (1959b). Psychodrama of a dream. In J. H. Masserman & J. L. Moreno (Eds.), *Progress in psychotherapy (Vol. 4) (pp. 193–211)*. New York: Grune & Stratton.

Moreno, J. L. (in collaboration with Z. T. Moreno), (1959c). *Psychodrama second volume, foundations of psychotherapy*. Beacon, NY: Beacon House.

Moreno, J. L. (1960a). Definitions of the tele-transference relation. *Group Psychotherapy*, 13, 52–56.

Moreno, J. L. (1960b). The principle of encounter. In J. L. Moreno (with H. H. Jennings, J. H. Criswell, L. Katz, R. R. Blake, J. L. Mouton, M. E. Bonney, M. L. Northway, C. P. Loomis, C. Proctor, R. Tagiuri & J. Nehnevajsa (Eds.), *The sociometry reader* (pp. 15–16). Glencoe, IL: Free Press.

Moreno, J. L. (1960c). Role. In J. L. Moreno (with H. H. Jennings, J. H. Criswell, L. Katz, R. R. Blake, J. L. Mouton, M. E. Bonney, M. L. Northway, C. P. Loomis, C. Proctor, R. Tagiuri & J. Nehnevajsa (Eds.), *The sociometry reader (80–86)*. Glencoe, IL: Free Press.

Moreno, J. L. (1960d). The social atom: A definition. In J. L. Moreno (with H. H. Jennings, J. H. Criswell, L. Katz, R. R. Blake, J. L. Mouton, M. E. Bonney, M. L. Northway, C. P. Loomis, C. Proctor, R. Tagiuri & J. Nehnevajsa (Eds.), *The sociometry reader (52–54)*. Glencoe, IL: Free Press.

Moreno, J. L. (1960e). Theory of interpersonal networks. In J. L. Moreno (with H. H. Jennings, J. H. Criswell, L. Katz, R. R. Blake, J. L. Mouton, M. E. Bonney,

M. L. Northway, C. P. Loomis, C. Proctor, R. Tagiuri & J. Nehnevajsa. (Eds.), *The sociometry reader (67–79)*. Glencoe, IL: Free Press.

Moreno, J. L. (1961a). Psychodrama and sociodrama of Judaism and the Eichmann trial. *Group Psychotherapy*, 14, 18–19.

Moreno, J. L. (1961b). The role concept, a bridge between psychiatry and sociometry. *American Journal of Psychiatry*, 118, 518–523.

Moreno, J. L. (1962). Role theory and the emergence of the self. *Group Psychotherapy*, 15, 114–117.

Moreno, J. L. (1964). *Psychodrama, first volume* (3rd Ed.). Beacon, NY: Beacon House.

Moreno, J. L. (1965a). Psychodrama in action. *Group Psychotherapy*, 18, 87–117.

Moreno, J. L. (1965b). Therapeutic vehicles and the concept of surplus reality. *Group Psychotherapy*, 18, 211–216.

Moreno, J. L. (1966a). Editor's foreword: Open letter to group psychotherapists. In J. L. Moreno (in association with A. Friedeman, R. Battegay & Z. T. Moreno) (Ed.), *The international handbook of group psychotherapy*. London: Peter Owen.

Moreno, J. L. (in association with A. Friedeman, R. Battegay & Z. T. Moreno). (Ed.). (1966b). *The international handbook of group psychotherapy*. London: Peter Owen.

Moreno, J. L. (1966c). Psychiatry of the twentieth century: Function of the universalia: Time, space, reality and cosmos. *Group Psychotherapy*, 19, 146–158.

Moreno, J. L. (1966d). Psychodrama of a marriage. *Group Psychotherapy*, 19, 49–93.

Moreno, J. L. (1968). The validity of psychodrama. *Group Psychotherapy*, 21, 3.

Moreno, J. L. (1969a). A case of paranoia. In J. L. Moreno (with Z. T. Moreno), *Psychodrama third volume, action therapy and principles of practice*. Beacon, NY: Beacon House.

Moreno, J. L. (1969b). The concept of the here and now, hic et nunc: Small groups and their relation to action research. *Group Psychotherapy*, 22, 139–140.

Moreno, J. L. (1969c). The Viennese origins of the encounter movement, paving the way for existentialism, group psychotherapy and psychodrama. *Group Psychotherapy*, 22, 7–16.

Moreno, J. L. (1970a). Is God a single person? My first encounter with a muse of high order, Zerka. *Group Psychotherapy and Psychodrama*, 23, 75–78.

Moreno, J. L. (1970b). The triadic system, psychodrama-sociometry-group psychotherapy. *Group Psychotherapy and Psychodrama*, 23, 16.

Moreno, J. L. (1972a). Introduction to the third edition. In J. L. Moreno, *Psychodrama, first volume* (3rd Ed.) pp i–xxii. Beacon, NY: Beacon House.

Moreno, J. L. (1972b). The religion of God–Father. In P. Johnson (Ed.), *Healer of the mind*. Nashville, TN: Abingdon Press.

Moreno, J. L. (1989a). The autobiography of J. L. Moreno, MD (Abridged). *Group Psychotherapy, Psychodrama & Sociometry*, 42, 1, 15–52, 124.

Moreno, J. L. (1989b). The autobiography of J. L. Moreno, MD (Abridged). *Group Psychotherapy, Psychodrama & Sociometry*, 42, 2, 59–125.

Moreno, J. L. (1993). *Who shall survive? First student edition*. Roanoke, VA: Royal Publishing Company.

Moreno, J. L. & Borgatta, E. F. (1951). An experiment with sociodrama and sociometry in industry. *Sociometry*, 14, 71–104.

Moreno, J. L. et al. (Eds.). (1960). *The sociometry reader*. Glencoe, IL: Free Press.

Moreno, J. L. & Jennings, H. H. (1938). Statistics of social configurations. *Sociometry*, 1, 342–374.

Moreno, J. L. & Moreno, F. B. (1944). Spontaneity theory of child development. *Sociometry*, 7, 89–128.

Moreno, J. L., Moreno, J. D. & Moreno, Z. T. (1963). The first psychodramatic family. *Group Psychotherapy*, 16, 203–249.
Moreno, J. L. & Whitin, E. S. (1932). *Application of the group method to classification*. New York: National Committee on Prisons and Prison Labor.
Moreno, J. L. & Zelany, L. D. (1961). Role theory and sociodrama. In J. S. Roucek (Ed.), *Contemporary sociology*. (pp. 642–654). Paterson, NJ: Littlefield, Adams & Co..
Moreno, Z. T. (1952). Psychodrama in a well-baby clinic. *Group Psychotherapy*, 4, 100–106.
Moreno, Z. T. (1954). Psychodrama in the crib. *Group Psychotherapy*, 7, 291–302.
Moreno, Z. T. (1958a). A note on spontaneous learning "in situ" versus learning the academic way. *Group Psychotherapy*, 11, 50–51.
Moreno, Z. T. (1958b). The reluctant therapist and the reluctant audience technique in psychodrama. *Group Psychotherapy*, 11, 278–282.
Moreno, Z. T. (1959). A survey of psychodramatic techniques. *Group Psychotherapy*, 12, 5–14.
Moreno, Z. T. (1965). Psychodramatic rules, techniques and adjunctive methods. *Group Psychotherapy*, 18, 73–86.
Moreno, Z. T. (1966a). Evolution and dynamics of the group psychotherapy movement. In J. L. Moreno (Ed.), *International handbook of group psychotherapy*.
Moreno, Z. T. (1966b). Sociogenesis of individuals and groups. In J. L. Moreno (Ed.), *International handbook of group psychotherapy*.
Moreno, Z. T. (1969a). Moreneans: The heretics of yesterday are the orthodoxy of today. *Group Psychotherapy*, 22, 1–6.
Moreno, Z. T. (1969b). Practical aspects of psychodrama. *Group Psychotherapy*, 22, 213.
Moreno, Z. T. (1971). Beyond Aristotle, Breuer and Freud: Moreno's contribution to the concept of catharsis. *Group Psychotherapy and Psychodrama*, 24, 34–43.
Moreno, Z. T. (1972). Note on psychodrama, sociometry, individual psychotherapy and the quest for unconditional love. *Group Psychotherapy and Psychodrama*, 25, 155–157.
Moreno, Z. T. (1978). The function of the auxiliary ego in psychodrama with special reference to psychotic patients. *Group Psychotherapy, Psychodrama & Sociometry*, 31, 163–166.
Moreno, Z. T. (1983). Psychodrama. In H. I. Caplan & B. J. Sadock (Eds.). *Comprehensive group psychotherapy*. Baltimore: Williams & Wilkins.
Moreno, Z. T. (1986). J. L. Moreno's concept of ethical anger. *Group Psychotherapy, Psychodrama & Sociometry*, 38, 145–153.
Moreno, Z. T. (1987). Psychodrama, role theory and the concept of the social atom. In J. K. Zeig (Ed.), *The evolution of psychotherapy*. New York: Brunner Mazel.
Moreno, Z. T. (1991). Time, space, reality and the family: Psychodrama with a blended (reconstituted) family. In P. Holmes & M. Karp (Eds.). *Psychodrama: Inspiration & technique*. London: Tavistock/Routledge.
Moreno, Z. T. (1994). Foreword. In P. Holmes, M. Karp & M. Watson (Eds.). *Psychodrama since Moreno*. London: Routledge
Moreno, Z. T. (1996). Introduction. In A. P. Hare & J. R. Hare, *J. L. Moreno*. London: Sage Publications.
Moreno, Z. T. (2000a). The function of "tele" in human relations. In J. Zeig (Ed.), *The evolution of psychotherapy: A meeting of the minds*. Phoenix, AZ: Erickson Foundation Pres.
Moreno, Z. T. (2000b). Introduction. In Z. T. Moreno, L. D. Blomkvist, & T. Rützel *Psychodrama, surplus reality and the art of healing*. London: Routledge.

Moreno, Z. T. (2006a). Comments, article 3. In T. Horvatin & E. Schreiber (Eds.), *The quintessential Zerka*. New York: Routledge.

Moreno, Z. T. (2006b). The function of tele in human relations. In T. Horvatin & E. Schreiber (Eds.), *The quintessential Zerka*. New York: Routledge.

Moreno, Z. T. (2006c). In the spirit of two thousand. In T. Horvatin & E. Schreiber (Eds.), *The quintessential Zerka*. New York: Routledge.

Moreno, Z. T. (2012). *To dream again*. Catskill, NY: Mental Health Resources.

Moreno, Z. T., Blomkvist, L. D. & Rützel (2000) *Psychodrama, surplus reality and the art of healing*. London: Routledge.

Murphy, G. (1951). Foreword. In J. L. Moreno, *Sociometry, experimental method and the science of society*. Beacon, NY: Beacon House.

Nichol, L. (1994). Foreword. In D. Bohm, *Thought as a system*. New York: Rutledge.

Nichol, L. (2003). *The essential David Bohm*. New York: Routledge.

Nichols, M. P. & Efran, J. S. (1985). Catharsis in psychotherapy: A new perspective. *Psychotherapy*, 22, 46–58.

Nichols, M. P. & Zax, M. (1977). *Catharsis in psychotherapy*. New York: Gardiner Press.

Nichols, S. (2011). Experimental philosophy and the problem of free will. *Science*, 331, 1401–1403.

Nolte, J. (1984). *Strategies of directing*. Paper presented at the Annual Meeting of the American Society of Group Psychotherapy and Psychodrama, Washington, DC, April.

Nolte, J. (2008). *The Psychodrama Papers*. Hartford, CT: Encounter Publications.

Northway, M. L. (1940). A method for depicting social relationships obtained by sociometric testing. *Sociometry*, 3, 144–150.

Peat, F. D. (1997). *Infinite potential*. New York: Addison-Wesley Publishing Co.

Penrose, R. (1989). *The emperor's new mind: Concerning minds, computers and the laws of physics*. Oxford: Oxford University Press.

Perrott, L. A. (1986). Using psychodramatid techniques in structural family therapy. *Contemporary Family Therapy*, 8, 279–290.

Perls, F. S. (1969). *Gestalt therapy verbatim*. New York: Bantam.

Powell, A. (1989). Object relations theory in the psychodramatic group. *Journal of the British Psychodrama Association*, 4, 5–16.

Pratt, J. H. (1917/1963). The tuberculosis class: An experiment in home treatment. In M. Rosenbaum & M. Berger (Eds.), *Group psychotherapy and group function*. New York: Basic Books.

Pratt, J. H. (1945). The group method in the treatment of psychosomatic disorders. *Sociometry*, 8, 85–93.

Remer, R. (1990). Family therapy inside out. *Group Psychotherapy, Psychodrama & Sociometry*, 43, 70–81.

Robbins, M. K. (1973). Psychodramatic children's warm-ups for adults. *Group Psychotherapy and Psychodrama*, 26, 67–71.

Rokeach, M. (1964). *The three Christs of Ypsilanti*. New York: New York Review Books.

Rosenbaum, M. & Berger, M. (Eds.) (1963). *Group psychotherapy and group function*. New York: Basic Books.

Roethlisberger, F.J. & Dickson, W.J. (1939) *Management and the worker: an account of a research program conducted by the Western electric company, Hawthorne works, Chicago*. Cambridge, MA: Harvard University Press,.

Sacks, J. M. (1967). Psychodrama: The warm up. *Group Psychotherapy*, 20, 118–122.

Sanderson, D. (1943). Discussion of sociometry. *Sociometry*, 6, 214–218.

Sappington, A. A. (1990). Recent psychological approaches to the free will versus determinism issue. *Psychological Bulletin*, 108, 19–29.

Scheff, T. J. (1979). *Catharsis in healing, ritual and drama*. The Hague: Mouton.

Schutz, W. C. (1971). *Here comes everybody*. New York: Harper & Row.

Sewell, W. H. (1942). The development of a sociometric scale. *Sociometry*, 5, 279–297.

Shoobs, N. E. (1943). The psychodramatic approach to classroom problems. *Sociometry*, 6, 264–265.

Siroka, R. W., Siroka, E. K. & Schloss, G. A. (1971). *Sensitivity training and group encounter*. New York: Grosset & Dunlap.

Smith, H. (2001). *Why religion matters*. New York: HarperCollins.

Sorokin, P. (1949). Concept, tests, and energy of spontaneity-creativity. *Sociometry*, 12, 215–224.

Sorokin, P. (1955). Remarks on J. L. Moreno's theory of spontaneity-creativity. *Sociometry*, 18, 374–392.

Spence, G. (1998). *Give me liberty: Freeing ourselves in the twenty-first century*. New York: St. Martin's Press.

Starr, A. & Weisz, H. S. (1989). Psychodramatic techniques in the brief treatment of inpatient groups. *Individual Psychology: Journal of Adlerian Theory, Research & Practice*, 45, 143–147.

Sternberg, P. & Garcia, A. (1989). *Sociodrama: Who's in your shoes?* Westport, CT: Praeger.

Stewart, J. Q. (1942). A measure of the influence of a population at a distance. *Sociometry*, 5, 63–71.

Sulloway, F. J. (1979). *Freud, biologist of the mind*. New York: Basic Books.

Synnot, E. (1992). The application of sociodrama in the training of middle management. *Australian & New Zealand Psychodrama Association Journal*, 1, 31–36.

Thorndike, E. L. (1942). The causes of inter-state migration. *Sociometry*, 5, 321–335.

Toeman, Z. (1945). Psychodramatic research of pre-marital couples. *Sociometry*, 8, 89.

Toeman, Z. (1946). Clinical psychodrama: Auxiliary ego, double, and mirror techniques. *Sociometry*, 9, 178–183.

Toeman, Z. (1948a). The "double" situation in psychodrama. *Sociatry*, 2, 436–466.

Toeman, Z. (1948b). How to construct a sociogram. *Sociatry*, 2, 407–419.

Toeman, Z. (1949). History of the sociometric movement in headlines. *Sociometry*, 12, 255–259.

Wampole, B. (2001). *The great psychotherapy debate*. Mahwah, NJ: Lawrence Erlbaum.

Warner, W. J. (1954). Sociology and psychiatry. *British Journal of Sociology*, 5, 228–237.

Weiner, H. B. & Sacks, J. M. (1969). Warm-up and sum-up. *Group Psychotherapy*, 22, 85–102.

Wiener, R. L. & Traynor, J. (1987–1988). The use of sociodrama in staff training in working with older people. *Practice*, 1, 332–338.

Wieser, M. (2013). *Bibliography of psychodrama*. Retrieved November 16, 2013, from http://www.pdbib.org/.

Williams, A. (1989). *The passionate technique: Strategic psychodrama with individuals, families and groups*. London: Tavistock/Routledge.

Yablonsky, L. (1953). An operational theory of roles. *Sociometry*, 16, 349–354.

Yablonsky, L. (1972). *Robopaths*. Indianapolis: Bobbs-Merrill Company.

Yablonsky, L. & Enneis, J. M. (1956). Psychodrama theory and practice. In F. Fromm-Reichman & J. L. Moreno (Eds.), *Progress in psychotherapy, Vol. 1.* New York: Grune & Stratton.

Yalom, I. D. (1985). *The theory and practice of group psychotherapy.* New York: Basic Books.

Young, D. & Moreno, J. L. (1955). Transfer of *Sociometry* to the American Sociological Society. *Sociometry,* 18, 177–180.

Znaniecki, F. (1945). Controversies in doctrine and method. *American Journal of Sociology,* 50, 514–521.

Index